Neonatology
at a Glance

Neonatology at a Glance

TOM LISSAUER, MB, BChir, FRCPCH
Hon Consultant Neonatologist
Imperial College Healthcare Trust
Consultant Paediatric Programme Director
Institute of Global Health
Imperial College
London UK

AVROY A. FANAROFF, MD, FRCPCH
Eliza Henry Barnes Chair of Neonatology
Rainbow Babies & Children's Hospital
Professor of Pediatrics and Reproductive Biology
Case Western Reserve University School of Medicine
Cleveland, Ohio, USA

Second edition

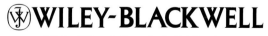
WILEY-BLACKWELL
A John Wiley & Sons, Ltd., Publication

Library of Congress Cataloging-in-Publication Data
Neonatology at a glance / [edited by] Tom Lissauer, Avroy A. Fanaroff. – 2nd ed.
     p. ; cm. – (At a glance)
  Includes bibliographical references and index.
    ISBN 978-1-4051-9951-3 (pbk. : alk. paper) 1. Neonatology–Outlines, syllabi, etc.
I. Lissauer, Tom. II. Fanaroff, Avroy A. III. Series: At a glance series (Oxford, England)
  [DNLM: 1. Infant, Newborn. 2. Infant Care. 3. Infant, Newborn, Diseases–therapy.
4. Neonatology–methods. WS 420]
  RJ251.N22 2011
  618.92'01–dc22

                  2010039147

A catalogue record for this book is available from the British Library.

Set in Times by Toppan Best-set Premedia Limited
Printed and bound in Malaysia by Vivar Printing Sdn Bhd

1 2011

Contents

Preface

This book provides a concise, illustrated overview of neonatal medicine. We have aimed to cover the breadth of neonatology in under 100 double pages, with major topics confined to one or two double pages. This has been a challenging exercise as it would have been easier to write a longer book, but this format has forced us to identify the most important points and omit unnecessary details. The book has been designed to make learning easier and more enjoyable. Modern education emphasizes visual impact and this is reflected in this book. The layout, photographs and illustrations have been chosen to assist learning and make the book attractive and interesting. In addition, there are specific aids to learning, with boxes to highlight key points and questions and answers.

The book covers the preterm infant and the wide range of common or important neonatal clinical conditions and their management. It also puts neonatology into context, with sections on its history, epidemiology, perinatal medicine and a global overview, together with the care of the normal newborn and how to recognize the sick infant. The challenging topics of ethical issues, research, quality assurance, evidence-based medicine, when a baby dies, autopsy and neonatal outcome are also considered. Practical procedures are described, including neonatal resuscitation and neonatal transport; a description of cranial ultrasound and echocardiography have been included to inform the practicing clinician about them even if they do not perform these procedures themselves.

The book is written for pediatric interns and residents, medical students, neonatal nurse practitioners, neonatal nurses, therapists and midwives who care for newborn babies either on a neonatal unit or with their mothers in the normal newborn nursery (postnatal wards). Whilst the book describes the salient features of intensive care, such as stabilizing the sick infant and respiratory support, it is not a manual of neonatal intensive care, of which there are many.

The book has been a collaborative project between editors and contributors from both North America and the UK. Where practices differ between the two sides of the Atlantic this has been acknowledged and described. This collaboration has been highly educational and hugely enjoyable for the editors and contributors as well as improving the book by forcing us to concentrate on the principles of practice instead of the details.

This new edition has allowed us to update and revise the book. We would like to thank the many doctors, nurses and therapists whose positive comments about the book encouraged us to produce this 2nd edition. We would also like to thank our families for allowing us to spend so much time over many years on this project.

Tom Lissauer and Avroy A. Fanaroff (Editors)

Contributors

The editors are indebted to the following for their contributions to the chapters listed below:

Mark Anderson
Consultant Paediatrician, Newcastle upon Tyne Hospitals NHS Trust, Newcastle upon Tyne, UK
Pharmacology

Cheryl Jones
Associate Professor & Sub Dean Research, Discipline of Paediatrics & Child Health, University of Sydney; Paediatric Infectious Diseases Consultant and Head, Centre for Perinatal Infection Research, The Children's Hospital at Westmead, Australia
Congenital infection, Neonatal infection, Specific bacterial infections, Viral infections

Mark Kilby
Professor of Fetal Medicine, School of Clinical & Experimental Medicine, The College of Medical & Dental Sciences, University of Birmingham; Department of Fetal Medicine, Birmingham Women's Foundation Trust, Birmingham, UK
Perinatal Medicine – Part 2

Joy Lawn
Senior Policy and Research Advisor, Saving Newborn Lives/Save the Children, USA
Epidemiology, Global overview

David Lissauer
Research Fellow, Department of Fetal Medicine, Birmingham Women's Foundation Trust, Birmingham, UK
Perinatal medicine – Part 2

Sam Lissauer
Specialist Pediatric Registrar, Heart of England Foundation Trust, Birmingham, UK
Intubation and chest drains, Common practical procedures, Umbilical catheters and intraosseous cannulation, Central venous catheters and exchange transfusions

Neil Marlow
Professor of Neonatal Medicine, UCL Institute for Women's Health, London, UK
Epidemiology, Outcome of very preterm infants, Follow-up of high-risk infants

Richard J. Martin
Director, Division of Neonatology, Drusinsky-Fanaroff Chair in Neonatology, Rainbow Babies & Children's Hospital, Cleveland, Ohio, USA
Lung development and surfactant, Respiratory distress syndrome, Apnea, bradycardia and desaturations, Bronchopulmonary dysplasia, Respiratory distress in term infants

Patrick McNamara
Staff Neonatologist and Director of Clinical Research, Hospital for Sick Children; Associate Professor, University of Toronto, Toronto, Canada
Patent ductus arteriosus, Echocardiography for the neonatologist

Sam Richmond
Consultant Neonatologist, Sunderland Royal Hospital, Sunderland, UK
Adaptation to extrauterine life, Neonatal resuscitation, Stabilizing the sick newborn infant

Irene Roberts
Professor of Paediatric Haematology, Imperial College, London
Anemia and polycythemia, Neutrophil and thrombotic disorders, Coagulation disorders

Inga Warren
Consultant Therapist in Neonatal Developmental Care, St Mary's Hospital, London, UK
Developmental care, Admission to the neonatal unit, Pain, Discharge from hospital

We would also like to thank those who assisted us with the revision and updating of the chapters:

Karel Allegaert
Assistant Professor, University Hospitals Leuven and Catholic University Leuven, Belgium
Pharmacology

Nancy Bass
Rainbow Babies & Children's Hospital, Cleveland, Ohio, USA
Cerebral hemorrhage and periventricular leukomalacia, Seizures and strokes, Neural tube defects and hydrocephalus, The hypotonic infant

Monica Bhola
Director of Neonatal Transport, Rainbow Babies & Children's Hospital, Cleveland, Ohio, USA
Intubation and chest drains, Common practical procedures, Umbilical catheters and intraosseous cannulation, Central venous catheters and exchange transfusions

Bernie Borgstein
Consultant Paediatric Audiological Physician, Imperial College Healthcare Trust, London UK
Hearing

Hugo Devlieger
Professor Emeritus, University Hospitals Leuven and Catholic University Leuven, Belgium
Pharmacology

Subarna Chakravorty
Clinical Research Fellow, Centre for Haematology, Hammersmith Hospital, Imperial College London
Anemia and polycythemia, Neutrophil and thrombotic disorders, Coagulation disorders

Jonathan Fanaroff
Associate Professor of Pediatrics, Associate Medical Director, Neonatal Intensive Care Unit; Director, Rainbow Center for Pediatric Ethics, Rainbow Babies & Children's Hospital/UH Case Medical Center, Cleveland, Ohio, USA
Ethics

Larissa Kerecuk
Consultant Paediatric Nephrologist, Royal Victoria Infirmary, Newcastle upon Tyne
Kidney and urinary tract disorders: antenatal diagnosis, Kidney and urinary tract disorders, Genital abnormalities

Simon Newell
Consultant and Senior Clinical Lecturer in Neonatal Medicine, St James' University Hospital, Leeds Teaching Hospitals, Leeds, UK
Growth and nutrition

Mary Nock
Associate Professor of Pediatrics; Director MacDonald Hospital For Women and Director Neonatal Fellowship Program, Rainbow Babies & Children's Hospital, Cleveland, Ohio, USA
Jaundice

Clare Roberts
Consultant Paediatric Ophthalmologist, Imperial College Healthcare Trust, London UK
Vision

Jonathan Stevens
Staff Neonatologist, Northern Alberta Neonatal Program, Edmonton, Alberta, Canada
Transport of the sick newborn infant

Robert Tulloh
Consultant in Paediatric Cardiology, Bristol Congenital Heart Centre, Bristol Royal Hospital for Children, Bristol Royal Infirmary, University Hospitals Bristol NHS Foundation Trust, Bristol, UK
Cardiac disorders

Qin Yao
Rainbow Babies & Children's Hospital, Cleveland, Ohio, USA
Neonatal resuscitation

We would like to thank contributors to the first edition whose work we have extensively drawn upon:

Ricardo J. Rodriguez – Associate editor

Michael Weindling – Associate editor

Paula Bolton-Maggs – *Anemia and polycythemia, Coagulation disorders*

George Haycock – *Kidney and urinary tract disorders: antenatal diagnosis, Kidney and urinary tract disorders*

Susan Izatt – *Neonatal resuscitation*

Helen Kingston – *Birth defects and genetic disorders*

Carolyn Lund – *Skin*

Hermione Lyall – *Congenital infection, Neonatal infection, Specific bacterial infections, Viral infections*

Neil McIntosh – *Ethics, Research and consent*

Maggie Meeks – *Common problems of term infants, Common practical procedures, Central venous catheters and intraosseous cannulation, Chest tubes and exchange transfusions*

Michael Reed – *Pain*

Jonathan Stevens – *Transport of the sick newborn infant*

Eileen Stork – *Bone and joint disorders*

Nim Subhedar – *Respiratory support, Lung development and surfactant, Respiratory distress syndrome*

Dharmapuri Vidyasagar – *Milestones in neonatology*

Deanne Wilson-Costello – *Outcome of very low birthweight infants, Follow-up of high-risk infants*

We would also like to thank Dr David Clark, Professor and Chairman, The Children's Hospital, Albany, New York, USA, and Dr Alan Spitzer, Senior Vice President and Director, The Center for Research and Education, Pediatric Medical Group, Sunrise, Florida, USA, for contributing photographs and Dr Carlos Sivit, Professor of Radiology and Director of Pediatric Radiology, Rainbow Babies & Children's Hospital, Cleveland, Ohio, USA, for providing the cranial ultrasound photographs for Chapter 78.

The care of newborn infants has evolved over the last century from simple and empirical care to modern, evidence-based, high-tech medicine. Neonatal mortality has correspondingly declined dramatically from 40/1000 live births in 1900 to <4/1000 in the US and UK. Improved obstetric care and maternal health and nutrition have also contributed. It was only in the 1950s that medical care of healthy and sick newborn infants was transferred from obstetricians to pediatricians. The specialty of neonatology developed only in the 1960s, and the first certifying examination for physicians in the US was held in 1975.

Thermal regulation

- 1890s: Tarnier in France showed that a warm, controlled environment reduced mortality of infants <2 kg from 66% to 38% (Fig. 1.1).
- 1893: Budin, Tarnier's student, established the first unit for premature babies in Paris, emphasizing thermal regulation and breast-feeding.
- Early 1900s: premature babies in incubators were exhibited in fairs around Europe and the US (Fig. 1.2).
- 1950s: Silverman in the US conducted elegant randomized controlled trials to confirm the beneficial effects of thermal control (including humidity) on mortality.
- 2000s: Heat loss at delivery of extremely preterm babies minimized by plastic wrapping.

Nutrition

- 1880s: Tarnier and Budin recommend early feeding and intragastric 'gavage' feeding via a rubber tube inserted through the mouth.

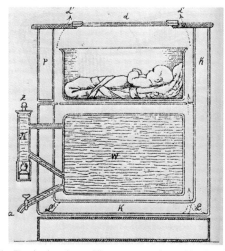

Fig. 1.1 The Tarnier incubator. The water was heated by the oil flame. The baby was kept warm by the heated air circulating around the incubator.

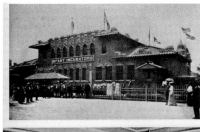
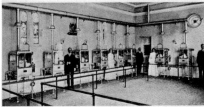

Fig. 1.2 Incubators with premature babies at the Pan-American Exposition, Buffalo, New York in 1901. (Source: Silverman WA. Incubator-baby side shows. *Pediatrics* 1979; **64**: 127. Courtesy of the American Academy of Pediatrics.)

- 1907: Rotch in US introduces infant formula. Breast-feeding declines as some believed formula was superior.
- 1940s: Gavage feeding via a nasogastric tube used in neonatal units.
- 1940s: Feeding of preterm infants delayed up to 4 days to avoid aspiration. Adverse effects (hypoglycemia, increased bilirubin and impaired development) recognized only in the 1960s, and early feeding reintroduced.
- 1960s: TPN (total parenteral nutrition) by central venous catheter introduced centrally, then via peripheral veins.
- 1960s: Infant formula associated with neonatal tetany from hypocalcemia and hemolysis from vitamin E deficiency.
- 1980s: Development of special formulas for very low birthweight infants.
- 1980s: Resurgence of use of breast milk. Human milk fortifiers developed for preterm infants.
- 2000s: Addition of long-chain polyunsaturated fatty acids (LCPUFA) to formula.

Rhesus hemolytic disease

Kernicterus, from bilirubin deposition in the brain from rhesus disease, was first described in 1938. Exchange transfusions became a common procedure in neonatal units and saved an estimated 8000 lives/year in the US alone.

- 1925: Hart describes first exchange transfusion – blood given via saphenous vein, removed from anterior fontanelle.
- 1940: Landsteiner discovers rhesus factor.
- 1945: Coombs develops Coombs test (direct antiglobulin test, DAT) to detect rhesus agglutinins.

Neonatology at a Glance, 2nd edition. Edited by Tom Lissauer & Avroy A. Fanaroff. © 2011 Blackwell Publishing Ltd.

- 1947: Diamond describes exchange transfusion via umbilical vein with rubber catheter.
- 1963: Liley introduces intrauterine transfusion.
- 1964: Freda and Clarke develop prophylaxis with anti-D immunoglobulin.
- 1968: Rho(D) immune globulin prophylaxis introduced. Rhesus disease now almost completely prevented.

Antibiotics

Before antibiotics, mortality from neonatal sepsis was almost 100%, but it declined markedly when penicillin was introduced in 1944. The organisms causing sepsis have changed (Fig. 1.3).

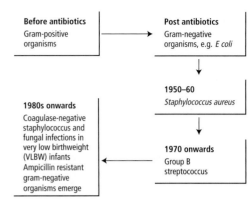

Fig. 1.3 Change with time of main organisms causing neonatal infection.

Respiratory distress syndrome (RDS)

Oxygen therapy, monitoring and respiratory support

Whereas about 25 000 infants died every year in the US from RDS in the early 1950s, by 2003 there were fewer than 500 such deaths. This has resulted from:
- understanding the pathogenesis of RDS, which enabled development of surfactant replacement therapy
- antenatal corticosteroids to induce surfactant and lung maturation
- developments in respiratory support:
  - oxygen therapy
  - continuous positive airway pressure (CPAP), introduced by Gregory
  - mechanical ventilators, first shown to improve survival by Swyer in Toronto and Reynolds in London (1965)
- ability to closely monitor vital signs and blood gases:
  - cardiorespiratory monitors for neonates
  - measurement of blood gases on small blood samples
  - umbilical/peripheral artery catheters
  - transcutaneous arterial O_2 and CO_2 monitors
  - non-invasive oxygen saturation monitors.

History of respiratory distress syndrome (surfactant deficiency)
- 1955: Pattle describes properties of surfactant.
- 1956: Clements isolates surfactant.
- 1959: Avery and Mead demonstrate lack of surfactant in preterm lungs.
- 1972: Liggins and Howie show that prenatal corticosteroids to the mother induce fetal lung maturity.
- 1980: Fujiwara – first surfactant replacement therapy.
- 1985: Multicenter clinical trials of natural and artificial surfactant replacement therapy.
- 1989: Surfactant therapy approved.

Key point

Since the 1950s RDS has been the major focus of research in neonatology. Understanding its pathophysiology and the biochemistry of surfactant has been the key to developing surfactant therapy and respiratory support, which have dramatically improved survival.

Development of neonatal intensive care

- 1922: First neonatal unit in US in Chicago by Hess; in UK by Crosse in Birmingham in 1945.
- 1960s and 1970s: Development of regional neonatal intensive care units with dedicated staff, introduction of CPAP and mechanical ventilation.
- 1970s: Ultrasound to identify intraventricular hemorrhage.
- 1970s: Ability to safely perform surgery in tiny infants.
- 1980s: Development of multicenter clinical trials, national and international.
- 1980s: ECMO (extracorporeal membrane oxygenation).
- 1990s: NO (nitric oxide) therapy for persistent pulmonary hypertension of the newborn.
- 2000s: Mild hypothermia shown to reduce morbidity of hypoxic–ischemic encephalopathy.

Challenges for the future

- Reduce prematurity, hypoxic–ischemic brain injury, neonatal infection, congenital abnormalities.
- Avoid complications of preterm infants: brain injury, necrotizing enterocolitis, bronchopulmonary dysplasia (chronic lung disease), retinopathy of prematurity.
- Practice evidence-based medicine.
- Improve quality assurance – reduce medication errors etc.
- Develop better non-invasive monitoring.
- Enhance nursery environment.
- Confront ethical dilemmas at the limit of viability.
- Improve/extend care at home of technology-dependent infants.
- Develop personalized medicine incorporating modern genetics.
- Global reduction of neonatal mortality, to achieve Millennium Development Goal target by 2015.

Epidemiology is the study of factors affecting disease or death. In perinatal medicine the focus is on the prevalence and causes of illness and death and long-term disability in mothers, the fetus and newborn infants.

Definitions

Newborn infant
- **Preterm:** *<37 completed weeks of gestation.*
- **Term:** *37–41 completed weeks of gestation.*
- **Post-term:** *≥42 completed weeks of gestation.*
- **Low birthweight (LBW):** *<2500 g.*
- **Very low birthweight (VLBW):** *<1500 g.*
- **Extremely low birthweight (ELBW):** *<1000 g.*

Mortality
- **Maternal mortality ratio:** *the number of maternal deaths (during pregnancy and within 42 days postpartum) per 100 000 live births.*
- **Stillbirth:** *Variable definitions. In US, fetal death (no signs of life) ≥20 weeks' gestation. In the UK, fetus born with no signs of life after 24 weeks. For international comparison, WHO recommend defining stillbirth rate as fetal deaths >1000 g or >28 completed weeks per 1000 total births.*
- **Perinatal mortality rate (PMR):** *stillbirths plus early neonatal deaths (up to 6 completed days of life) per 1000 live and stillbirths (adjusted as above for international comparisons).*
- **Neonatal mortality rate (NMR):** *deaths in the first 4 weeks (27 completed days) of life per 1000 live births.*
- **Post-neonatal mortality rate:** *deaths from 28 days until 1 year per 1000 live births.*
- **Infant mortality rate:** *deaths in the first year of life per 1000 live births.*

These indicators are valuable as measures of the health of a region or country and allow comparisons between them and monitoring of changes over time.

Births

There are 4.3 million births per year in the US and 790 000 in the UK. The average age of a mother giving birth has risen to 25 years in the US and to 29 years in the UK (average age at first child 27 years). There has been a steady rise in the birth rate for women in their thirties and forties.

Maternal mortality

The huge reduction in maternal mortality is one of the most dramatic improvements in health outcomes in high income countries. In the US, maternal mortality declined from 582/100 000 live births in 1936 to 11.5/100 000 in 1990. This is due to reduced mortality from puerperal sepsis following the development of antibiotics, improved obstetric care, availability of blood and blood products, and better maternal health, including fewer pregnancies per woman. However, maternal mortality in the US has not continued to fall – it was 16.7/100 000 in 2008 (8 in the UK).

Perinatal mortality

The causes of perinatal mortality are shown in Fig. 2.1. The risk to the infant of perinatal death is about 100 times that for the mother. In the US, the perinatal mortality fell from 13/1000 live and stillbirths in 1980 to 6.6/1000 in 2005. The decline has occurred not only because of advances in neonatal care, but also from improved maternal health and nutrition and obstetric care.

Neonatal mortality

Neonatal mortality has declined steadily over the last 25 years (Fig. 2.2).

Gestational age and birthweight are the main risk factors for neonatal death. Rates of preterm birth vary widely between countries. The neonatal mortality rate is therefore largely determined by proportion of preterm deliveries, the birthweight distribution and gestation- or birthweight-specific mortality rates (Table 2.1). As mortality has been reduced, there is increased focus on survival at very low

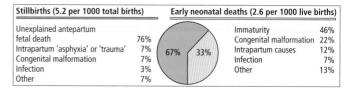

Fig. 2.1 Causes of perinatal mortality in UK (Confidential Enquiry into Maternal and Child Health, 2009).

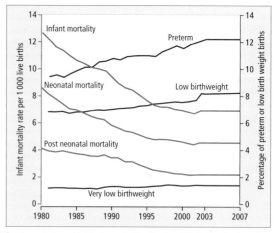

Fig. 2.2 Neonatal and infant mortality in the US have declined markedly since 1980. This is in spite of an increase in the proportion of infants born preterm or with low birth weight, mainly from the rise in maternal age and assisted reproduction. However, the proportion of very low birthweight (VLBW) infants has remained unchanged. (Source: Annual Summary of Vital Statistics – 2007; Heron M *et al. Pediatrics* 2009; **125**: 1–14.)

Table 2.1 Birthweight distribution and neonatal mortality (US, 2006).

Birthweight	Births (%)	Neonatal mortality rate (per 1000 live births)
>2500 g	91.7	0.8
2000–2499 g	5.2	5.6
1500–1999 g	1.6	17
<1500 g	1.5	209

gestational ages (22 to 25 weeks) and on non-fatal outcomes such as long-term disability (Fig. 2.3a, b, c). Now, half of babies born at 25 weeks' gestation are expected to survive and around half of these will have no or only mild impairment during childhood.

For information on global neonatal mortality see Chapter 72.

Epidemiologic data collection

Neonatal epidemiologic data are gathered through several systems including national vital registration (death certificates), rapid reporting audit systems and special neonatal databases such as the Vermont–Oxford Neonatal Network and NICHD (National Institute of Child Health and Human Development) Neonatal Research Network, which collect clinical data from a large number of neonatal units. Particularly informative are the population-based databases (Fig. 2.3a, b), and some combine obstetric and neonatal data with outcome data.

Infant mortality

The marked reduction in infant mortality since 1980 is shown in Fig. 2.2. With the decline in deaths from infectious diseases since the 1900s and more recently from sudden infant death syndrome,

over two-thirds of infant deaths are in the neonatal period, and even after the first month of life many deaths are related to neonatal problems (Fig. 2.4). Sixty-six percent of all infant deaths occur in the 8.3% of infants born with low birthweight; 52% of infant deaths are among the 1.5% very low birthweight infants. Complications of preterm birth and congenital abnormalities are the largest contributors to both neonatal and infant deaths.

In 2007 the infant mortality rate was 6.8 per 1000 live births in the US and 5.0 in the UK. Compared with other countries, the US had only the 45th lowest infant mortality rate in 2007; the UK had the 36th lowest. A major reason for this relatively poor performance is the higher percentage of preterm infants born in the US (13%) compared to many other developed countries (5% in northern Europe). The preterm birth rate in the UK is rising and is now almost 10%. Both preterm birth prevalence and mortality risk in the US are influenced by ethnicity; the infant mortality of infants of black mothers is over twice that of infants of white or Hispanic mothers. The difference in the UK is similar.

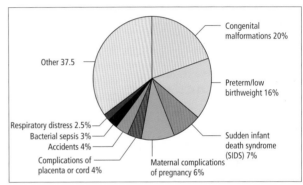

Fig. 2.4 Causes of infant mortality in the US, 2007 (source: www.cdc.gov/nchs/nvss/mortality_tables.htm).

The EPICure Studies

Two country-wide epidemiological studies of very preterm birth have been undertaken – the first in babies <26 weeks of gestation in the UK in 1995 and the second in babies born <27 weeks in England during 2006.

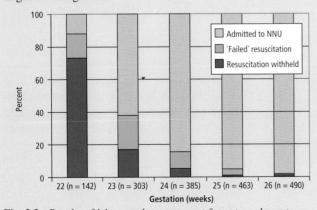

Fig. 2.3a Results of labor ward management for extremely preterm births, England 2006 (source EPICure 2; www.epicure.ac.uk).

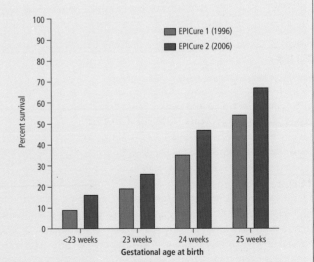

Fig. 2.3b Gestation-specific mortality rates for babies admitted for neonatal intensive care in England in 1995 and 2006 (sources Costeloe *Pediatrics* 2000; **106**: 659–671; www.epicure.ac.uk).

The concept of perinatal care evolved from the development of maternal–fetal medicine (fetal medicine and high-risk obstetrics) linked to neonatal intensive care and associated pediatric specialties. This should allow a 'seamless' care plan for the baby extending from before birth to the newborn period for mothers or babies with complex problems. This requires expertise which is highly specialized, rapidly advancing and multidisciplinary. Such care is usually provided centrally as a tertiary service, though some services may be available locally (Fig. 3.1). The establishment of 'Pregnancy/Newborn Networks' allows experience and management protocols to be cascaded from the tertiary care center to other units to enhance collaborative working and minimize geographical variations in care.

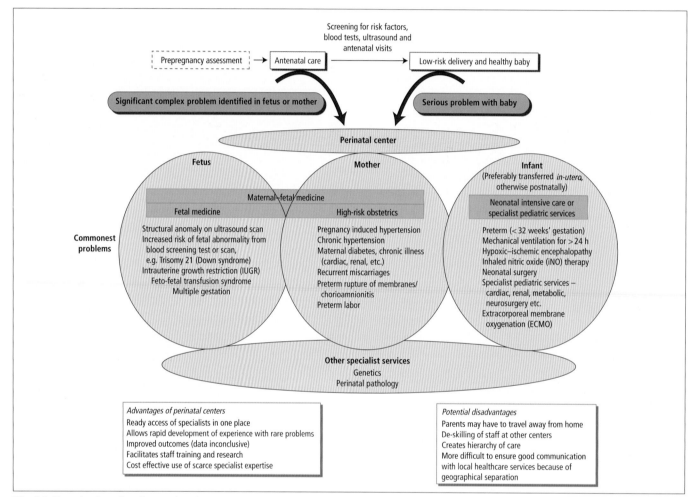

Fig. 3.1 Organization of tertiary perinatal care.

Neonatal involvement in perinatal care

An increasing number of neonatal conditions requiring neonatal intensive care or specialist pediatric services are recognized antenatally. This allows counseling (both obstetric and pediatric), multidisciplinary discussion and transfer, if necessary, before birth to a perinatal center (Fig. 3.2). Parents require information about their baby's condition and management options. Neonatologists, specialist pediatricians and pediatric surgeons are involved to provide information before the baby is born. In particular, interpretation of antenatal ultrasound scans may be difficult and may require input from fetal medicine specialists and specialist radiologists as prognosis may be difficult to define. Specialist assessment and counseling needs to be particularly prompt and within national legal boundaries if termination of pregnancy is considered.

Information about problems identified antenatally needs to be communicated to the neonatology and specialist pediatric teams so that appropriate assessment and follow-up are arranged postnatally.

Neonatology at a Glance, 2nd edition. Edited by Tom Lissauer & Avroy A. Fanaroff. © 2011 Blackwell Publishing Ltd.

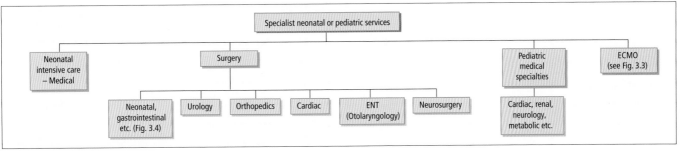

Fig. 3.2 Specialist neonatal care.

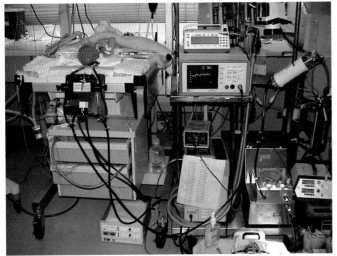

Fig. 3.3 An infant on extracorporeal membrane oxygenation (ECMO), which is provided at only a relatively small number of specialist centers.

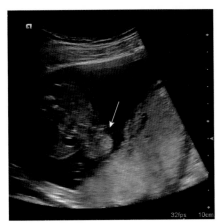

Fig. 3.4 Significant fetal abnormalities detected on prenatal ultrasound screening, such as the omphalocele (arrow) shown here, will need to be assessed in a perinatal center to allow review by fetal medicine specialist, parental counseling, consultation with pediatric surgeon by both doctors and parents and planning for delivery and treatment.

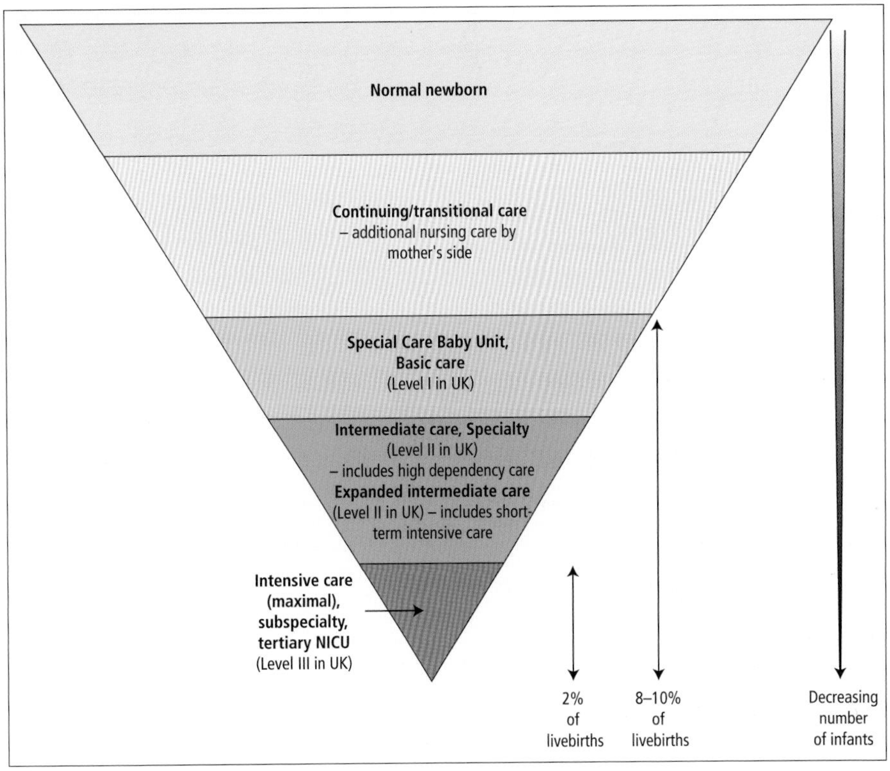

Key point

It is not always possible to provide all these specialist services in a single center on one site. Collaboration between specialties is essential.

Levels of neonatal care

The different levels of care required by newborn infants are shown in Fig. 3.5.

Fig. 3.5 Levels of neonatal care.

Prepregnancy care

Provide advice for all mothers to optimize chances of healthy baby:
- Attend clinic for prenatal care.
- Avoid maternal smoking, alcohol, drug misuse, medication (unless essential).
- Toxoplasmosis exposure – avoid eating undercooked meat (and wear gloves when handling cat litter).
- *Listeria* infection – avoid unpasteurized dairy products and soft ripened cheeses, e.g. brie.
- Folic acid supplements preconceptually to 12 weeks – to reduce risk of neural tube defects and cardiac malformations in countries without folic acid fortification of foods, as in UK. Higher dose of folic acid if woman has had previous baby with neural tube defect.
- Check management of pre-existing maternal medical conditions.

Identify pregnancies at increased risk of fetal abnormality:
- previous child with congenital anomaly
- family history of an inherited disorder
- consanguineous relationship
- parents known carriers of an autosomal recessive disorder, e.g. thalassemia
- parents from ethnic group with specific risk, e.g. African American (sickle cell disease), Ashkenazi Jews (Tay–Sachs disease, a neurodegenerative disorder)
- parent with known chromosomal rearrangement.

Prenatal screening

Maternal blood
The routine screening tests vary geographically, but include:
- maternal blood group, antibodies for rhesus (D) and other red cell incompatibilities
- hepatitis B
- syphilis
- rubella
- HIV infection
- neural tube defects – by maternal serum alphafetoprotein (MSAFP), in some areas
- screening for chromosomal anomalies (see below)
- hemoglobin electrophoresis.

Chlamydia screening – US only

Ultrasound
Ultrasound screening recommended for all mothers before 20 weeks. Allows:

Gestational age calculation, optimal if 11–14 weeks' gestation.

Multiple pregnancy to be identified – number of viable fetuses and chorionicity determined.

Structural malformations detected – in up to 80% of major congenital malformations (first and second trimester).

Screening for trisomy 21 (Down syndrome). First trimester – nuchal translucency thickness combined with serum maternal hormones. Second trimester – four fetoplacental and maternal hormones in serum, adjusted for maternal age. Confirmed on amniocentesis or chorionic villous sampling. Detects 90% of babies with trisomy 21 for a 2.5% risk of fetal loss.

Fetal growth monitoring – by serial measurement of fetal head size (biparietal diameter and head circumference), abdominal circumference and femur length.

Amniotic fluid volume assessment to identify:
(i) oligohydramnios
    – from reduced fetal urine production, placental insufficiency and from prolonged rupture of the membranes
    – may cause pulmonary hypoplasia and limb and facial deformities from pressure on the fetus
(ii) polyhydramnios – associated with maternal diabetes, fetal bowel obstruction, CNS anomalies and multiple births.

Doppler ultrasound measurement of flow/velocity waveforms – maternal and fetal circulation (if indicated).

Examples of structural malformations identified on ultrasound (Figs 4.1–4.3)

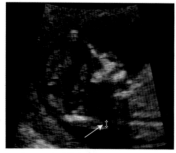

Fig. 4.1 Nuchal translucency (thickened fat pad at back of neck) associated with trisomy 21 (Down syndrome).

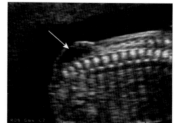

Fig. 4.2 Sacral myelocele. (Courtesy of Dr Venkhat Rahman.)

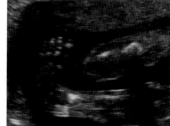

Fig. 4.3 Talipes equinovarus. (Courtesy of Dr Venkhat Rahman.)

Neonatology at a Glance, 2nd edition. Edited by Tom Lissauer & Avroy A. Fanaroff. © 2011 Blackwell Publishing Ltd.

Fetal medicine

Fetal medicine (Fig. 4.4) may allow:
- identification of congenital anomalies
- option of termination of pregnancy to be offered for severe disorders
- therapy to be given for a limited but increasing number of conditions, e.g. fetal arrhythmias, intrauterine blood transfusion for rhesus disease

- optimal multidisciplinary discussion to impart information on prognosis and perinatal care
- optimal obstetric management of the fetus, e.g. timing of delivery
- neonatal management to be planned in advance, e.g. counseling and transfer to specialty center.

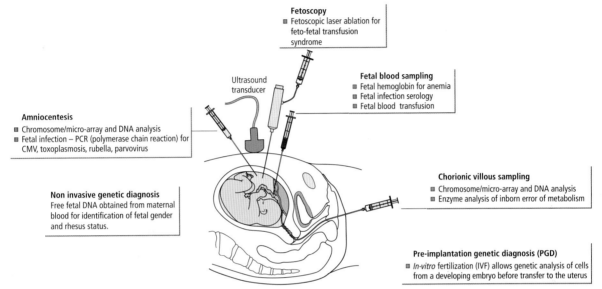

Fetoscopy
- Fetoscopic laser ablation for feto-fetal transfusion syndrome

Ultrasound transducer

Fetal blood sampling
- Fetal hemoglobin for anemia
- Fetal infection serology
- Fetal blood transfusion

Amniocentesis
- Chromosome/micro-array and DNA analysis
- Fetal infection – PCR (polymerase chain reaction) for CMV, toxoplasmosis, rubella, parvovirus

Chorionic villous sampling
- Chromosome/micro-array and DNA analysis
- Enzyme analysis of inborn error of metabolism

Non invasive genetic diagnosis
Free fetal DNA obtained from maternal blood for identification of fetal gender and rhesus status.

Pre-implantation genetic diagnosis (PGD)
- *In-vitro* fertilization (IVF) allows genetic analysis of cells from a developing embryo before transfer to the uterus

Fig. 4.4 Techniques in fetal medicine and their indications.

Fetal surgery

Creates media headlines as cutting-edge technology. However, the results are mostly poor as the malformations justifying fetal surgery are so severe and risk of premature labor is high. Now practiced only in a few centers and mainly restricted to randomized trials. Cases must be carefully selected and detailed follow-up results collected and published.

Open fetal surgery
Hysterotomy (uterus opened at 19–25 weeks' gestation) for open neural tube defects in the US. Randomized trial. May precipitate preterm delivery, outcome disappointing.

Fetoscopic/minimally invasive fetal surgery
In Europe, trial of fetal treatment of diaphragmatic hernia is being undertaken. As tracheal obstruction promotes lung growth, this is produced in the fetus by inflating a balloon in the trachea, inserted by tracheal intubation at fetoscopy.

Catheter shunts
Fetal pleural effusions, usually a chylothorax (lymphatic fluid) – inserted under ultrasound guidance (Fig. 4.5). One end of a looped catheter lies in the chest, the other end in the amniotic cavity. Neonatal course often satisfactory.

Congenital bladder neck obstruction – vesicoamniotic shunting. Controversial. Cohort studies indicate may be beneficial but a significant number of babies have chronic renal impairment and severe bladder dysfunction. Randomized controlled trial is being undertaken.

Dilatation of stenotic heart valves
Percutaneous catheter insertion under ultrasound guidance into the fetal heart. Experimental.

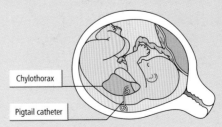

Chylothorax

Pigtail catheter

Fig. 4.5 Fetus with pigtail catheter to drain a pleural effusion.

Diabetes mellitus

Fetal mortality and morbidity are increased with maternal insulin-dependent diabetes (type 1), mainly from congenital malformations and intrauterine death. Good diabetic control, from preconception onwards, reduces malformations and mortality. This requires multidisciplinary management and close prenatal surveillance. The aim is for delivery at approximately 38 weeks, by induction if necessary.

Fetal problems

- Congenital malformations. Risk 6%, four times normal. Wide spectrum of malformations but specific increased risk of cardiac malformations and caudal regression syndrome (sacral agenesis).
- Macrosomia (Fig. 5.1). Maternal hyperglycemia results in fetal hyperinsulinemia, which promotes growth. Depending upon pre-pregnancy and gestational control of blood glucose; up to 25% of infants of diabetic mothers are macrosomic, with a birthweight >4 kg, compared with 8% of infants of non-diabetic mothers.
- Macrosomia predisposes to cephalopelvic disproportion and increased risk of delivery-related complications, both to the mother (cesarean section and forceps delivery) and the fetus; including birth injuries.
- Intrauterine growth restriction (IUGR). Threefold increase. Usually associated with maternal vascular disease.
- Polyhydramnios.
- Preterm labor. Occurs in 10%, either natural or induced.
- Intrauterine death – sudden, in third trimester. Less common with good diabetic control and induction at 38 weeks.

Neonatal problems

- Check for malformations and birth injuries.
- Hypoglycemia – common in first 48 hours due to hyperinsulinism. Monitor blood glucose before feeds until >45 mg% (>2.6 mmol/L). Hypoglycemia is prevented by early, frequent feeding, but may require gavage (nasogastric) feeds or intravenous glucose. Hypocalcemia and hypomagnesemia are often present.
- Polycythemia – plethoric appearance. Occasionally requires partial exchange transfusion.
- Hyperbilirubinemia.
- Respiratory distress syndrome – increased risk from delayed maturation of surfactant.
- Hypertrophic cardiomyopathy – uncommon. Asymptomatic or poor cardiac output (may be treated with β-blockers) for several weeks.
- Renal vein thrombosis – rare.

Type 2 and gestational diabetes

Prevalence of type 2 diabetes is increasing and is associated with perinatal complications. Glucose intolerance from gestational diabetes complicates 1–2% of pregnancies and may require dietary or insulin treatment. May cause neonatal macrosomia, hypoglycemia and polycythemia. Also increases future risk of diabetes in later life.

Maternal red blood cell alloimmunization

Maternal antibody is formed to fetal red blood cell antigens, e.g. rhesus D, anti-Kell and anti-c. Before prophylaxis, rhesus disease was a major cause of fetal and neonatal morbidity and mortality.

Rhesus hemolytic disease

Etiology
See Fig. 5.2.

Presentation
- Antibodies found on routine antenatal antibody screen at first visit, 28 and 34 weeks.
- Previous pregnancy affected with hemolytic disease.
- Fetal hydrops on ultrasound.
- Detection of fetal anemia using ultrasound (middle cerebral artery blood flow increased for gestational age).
- Maternal polyhydramnios.
- Infant – jaundice, anemia, hydrops, hepatosplenomegaly.

Management
PRENATAL
- Increasing antibody levels on maternal blood screening – refer to specialist center if necessary.
- Fetal rhesus genotyping can be determined non-invasively through free fetal DNA detection in maternal plasma.
- Monitor with serial ultrasound for fetal anemia (usually by middle cerebral artery blood flow) and signs of hydrops.
- Amniocentesis – for amniotic fluid optical density (450 nm); rarely used as superseded by cerebral Doppler blood flow for anemia.
- Measure fetal hematocrit (from cordocentesis).

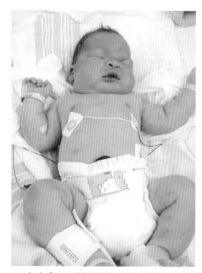

Fig. 5.1 Macrosomic infant with birthweight 4.8 kg at 38 weeks' gestation. There is excess fat and organomegaly (liver and heart).

Neonatology at a Glance, 2nd edition. Edited by Tom Lissauer & Avroy A. Fanaroff. © 2011 Blackwell Publishing Ltd.

Etiology

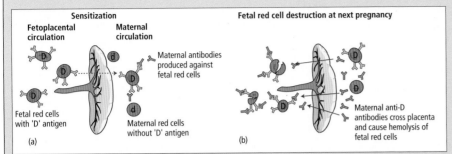

Fig. 5.2 (a) A small number of fetal red cells enter the maternal circulation and antibodies are formed. This usually occurs at delivery, but also at miscarriages, placental abruption, from blood transfusions and occasionally during normal pregnancies. (b) Maternal antibodies on re-exposure to fetal red cells at subsequent pregnancy cross the placenta and bind to fetal cells, causing hemolysis (see Table 5.1).

Table 5.1 Effect of hemolysis.

Fetus	Infant
Anemia – progressive	Anemia
Hepatosplenomegaly	Hyperbilirubinemia
Hydrops (edema, ascites)	
Death	

Key point

Over 50% of maternal red cell alloimmunization is now due to rarer red cell antigens (Kell and c).

- Intrauterine blood transfusion.
- Deliver preterm if necessary.

POSTNATAL
- Check cord blood for blood type, hemoglobin, bilirubin and direct antibody test (DAT).
- Monitor bilirubin closely as level may increase rapidly and cause high-frequency deafness or kernicterus.
- Start intensive phototherapy, adequate fluid balance and give IVIG (immunoglobulin) and perform an exchange transfusion if severe anemia or rapidly rising bilirubin concentration.
- May need 'top up' blood transfusion for anemia within first three months of age until endogenous hemopoiesis is normal.

Prevention
Anti-D gammaglobulin has almost eliminated rhesus disease. It is given to rhesus-negative mothers during pregnancy, after potentially sensitizing events, and after delivery.

Fifteen percent of white women are rhesus-negative; less than 2% of them become sensitized from inadequate or failed prophylaxis.

Perinatal alloimmune thrombocytopenia

Analogous to rhesus disease – maternal antibodies (HPLA1 in 80%) directed against fetal platelets cross the placenta. Affects 1 in 5000 births. May occur in first pregnancy. Intracranial hemorrhage secondary to fetal thrombocytopenia occurs in up to 25%, occasionally antenatally (at 20–24 weeks or during birth). If identified from a previously affected infant, prevention is by repeated maternal infusions of intravenous immunoglobulin (IVIG) and intrauterine platelet transfusions.

Thrombocytopenia after birth is treated with platelets that are negative for the platelet antigen. The role of IVIG postnatally is uncertain. The thrombocytopenia may persist for several weeks.

Other maternal medical conditions (Table 5.2)

Table 5.2 Other maternal medical conditions that may affect the infant.

Maternal condition	Significance for the infant
Maternal hyperthyroidism	If mother is controlled on treatment, fetus and infant are usually unaffected. Rarely causes:
	Transient hyperthyroidism – fetal tachycardia, and neonatal hyperthyroidism (1–3%) – tachycardia, heart failure, vomiting, diarrhea and failure to thrive (despite good intake), jitteriness, goiter and exophthalmos (protuberant eyes). Treated for 2–3 months
	Transient hypothyroidism – from maternal drug therapy
Maternal hypothyroidism	Worldwide; commonest cause is iodine deficiency. Important cause of congenital hypothyroidism, leading to short stature and severe learning difficulties. Rarely seen in the US or UK
	Mothers treated with thyroxine; neonatal problems are rare
Autoimmune thrombocytopenic purpura (AITP)	Maternal autoantibodies against platelet surface antigens cross the placenta and cause fetal thrombocytopenia. Most fetuses unaffected. Rarely requires treatment *in utero* with repeated intrauterine platelet transfusions. If severe, may cause cerebral hemorrhage before birth or from birth trauma, but this is rare. Infants with severe thrombocytopenia or petechiae at birth should be given intravenous immunoglobulin. Platelet transfusions are reserved for platelet count <20000 mm³ (20 × 10⁹/L) or active bleeding because of the anti-platelet antibodies. The platelet count declines over the first few days before increasing

Importance

The prenatal identification of the intrauterine growth restriction (IUGR) is important because it allows:
- timely delivery of the fetus with chronic hypoxia, who is at risk of intrauterine death
- early identification of serious fetal abnormalities and fetal infection.

The neonate is at risk of:
- preterm delivery
- birth asphyxia
- hypoglycemia because of poor reserves of glycogen and other energy sources, e.g. fat
- polycythemia from intrauterine hypoxia
- hypothermia
- increased mortality.

During childhood most show catch-up growth, but some remain short and thin. There is a slight increase in risk of learning difficulties with IUGR, depending upon underlying etiology.

Definition

IUGR is the failure of a fetus or infant to achieve his or her genetic growth potential. Most will also be small for gestational age (SGA), although the two terms are not synonymous.

SGA means that the infant is below a particular weight centile for gestation; the 10th centile is most often chosen, but the 3rd or other centiles are also used (Fig. 6.1). The higher the centile chosen, the higher the proportion of infants included who are normal but small; the lower the centile used the higher the proportion with a pathologic cause, but more will be missed. The fetus may have growth failure but may not be SGA as their weight is still above the 10th centile. For this reason a prenatal combination of ultrasound features are utilized to identify this condition:
(a) estimated fetal weight of less than 10th centile for gestation
(b) a 'reduced' fetal growth velocity (change in abdominal circumference <1 standard deviation over 14 days)
(c) the presence of oligohydramnios
(d) abnormal Doppler waveform in the middle cerebral artery (MCA) compared with the umbilical artery (UA).

'Pathologic IUGR' – three or more ultrasound features present.

Etiology

Fetal

- Chromosomal disorders, e.g. trisomy 18 and other genetic syndromes.
- Structural malformations.
- Congenital infection – CMV, toxoplasmosis, rubella.

Maternal

- Undernutrition, e.g. famine in developing countries, eating disorders.
- Maternal hypoxia, e.g. cyanotic heart disease, chronic respiratory disease, altitude.
- Drugs, e.g. cigarettes (Fig. 6.2), alcohol, illicit drug use.

Placental

- Reduced maternal uterine vascular supply – pre-eclampsia, chronic maternal disease, e.g. hypertension, diabetes mellitus, renal disease.

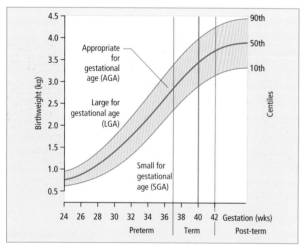

Fig. 6.1 Chart showing increase in birthweight with gestational age. Most small for gestational age fetuses or infants are constitutionally small.

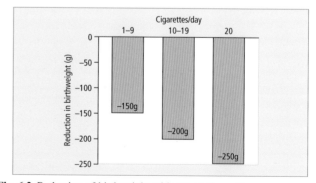

Fig. 6.2 Reduction of birthweight with maternal smoking.

Neonatology at a Glance, 2nd edition. Edited by Tom Lissauer & Avroy A. Fanaroff. © 2011 Blackwell Publishing Ltd.

- Placental vascular thrombosis and/or infarction, e.g. maternal lupus anticoagulant, antiphospholipid syndrome, sickle cell disease.
- Unequal sharing of uteroplacental vascularity – multiple gestation.

Pathophysiology

Traditionally, IUGR has been classified as symmetric or asymmetric, though in clinical practice there is considerable overlap and this distinction is no longer important prenatally.
- **Symmetric** – growth failure affecting weight, head and length. Caused by fetal factors, e.g. chromosomal disorders, syndromes or congenital infection. May be accompanied by polyhydramnios if there is reduced fetal swallowing of amniotic fluid, e.g. trisomy 21 (Down syndrome), gastrointestinal obstruction. The infant is likely to continue to be small throughout childhood.
- **Asymmetric** – growth failure with head (reflecting brain) growth relatively preserved. Classically caused by uteroplacental insufficiency with reduced oxygen transfer to the fetus. Fetal adaptation to hypoxia is to preserve blood supply to the vital organs, i.e. the brain, myocardium and adrenal glands, at the expense of the kidney, gastrointestinal tract and liver, limbs and subcutaneous tissues. This is reflected in maintained head growth but reduced abdominal circumference from reduced glycogen stores in the liver and oligohydramnios from reduced urine production. If it progresses, it results in fetal acidemia and fetal death.

Management

Management is intensive fetal surveillance to maximize gestation without compromising the fetus (Fig. 6.3).

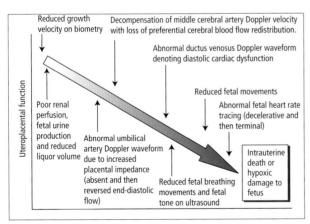

Fig. 6.3 Consequences of progressive uteroplacental failure with increasing base excess and worsening fetal blood pH (acidemia) which may result in intrauterine death. Progression may not follow sequentially.

Antenatal

- Establish if there is a fetal cause by detailed ultrasound scanning for fetal anomalies and karyotype if indicated.
- Monitor fetal growth and well-being from measurements of growth parameters, biophysical profile (amniotic fluid volume, fetal movement, fetal tone, fetal breathing movements, fetal heart activity) and Doppler blood flow velocity (umbilical and middle cerebral artery). Deliver, depending on gestational age, if growth ceases or there is an abnormal biophysical profile or significant abnormality of the Doppler flow velocity waveform (Fig. 6.4).

Postnatal

- After birth, the infant is monitored for hypoglycemia and polycythemia and examined for evidence of dysmorphic features or congenital infection.

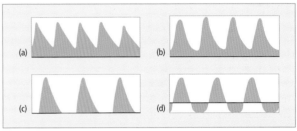

Fig. 6.4 Umbilical Doppler waveform. Normal (a), end-diastolic flow velocity reduced (b), absent (c), reversed (d). Doppler signals from the umbilical artery give information about fetoplacental blood flow. Increased blood flow velocities in the fetal middle cerebral artery and absent or reversed flow in diastole in the fetal aorta indicates fetal hypoxia. Reversed flow during atrial contraction in the ductus venosus indicates fetal myocardial insufficiency and the need for delivery.

Question

What is the significance of birthweight in adult life?

There is evidence that infants of low birthweight are at higher risk of NIDDM (non-insulin-dependent diabetes mellitus, type 2), coronary heart disease, hypertension and stroke (Barker hypothesis). However, postnatal environmental factors are complex and incompletely understood.

Preterm delivery

About 7–12% of deliveries in developed countries are preterm (12% in US, 10% in UK). The proportion of infants born preterm has increased as a result of assisted reproductive technology, increasing maternal age and medical intervention for fetal or medical reasons.

The causes of preterm delivery are shown in Fig. 7.1. The aim is to prolong pregnancy for as long as possible while ensuring the safety of the mother and fetus. The decision to deliver preterm is most difficult at the limit of viability, at 23–26 weeks of gestation, and should involve the obstetrician, neonatologist and parents. Decision-making is helped by a detailed assessment of fetal well-being, including assessment of liquor volume, fetal heart rate monitoring and Doppler studies, fetal growth, gestation and predicted birthweight (with estimates of their accuracy). This should also be informed by knowledge of the morbidity and mortality at these early gestational ages. National data are available, but will need to be modified according to the outcomes for each individual neonatal unit.

Key points

- Corticosteroids should be given to mothers at 24–34 weeks of gestation if at high risk of preterm labor to promote fetal lung maturation.
- Tocolytics are sometimes given to the mother to attempt to delay delivery to allow the corticosteroids to work or to facilitate *in utero* transfer to a perinatal center.
- Delivery of high-risk infants should preferably occur at a specialty center to avoid subsequent transfer and separation of the infant and mother.
- Neonatal care of preterm infants is very expensive. The typical cost of intensive care is $2400 (£1300) per day, basic (special) care $1500 (£800) per day. Preterm infants are likely to be in hospital until about 2 weeks before their expected date of delivery, but sometimes considerably longer.
- 25% of infants of birthweight <1500 g are multiple births (NICHD Neonatal Research Network, 2007).

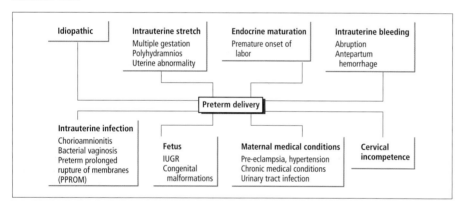

Fig. 7.1 Causes of prematurity. IUGR, intrauterine growth restriction; PPROM, preterm prolonged rupture of the membranes.

Multiple births

The incidence of spontaneous multiple gestation in white populations is:

- 1 in 89 for twins
- 1 in 89^2 (1 in 8000 for triplets)
- 1 in 89^3 (1 in 700 000 for quadruplets).

However, the number of multiple gestations has increased because of the older age of childbearing and fertility enhancing therapies. As a result, 1 in 34 births is now a multiple birth. The high number of triplets and higher-order births has declined in the UK as the maximum number of embryos transferred has been restricted to two, with one recommended (Fig. 7.2). In the US, the rate of twin pregnancies rose 70% between 1980 and 2004, but has plateaued (32 per 1000 births in 2007). Whereas the rate of triplet and higher-order multiple births climbed 400% from 1980 to a peak in 1998, they have since declined 21% to 1.5 per 1000 births in 2007 following recommendations that they should be avoided.

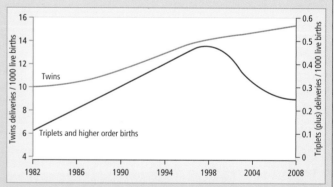

Fig. 7.2 The number of twin deliveries has increased markedly in the UK since 1982; the number of triplets and higher order deliveries increased until 1998 but has subsequently decreased.

Neonatology at a Glance, 2nd edition. Edited by Tom Lissauer & Avroy A. Fanaroff. © 2011 Blackwell Publishing Ltd.

Pregnancy complications

Twins may:
- have their own chorionic sac and placenta (dichorionic, 67%)
- share a chorionic sac and placenta (monochorionic, 33%).

Only 'chorionicity' can be allocated using ultrasound, i.e. if they share a placenta, not their zygosity, i.e. if they are identical; 20% of dichorionic twins are monozygotic.

The main pregnancy complications of twins are:
- **Preterm delivery.** The increased prematurity rate (Fig. 7.3) is responsible for the increase in perinatal mortality, which for twins is six times that of singletons. In very high order pregnancies selective fetal reduction reduces the rate of preterm delivery and perinatal mortality.
- **Intrauterine growth restriction (IUGR).** Severe IUGR, with inter-twin estimated fetal weight difference of >25%, affects 20% of dichorionic twins and 40% of monochorionic twins. If one twin has IUGR, the potential benefits of early delivery of that twin have to be weighed against the prematurity-related complications of the normally grown twin. Intrauterine death of a twin may result in neurologic impairment or death of the surviving twin if monochorionic.
- **Congenital abnormalities.** In dichorionic twins the risk is two times normal, as there are two infants. However, in monochorionic twins the risk is four times normal. Anomalies may be discordant or concordant. There is a particularly high risk of congenital heart disease.
- **Twin–twin transfusion syndrome (TTTS).** This occurs in approximately 15% of monochorionic twin pregnancies across placental arteriovenous anastomoses. The 'donor' has low perfusion pressures, growth restriction, oliguria and oligohydramnios. The other twin (the recipient) experiences hypervolemia, which may result in high-output cardiac failure, polyuria and polyhydramnios. Before 26 weeks' gestation, this may result in preterm labor or intrauterine death in up to 90% if untreated. Potential *in utero* treatment includes fetoscopic laser therapy to coagulate the placental blood vessels or periodic drainage of the amniotic fluid (amniodrainage). The latter is utilized in relatively mild disease presenting after 26 weeks' gestation. Such cases require prenatal evaluation in a perinatal center by a fetal medicine subspecialist. Even in treated cases, survivors may have neurologic morbidity in 5–10% of cases.

- **Death of a fetus.** Intrauterine death of a twin may result in preterm labor. In monochorionic twins, there may be blood loss from the live to the dead twin, leading to hypovolemia, severe anemia, neurologic impairment or death of the surviving twin.

Neonatal complications

For multiple preterm births, the immediate problem may be to find sufficient intensive care beds and staff. Every effort should be made to avoid sending the infants to different units.

Apart from prematurity, other immediate medical problems may be from twin–twin transfusion syndrome (anemia may require blood or exchange transfusion; polycythemia may require exchange transfusion), intrauterine growth restriction and congenital malformations. It is more difficult, but often possible, to fully breast-feed twins but is usually not possible for higher-order births.

Families of multiple births may need additional assistance and support:
- practical – with their care and housework (requires about 200 hours/week for triplets in infancy!); may require help to be able to leave the house (Fig. 7.4)
- emotional – exhausting to provide care
- privacy – loss of privacy as a couple, and increased rate of separation and divorce
- financial – considerable additional costs (cannot hand down clothes or equipment), may need rehousing
- increased incidence of parental depression, especially if there was fetal or neonatal loss (when every birthday or other achievement of the survivor is a reminder that the co-twin died)
- behavioral – problems in other siblings is increased threefold
- development – reduced opportunities for mother–infant interaction, as mothers are busy and often tired. Increased risk of delayed language development and poor attention span. While multiple births may provide companionship, affection and stimulation between each other, they may also engender domination, dependency and jealousy.

There are local and national support groups for parents of multiple births.

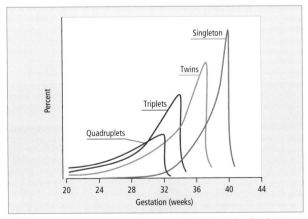

Fig. 7.3 Schematic diagram to show gestational age distribution at delivery of multiple births.

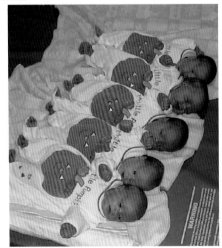

Fig. 7.4 Quintuplets. Multiple births look endearing but families may need assistance with their care.

The underlying etiologies of congenital anomalies and mechanisms by which they arise are shown in Table 8.1 and Figure 8.1. When confronted with a neonate with a congenital anomaly, there are a number of questions one needs to ask (Table 8.2), features one needs to look for (Table 8.3) and investigations to consider (Table 8.4). This evaluation process to establish a diagnosis is also appropriate when congenital anomalies are identified prenatally on antenatal ultrasound.

Table 8.1 Causes of congenital anomalies.

Teratogenic	Environmental agents during pregnancy – infections, drugs (particularly anticonvulsants), alcohol and radiation
Sporadic or multifactorial	Many single birth defects occur as isolated cases with low recurrence risk. These may be polygenic or due to faults in developmental pathways
Single-gene disorders	May be family history and previous pregnancy losses. Many multiple malformation syndromes follow autosomal recessive inheritance, but consider X-linked recessive disorders in males and new dominant mutations in isolated cases
Chromosomal	Usually cause multiple congenital malformations and learning difficulties

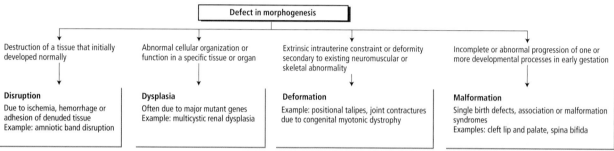

Fig. 8.1 Mechanisms of birth defects.

Table 8.2 What to ask about.

Parental age and health
Previous reproductive history
Family history of congenital anomalies
Consanguinity
Exposure to potential teratogens
Complications during pregnancy
Ultrasound screening and further investigations

Table 8.3 What to look for.

Growth parameters	Intrauterine growth restriction, overgrowth, microcephaly
Movement and posture	Hypotonia, contractures, seizures
Minor anomalies	Features with little cosmetic or functional significance. The presence of 2 or more should prompt a search for major anomalies
Major birth defects	May represent an association (defects occurring together more often than by chance alone), e.g. VACTERL (vertebral, anal atresia, cardiac, tracheo-esophageal fistula, renal and limb)
	May represent a sequence (one initial malformation resulting in the development of others, e.g. renal agenesis resulting in Potter sequence)
	May represent a syndrome (defects occurring together which have a common, specific etiology)
Dysmorphic features	Unusual or distinctive external appearance of the face, hands, feet, etc.

Table 8.4 Investigations to consider.

Clinical photographs	Provide a valuable record, especially if the phenotype changes with time
Chromosome analysis	Order chromosome analysis (karyotype) in all babies with multiple malformations or dysmorphic features. Consider requesting FISH (fluorescence in situ hybridization) tests for specific disorders, such as Williams syndrome, if appropriate
Biochemical analysis	Examples are calcium (for suspected Williams syndrome or DiGeorge syndrome) and creatine kinase (for suspected congenital muscular dystrophy)
Skeletal survey	Suspected skeletal dysplasia, such as achondroplasia
Echocardiography	Suspected congenital heart disease
Renal ultrasound	If renal anomalies suspected, e.g. in some chromosomal disorders
Brain CT/MRI/ultrasound scan	Suspected CNS malformation
Molecular analysis	Specific disorders, e.g. cystic fibrosis, spinal muscular atrophy type 1

Neonatology at a Glance, 2nd edition. Edited by Tom Lissauer & Avroy A. Fanaroff. © 2011 Blackwell Publishing Ltd.

Chromosomal disorders

As well as trisomies 21,18 and 13 and the many hundreds of well-described chromosomal disorders, subtle chromosomal rearrangements are being diagnosed using new techniques such as focused or high-resolution microarrays to examine fetal or neonatal DNA.

Trisomy 21 (Down syndrome)

Incidence is 1 in 650 live births. Most cases (94%) are due to non-disjunction of chromosome 21 during meiosis in the formation of eggs or sperm (Fig. 8.2). The risk increases with maternal age (Table 8.5).

Approximately 5% of cases are due to translocation, in which chromosome 21 is relocated onto another chromosome (usually onto chromosome 14). The risk of trisomy 21 is about 10% when the balanced translocation is carried by the mother.

Clinical features

Trisomy 21 is not always identified on prenatal screening with ultrasound or maternal blood testing. The facial appearance (Fig. 8.3a) and other clinical signs (Fig 8.3b, c) are usually recognizable at birth but diagnosis needs to be confirmed by chromosome analysis. Associated malformations include congenital heart disease, duodenal atresia and Hirschsprung disease.

Subsequently there is increased risk of:
- learning difficulties
- small stature
- secretory otitis media and hearing impairment
- visual impairment
- leukemia
- hypothyroidism
- Alzheimer disease.

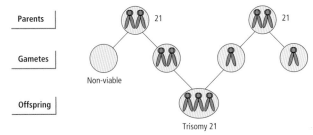

Fig. 8.2 Trisomy 21 due to non-disjunction.

Table 8.5 Risk of trisomy 21 in liveborn infants by maternal age.

Maternal age at delivery (years)	Risk
All ages	1 in 650
30	1 in 900
35	1 in 400
37	1 in 250
40	1 in 100
44	1 in 40

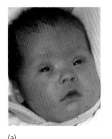
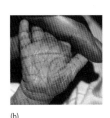
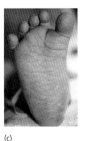

Fig. 8.3 Trisomy 21 (Down syndrome). (a) Facial features – upward slant of eyes, epicanthic folds, low set simple ears, flat occiput, third fontanelle, short neck. (b) Hands – single palmar crease and short little finger. (c) Feet – wide gap between first and second toes. Other features – hypotonia.

Trisomy 18 (Edwards syndrome)

Incidence is 0.1/1000 live births.

Most infants have intrauterine growth restriction (birth weight 1.5–2.5 kg at term). Dysmorphic features include prominent occiput, narrow forehead, small mouth and jaw, short sternum, clenched hands with overlapping digits (Fig. 8.4a), prominent heels and rocker-bottom feet (Fig. 8.4b). Major malformations include heart defects, neural tube defects, omphalocele, esophageal atresia and radial defects. Most die shortly after birth.

Trisomy 13 (Patau syndrome)

Incidence is around 0.7/1000 live births.

Dysmorphic features include scalp defects (Fig. 8.5a), broad nasal tip and polydactyly. Major malformations include holoprosencephaly (brain is a single hemisphere), microcephaly, ocular malformations, cleft lip and palate (Fig. 8.5b), heart defects and renal abnormality. Most babies die within 1 month.

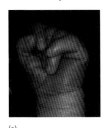
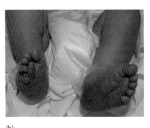

Fig. 8.4 Characteristic abnormalities of trisomy 18 (Edwards syndrome). (a) Typical clenched hand with overlying digits. (b) Rocker-bottom feet.

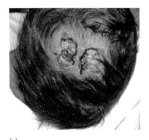
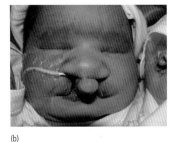

Fig. 8.5 Characteristic abnormalities of trisomy 13 (Patau syndrome). (a) Scalp defect. (b) Cleft lip and palate.

Almost all fetuses are exposed to one or more of the following potential toxins:
- over-the-counter medications
- prescription drugs
- diagnostic agents (e.g. X-rays)
- recreational drugs, e.g. cigarettes, alcohol or illicit drugs
- herbal and vitamin supplements
- environmental exposure (e.g. pollutants).

The potential consequences for the fetus are listed in Table 9.1.

Table 9.1 Potential consequences for the fetus of perinatal drug exposure.

Intrauterine growth restriction
Intrauterine death or abortion
Recognizable patterns of congenital anomalies
Maladaptation to extrauterine life
Neonatal withdrawal syndrome
Toxic effects due to passage of drugs into breast milk
Delayed effects on neurodevelopment and behavior

Maternal smoking

In the fetus, maternal cigarette smoking is associated with:
- increased risk of miscarriage, abruption and stillbirth
- reduction in birthweight, with increase in intrauterine growth restriction (IUGR) related to number cigarettes smoked per day, with average birth weight reduction of 170 g at term.

In the infant it is associated with:
- increased risk of sudden infant death syndrome (SIDS)
- increased wheezing in childhood.

Alcohol

Severe prolonged maternal alcohol ingestion is associated with fetal alcohol syndrome (FAS) (Fig. 9.1). Advice to pregnant women from the American Academy of Pediatrics and the Department of Health in the UK is to avoid alcohol whilst pregnant although the effect of occasional, mild alcohol ingestion or occasional binge drinking is not known.

Figure 9.1 shows features of fetal alcohol syndrome.

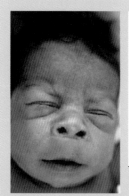

Features of fetal alcohol syndrome:
- Characteristic facies
  - saddle-shaped nose
  - maxillary hypoplasia
  - absent philtrum (ridges between the nose and upper lip)
  - thin upper lip
- Symmetric growth failure – severe, persistent
- Cardiac defects (40–50%)
- Behavior problems – irritable in infancy, hyperactive in childhood
- Developmental delay – average I.Q. 63

Fig. 9.1 Features of fetal alcohol syndrome. (Photograph courtesy of Dr David Clark.)

Neonatal withdrawal (abstinence) syndrome

- Serious problem because of widespread use of narcotics and other drugs of dependency.
- Situation often complicated by multiple drug use.
- Mothers on heroin are usually encouraged to change to methadone.
- Increased risk of hepatitis B and C and HIV infection if intravenous drug user.
- Onset of withdrawal:
  - heroin <2 days
  - methadone <2 days but can be delayed up to 2 weeks.
- Cocaine does not cause problems from withdrawal but from direct transfer of the drug:
  - placental infarction which may lead IUGR or placental abruption and antepartum hemorrhage or fetal death
  - rarely, cerebral infarction *in utero* and neonatal seizures.

Clinical assessment

This must be done systematically and repeatedly (6-hourly) (Table 9.2). This is facilitated by using a scoring system (e.g. Finnegan's

Table 9.2 Clinical features of opiate withdrawal.

Irritability	Vomiting
Scratching	Diarrhea
Wakefulness	Yawning
Shrill cry	Hiccoughs
Tremors	Salivation
Hypertonicity	Stuffy nose
Seizures	Sneezing
Unexplained pyrexia >38°C	Sweating
Tachypnea (rate >60/min)	Dehydration

Neonatology at a Glance, 2nd edition. Edited by Tom Lissauer & Avroy A. Fanaroff. © 2011 Blackwell Publishing Ltd.

score) to determine whether therapy is required. In some centers, analysis of meconium is performed to determine drug exposure during pregnancy.

Treatment

Usually with oral morphine sulfate, aiming to wean by titration of dose with score.

Medical and social services discharge planning meetings are often required during pregnancy and after birth as the lifestyle of many drug users is not conducive to the care of babies and children.

Medicines

Relatively few medicines produce recognizable patterns of malformation in the fetus (Table 9.3). Adverse effects may not be recognized if they are subtle or have delayed presentation, e.g. diethylstilbestrol (DES) given for threatened miscarriage in the mother and subsequent association with clear-cell adenocarcinoma of the vagina and cervix in female offspring, evident only during adolescence or early adult life.

Pregnant women should avoid taking both prescribed and over-the-counter medications whenever possible. For prescribed drugs, the benefits must outweigh the risks and appropriate maternal and fetal surveillance should be undertaken.

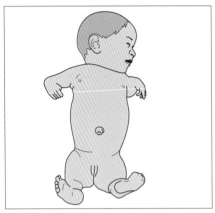

Fig. 9.2 Severe limb shortening (phocomelia, 'like a seal') from maternal thalidomide therapy, which was widely marketed (not in US) for morning sickness from 1957. Teratogenic effects only recognized several years later.

Table 9.3 Some recognizable patterns of malformation or neonatal problems following maternal drug ingestion.

Time in pregnancy	Drug	Malformations/problems	Drug	Malformations/problems
Organogenesis (<8 weeks' gestation)	**Thalidomide**	Short limbs (Fig. 9.2) Absent auricles, deafness	**Folic acid inhibitors** (methotrexate) as cytotoxic therapy	Fetal syndrome – microcephaly, neural tube defects, short limbs
	Anticonvulsants: • carbamazepine • valproic acid (sodium valproate) • hydantoins (phenytoin)	Fetal carbamazepine/ valproate/hydantoin syndrome – midfacial hypoplasia, CNS, limb and cardiac malformations Developmental delay	**Coumarin** (warfarin)	Fetal coumarin (warfarin) syndrome – nasal hypoplasia, microcephaly, hydrocephalus, optic atrophy, congenital heart defects, stippled epiphyses, purpuric rash
Pregnancy (>8 weeks' gestation)	**Antithyroid drugs** (iodides, propylthiouracil)	Goiter Congenital hypothyroidism	**Tetracyclines**	Hypoplasia of tooth enamel, yellow–brown staining of teeth
	Androgens **Aspirin/non-steroidal anti-inflammatory drugs**	Masculinization of female Closure of ductus arteriosus in fetus	**β-blockers and hypoglycemic agents**	Neonatal hypoglycemia Poor fetal growth
Labor and delivery	**Opiate analgesia**	Respiratory depression at birth		

The term 'congenital infection' applies to infections acquired *in utero* (Fig. 10.1) whereas 'neonatal infection' is acquired shortly before or at delivery or postnatally (see Chapter 41).

Most congenital infections are viral, but other significant causes include toxoplasmosis and syphilis.

Maternal infection is usually primary, i.e. it is a first infection, when there is lack of maternal immunity. Risk of infection from recurrent maternal infection (e.g. with CMV or HSV) is usually lower than from a primary infection. Maternal infection may be asymptomatic or associated with mild symptoms.

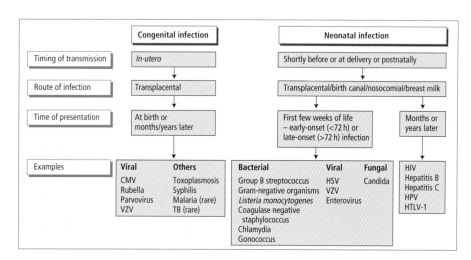

Fig. 10.1 Congenital and neonatal infections. (CMV – cytomegalovirus; VZV – varicella-zoster virus; HSV – herpes simplex virus; HPV – human papilloma virus; HTLV-1 – human T-cell leukemia virus 1.)

Diagnosis (Table 10.1)

Table 10.1 Diagnosis of congenital infection.

Antenatal	Postnatal
Maternal	
History (e.g. rash, 'flu-like' illness, contact)	
Screening serology – seroconversion (IgG, IgM, IgA), or low avidity IgG to identify if infection was recent	
Culture/PCR of lesion, e.g. cervical herpes, blood, urine	
Fetal	**Placenta**
Ultrasound or fetal MRI scanning for anomalies	Histology/microscopic dark-field examination for spirochetes in syphilis
Amniocentesis for fluid or fetal blood sample for serology/platelet count/PCR	Culture/PCR
	Infant
	Culture/PCR – blood, urine, CSF, stool, nasopharyngeal aspirate, skin lesions
	CT or MRI head for calcification, microcephaly
	Ophthalmologic assessment – for retinitis
	Early serology may not help, as seroconversion may be delayed

PCR, polymerase chain reaction.

Neonatology at a Glance, 2nd edition. Edited by Tom Lissauer & Avroy A. Fanaroff. © 2011 Blackwell Publishing Ltd.

Clinical features

Congenital infections may precipitate pregnancy loss or preterm delivery. The clinical features of the symptomatic infant are shown in Fig. 10.2.

Key point

It is not possible to reliably tell clinically if the cause is CMV, toxoplasmosis, rubella or syphilis either using ultrasound prenatally or by physical examination in the neonate.

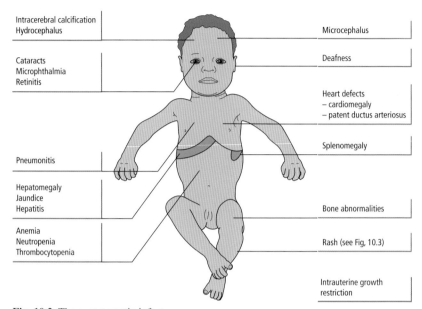

Intracerebral calcification
Hydrocephalus

Microcephalus

Cataracts
Microphthalmia
Retinitis

Deafness

Heart defects
– cardiomegaly
– patent ductus arteriosus

Splenomegaly

Pneumonitis

Hepatomegaly
Jaundice
Hepatitis

Bone abnormalities

Anemia
Neutropenia
Thrombocytopenia

Rash (see Fig, 10.3)

Intrauterine growth restriction

Fig. 10.2 The symptomatic infant.

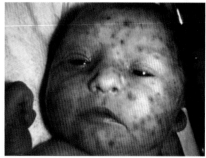

Fig. 10.3 Blueberry muffin rash.

Congenital cytomegalovirus (CMV) infection

- Commonest congenital infection in the US and UK (0.5–1/1000 live births).
- 1–2% of mothers seroconvert during pregnancy.
- Overall mother-to-infant transmission rate is 40%.
- May be transmitted in breast milk or blood transfusions.

Infected infants

- 5–10% severely affected (Fig. 10.2). Poor prognosis if abnormalities detectable on postnatal CT or MRI scan – microcephaly, periventricular calcification (Fig. 10.4), CNS translucencies.
- 80–90% asymptomatic at birth, but 10% of them are at risk of sensorineural hearing loss.
- Most common infectious cause of sensorineural hearing loss.

Diagnosis

- Viral isolation from infant's urine, saliva collected at less than 3 weeks of age, or amniotic fluid prenatally.
- Viral DNA (by PCR amplification) from amniotic fluid, fetal blood, or infant's blood, urine, CSF collected at less than 3 weeks of age.

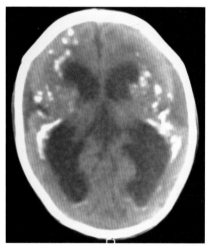

Fig. 10.4 Postnatal CT scan of the brain showing intracranial calcification from congenital CMV infection. The calcification may be identified on antenatal ultrasound.

Treatment

For severely affected newborn:
- Ganciclovir (intravenous) will improve acute organ disease (eye, liver, bone marrow, lungs), but controversial whether it has long-term benefit to prevent CNS damage.

Question

Should babies with congenital CMV infection be isolated when on the neonatal unit?

No. About 1% of infants in newborn nurseries excrete CMV, but most are asymptomatic. Pregnant staff are potentially at risk, though most are immune. Attention to hand-washing is the key to preventing infection of caregivers, and should be strictly adhered to when touching any baby.

Other points

• No vaccine yet for seronegative mothers.
• Infected infants may excrete CMV in urine for many months.
• All infected infants should be followed for late-onset sensorineural hearing loss until school age.

Congenital toxoplasmosis

• Usually after primary maternal infection in pregnancy.
• Seronegative mothers are most at risk from poorly cooked meat. Small risk from handling feces of recently infected cats or ingesting contaminated soil from unwashed vegetables.
• The transmission rate and treatment are shown in Table 10.2. The earlier in pregnancy the mother is infected the more severely the fetus is affected.
• The clinical features of the symptomatic infant are shown in Fig. 10.2. Subclinical disease includes retinitis (Fig. 10.5), epilepsy and learning difficulties.
• Treatment of infants with congenital infection – pyrimethamine and sulfadiazine, plus folinic acid for prolonged duration.

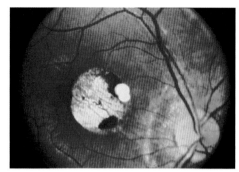

Fig. 10.5 Retinitis from toxoplasmosis. This may present many years later.

Rubella

• Prevented by maternal vaccination. Now very rare in immunized populations.
• The earlier in pregnancy the mother is infected the more severely the fetus is affected.
• Clinical features are shown in Fig. 10.2.
• There is no effective treatment.

Congenital syphilis

In the US, a marked increase in incidence occurred in the 1980s, especially among drug users, but it has since declined. In the UK it is extremely rare. Antenatal screening on maternal blood is performed routinely. If active infection is diagnosed or suspected, the mother should be treated. Treatment more than 4 weeks before delivery prevents congenital infection.
• Transmission rate during primary infection in pregnancy is 100%.
• Without treatment there is 40% abortion/stillbirth/perinatal death.
• Prenatally, is associated with severe IUGR in developing countries.
• Clinical features are shown in Fig. 10.2. Those specific to congenital syphilis include a characteristic rash on the soles of the feet (Fig. 10.6) and hands (Fig. 10.7) and bone lesions (Fig. 10.8).

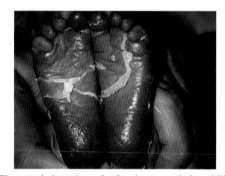

Fig. 10.6 Characteristic rash on the feet in congenital syphilis. (Courtesy of Dr Hermione Lyall.)

Table 10.2 Transmission rate and treatment of toxoplasmosis.

Trimester	Transmission rate	Clinical features	Treatment
First	15%	35% die before birth, 40% severely affected	Preventative – maternal spiramycin <18 weeks
Second Third	40% 60%	90% subclinical disease at birth; clinical manifestations may present years later	If severely affected – with antibiotics (pyrimethamine and sulfadiazine) and folinic acid

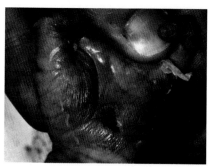

Fig. 10.7 Characteristic rash on hands in congenital syphilis. (Courtesy of Dr Hermione Lyall.)

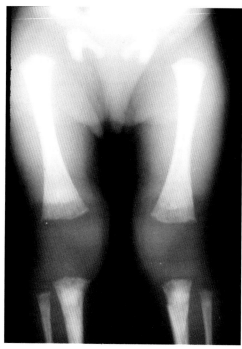

Fig. 10.8 X-rays in congenital syphilis showing bilateral metaphyseal lucency of the long bones and destruction of the medial proximal metaphysis of the left tibia.

• Treatment antenatally and/or postnatally is with penicillin. Effectiveness of treatment is monitored serologically.
• If the mother has not received adequate treatment or if there is physical, laboratory or radiographic evidence of disease, treat. If there is any doubt, treat directly.

Varicella: chickenpox, varicella zoster virus (VZV) infection

Primary maternal infection in pregnancy is uncommon as more than 90% of mothers are immune.

Early in pregnancy

• Intrauterine infection is rare (2% risk).
• Can lead to eye and CNS damage, skin scarring (Fig. 10.9) and limb hypoplasia.
• 1% risk of herpes zoster (shingles) in infancy.

Late in pregnancy

Infants born to mothers who develop chickenpox between 5 days before or 2 days after delivery should be given varicella zoster immune globulin (VZIG). This reduces but does not eliminate the risk of neonatal varicella zoster virus (VZV).

They should be closely monitored, and should be started on aciclovir (intravenous) if any signs of infection develop.

Parvovirus B19

• 50% of pregnant women are susceptible to infection.
• Transmission rate is 20–30%.
• In most cases there is a normal outcome of pregnancy but rarely:
  – infection in early pregnancy can lead to fetal loss
  – infection in pregnancy may lead to severe fetal anemia (aplastic anemia), causing hydrops fetalis (edema and ascites from heart failure) and is associated with an abnormal middle cerebral artery waveform on Doppler ultrasound. May require an intrauterine transfusion for the severe anemia.

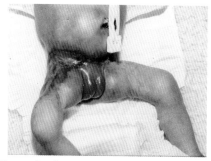

Fig. 10.9 Skin scarring from maternal VZV infection early in pregnancy. This is rare.

11 Adaptation to extrauterine life

The transition from intrauterine to extrauterine life involves a complex sequence of physiologic changes that begin before birth. Remarkably, although infants experience some degree of intermittent hypoxemia during labor, most undergo this transition smoothly and uneventfully. If not, cardiorespiratory depression requires prompt and appropriate resuscitation.

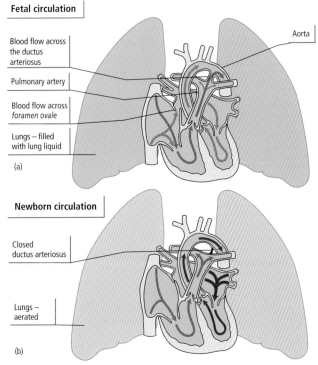

Fig. 11.1 Changes in the circulation at birth. (a) Fetal circulation. (b) Newborn circulation.

Physiologic changes in fetal–neonatal transition

- Before birth, the lungs are filled with fluid. Oxygen is supplied by the placenta. On reaching the right atrium, some of the oxygenated blood from the placenta flows directly to the left atrium via the patent foramen ovale, bypassing the lungs. In addition, the blood vessels that supply and drain the lungs are constricted (providing high pulmonary vascular resistance), so most blood from the right side of the heart bypasses the lungs and flows through the ductus arteriosus into the aorta (Fig. 11.1a).
- Shortly before and during labor, lung liquid production is reduced.
- During descent through the birth canal, the infant's chest is squeezed and some lung liquid exudes from the trachea.
- Multiple stimuli (thermal, chemical, tactile) initiate breathing. Serum cortisol, ADH (antidiuretic hormone), TSH (thyroid-stimulating hormone) and catecholamines dramatically increase.
- The first gasp is usually within a few seconds of birth. A negative intrathoracic pressure is generated to achieve this. Most lung liquid is absorbed into the bloodstream or lymphatics within the first few minutes of birth.
- Aeration of the lungs is accompanied by increased arterial oxygen tension; the pulmonary artery blood flow increases and the pulmonary vascular resistance falls.
- Contraction of the umbilical arteries restricts access to the low resistance placental circulation. This results in increased peripheral vascular resistance and an increase in systemic blood pressure.
- The fall in pulmonary vascular resistance and the rise in systemic vascular resistance result in near equalization of pressures across the duct and virtual cessation of ductal flow (Fig. 11.1b).

Abnormal transition from fetal to extrauterine life

The transition may be altered by a variety of antepartum or intrapartum events, resulting in cardiorespiratory depression, asphyxia or both (Table 11.1). The consequences may include hypoxic

Table 11.1 Conditions associated with abnormal neonatal adaptation to extrauterine life.

Fetal	Maternal	Placental
Preterm/post-dates	General anesthetic	Chorioamnionitis
Multiple birth	Maternal drug therapy	Placenta previa
Forceps or vacuum-assisted delivery	Pregnancy-induced hypertension	Placental abruption
Breech or abnormal presentation	Chronic hypertension	Cord prolapse
Shoulder dystocia	Maternal infection	
Emergency cesarean section	Maternal diabetes mellitus	
Intrauterine growth restriction (IUGR)	Polyhydramnios	
Meconium-stained amniotic fluid	Oligohydramnios	
Abnormal fetal heart rate trace		
Congenital malformations		
Anemia		
Infection		

Neonatology at a Glance, 2nd edition. Edited by Tom Lissauer & Avroy A. Fanaroff. © 2011 Blackwell Publishing Ltd.

ischemic encephalopathy, persistent pulmonary hypertension and multi-organ system failure.

The Apgar score

The Apgar score, named after Virginia Apgar, an anesthesiologist, is used to describe an infant's condition during the first few minutes of life (Table 11.2). It is assigned at 1 and 5 minutes of life. If the score is still below 7 or the infant is requiring resuscitation, it is continued every 5 minutes until normal or 20 minutes of age. Although often assigned, few babies truly attain a score of 10, because it is uncommon for the baby to be pink all over. The Apgar score is useful as a guide in rapidly assessing respiration, circulation and the nervous system, and as a record of the infant's condition shortly after birth.

Table 11.2 Apgar score.

	Apgar score		
	0	1	2
Heart rate	Absent	Slow (<100 beats/ minute)	>100 beats/ minute
Respiration	Absent	Slow, irregular	Good, crying
Muscle tone	Limp	Some flexion of extremities	Active motion
Reflex irritability (response to stimulation)	No response	Grimace	Cough, sneeze, cry
Color	Blue or pale	Body pink, blue extremities	Pink

Key points

The Apgar score is not used to determine the need for resuscitation.

Evaluation for resuscitation is made second by second and is based on the three most important signs:
- respiration
- heart rate
- color.

Questions

How does resuscitation affect the Apgar score?

The Apgar score is assigned irrespective of resuscitation being performed.

Can one determine Apgar scores in preterm infants?

Yes. However, the extremely preterm infant's maximum score is reduced by poor muscle tone and weaker response to stimulation than term infants.

Asphyxia

Sustained, severe asphyxia (Fig. 11.2) *in utero* or during labor results in the infant making increased respiratory effort, followed by a period of apnea (primary apnea). During primary apnea the heart rate falls to about half its normal rate but the blood pressure is initially maintained.

With continuing asphyxia, the infant starts to gasp, the heart rate slowly falls, as does the blood pressure. After several minutes, after a last gasp, there is secondary apnea. To recover, positive pressure ventilation, if necessary accompanied by cardiac compressions, is required.

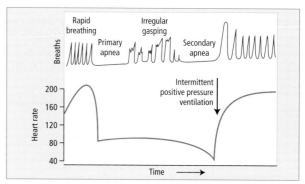

Fig. 11.2 Effect of asphyxia.

Question

What is the long-term significance of a low Apgar score (3 or less)?

An infant with a low Apgar score at 1 minute but responding rapidly to resuscitation has an excellent prognosis.

An infant with a low Apgar score beyond 10 minutes of age in spite of adequate resuscitation is at increasing risk of neurologic injury resulting in cerebral palsy the longer the score remains low.

12 Neonatal resuscitation

Neonatal resuscitation is a rapid sequence of steps to be initiated if a baby's breathing or circulation is impaired (Fig. 12.1). The aim is to optimize the airway, breathing and circulation as quickly as possible.

Approximately 6–10% of all deliveries receive some form of resuscitation. Ventilation, i.e. lung inflation, is the key. Only 0.1% of newborns of any gestation appear to need chest compressions and medications during delivery room resuscitation.

Preparation

The presence of antepartum and intrapartum risk factors will usually allow the need for resuscitation to be anticipated. This enables health-care professionals skilled in neonatal resuscitation to be present. However, the need for neonatal resuscitation cannot always be predicted. All health-care professionals in maternity or neonatal units should be skilled in airway management, mask ventilation and cardiac compressions. Staff skilled in intubation and drug administration must be available at all times.

Before delivery

- Introduce yourself to the parents and explain why present.
- Review obstetric records.
- Wash hands and put on gloves.
- Turn on radiant warmer.
- Check equipment is present and functional:
  - clock
  - gas supply and delivery system – mask with T-piece connected to a pressure-limited circuit or bag and mask or Neopuff® (provides pressure-limited gas supply)
  - airway adjuncts (oropharyngeal (Guedel) airway)
  - suction apparatus
  - laryngoscope, tracheal tube and introducer
  - stethoscope
  - venous access equipment and drugs
  - pulse oximeter.
- Warm towels available.

Specific questions to consider

- Will you need help?
- Is neonatal transport going to be needed?

Warmth/stimulation

Why important

Hypothermia may contribute to hypoglycemia, acidosis and even mortality, especially in VLBW (very low birthweight) infants.

Action

- Keep resuscitation area warm and draft-free.
- Perform resuscitation under radiant warmer.
- Dry infant, remove wet towel, then use dry towel.
- For extremely preterm infants, place infant in plastic wrapping with only face exposed.
- Start the clock or note the time.
- Stimulate if necessary – by drying with the towel.

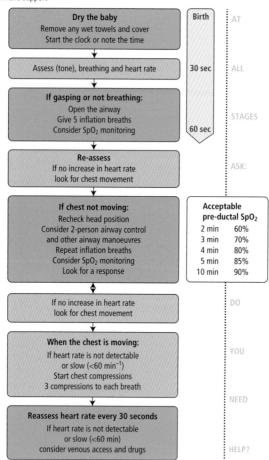

Fig. 12.1 Algorithm for newborn life support. (Resuscitation Council UK, 2010 and Pediatrics DOI:10.1542/peds.2009-1510.)

Initial assessment at birth (Fig. 12.2)

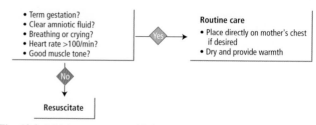

Fig. 12.2 Initial assessment at birth.

Neonatology at a Glance, 2nd edition. Edited by Tom Lissauer & Avroy A. Fanaroff. © 2011 Blackwell Publishing Ltd.

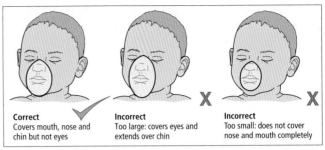

Fig. 12.5 Correct size and position of face mask. It should cover the mouth, nose and chin.

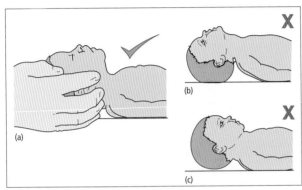

Fig. 12.3 Head position, the key to airway management. (a) Head in correct neutral position. (b) Head overextended – incorrect. (c) Head flexed – incorrect.

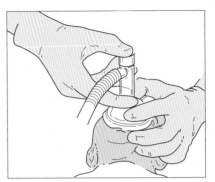

Fig. 12.6 Mask ventilation via T-piece connected to oxygen from a pressure-limited circuit, e.g. a mechanical ventilator or a Neopuff®.

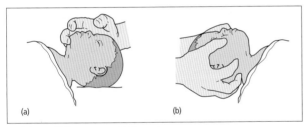

Fig. 12.4 (a) Chin support. (b) Jaw thrust.

Airway

If gasping or not breathing – open airway:
- **Position** – head in neutral position (Fig. 12.3), using towel beneath shoulders if desired, chin support (Fig. 12.4a) or jaw thrust (Fig. 12.4b).
- **Patency** – remove any meconium or blood if obstructing the airway. Not necessary to remove amniotic fluid.
- **Rare causes of airway obstruction** – choanal atresia, micrognathia (small jaw) or macroglossia (large tongue) – oral airway.
- If cyanosed but breathing – **give oxygen**.

Breathing

Assessment

- Look for chest movement.
- Listen and feel for airflow. Attach oxygen saturation monitor if necessary.

Action

Initiate ventilation with a mask (Fig. 12.5) attached to a mechanical ventilator via a T-piece or a Neopuff® or a ventilation bag (Fig. 12.6) if:
- no or inadequate respiratory effort
- heart rate <100 beats/minute
- centrally cyanosed in spite of facial oxygen.

Mask ventilation

Most babies will respond to lung inflation.
- Term babies – use air. Only give oxygen if oxygenation, judged by oximetry, remains inadequate despite good ventilation. Avoid hyperoxaemia as damaging.
- Preterm infants – use air/oxygen blender and pulse oximetry. Use minimum oxygen for pre-ductal saturation of 80–90% by 10 minutes of age. Avoid SpO2 >95%.

Inflation breaths

- Initially, for a term infant, give five breaths at an inflation pressure of 30 cm water for 2–3 seconds each. This will usually expand the lungs.
- If the heart rate has improved move to ventilation breaths described below. If not:
- Assess chest movement. If no chest movement recheck airway position and patency.

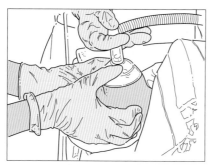

Fig. 12.7 Two-person airway control – consider if mask inflation ineffective. One person holds the head in the correct position, applies jaw thrust and holds the mask in place, the assistant operates the T-piece to provide lung inflation.

- If still no chest movement consider using two person airway control – see Fig. 12.7. Repeat inflation breaths.
- Monitor oxygen saturation, right hand (Fig. 12.1).

Ventilation breaths

- After inflation breaths, continue at 30–40 breaths/min. Use correct size mask and position, ventilating sufficiently to maintain a good heart rate.
- Assess heart rate after 15–30 seconds.
- Stop when heart rate remains >100 breaths/minute and breathing effectively.

Intubation

Indications

- Mask ventilation ineffective (apnea or heart rate <100 beats/minute), i.e. after checking baby's head in neutral position, chin tilt/jaw thrust applied, longer inflation time given.
- Tracheal suction needed for meconium.
- Congenital upper airway abnormality.
- Prolonged ventilation needed.
- Extreme prematurity – delivery of surfactant.
  But:
- **Limit attempts to 20–30 seconds!**
- Mask-ventilate infant between attempts.

Circulation

- Assess heart rate with stethoscope or feel at the base of the umbilical cord.
- Initiate chest compressions (Fig. 12.8) if:
  – lung aeration has been achieved **and** heart rate <60 beats/minute.

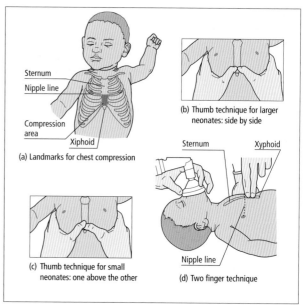

Fig. 12.8 (a) Apply pressure to lower third of sternum, just below imaginary line joining the nipples. Avoid the xiphoid. Depress to reduce anteroposterior diameter of the chest by one-third (1–1.5 cm, ½ to ¾ inches) with no bounce. The thumb technique (b and c) is more effective than the two-finger technique and is recommended (d), but the two-finger technique is easier if you are alone or have small hands.

Give three compressions to one breath to achieve 90 compressions and 30 breaths (i.e. 120 events) in 1 minute. Stop and recheck heart rate every 30 seconds. Stop compressions when heart rate >60 beats per minute.

Key points

- Are the lungs inflated, i.e. good chest movement (and exhaled CO_2 detected, if measured)? In neonates chest compressions will have no effect if the lungs have not been inflated.
- Call for help – giving chest compressions is easier with two people.

Drugs (Table 12.1)

Only use if no response in spite of:
- effective ventilation
- effective cardiac compression.

Key point

In neonates, drugs are useless unless ventilation is effective.

Table 12.1 Drugs for neonatal resuscitation.

Medication	Concentration	Dosage/route	Indications
Epinephrine (adrenaline)	1 : 10 000	IV: 0.1–0.3 mL/kg ET: 0.3–1 mL/kg	Heart rate <60 beats/minute after effective ventilation with 100% oxygen and chest compressions
Volume expander	Normal saline Whole blood	10 mL/kg IV	Suspected acute blood loss and/or signs of hypovolemia (poor perfusion, weak pulses, pallor)
Dextrose	10%	2.5 mL/kg (250 mg/kg) IV	Hypoglycemia
Sodium bicarbonate	0.5 mEq/mL (0.5 mmol/mL) (4.2% solution)	1–2 mEq/kg (1–2 mmol/kg) (2–4 mL/kg 4.2%) IV, slowly	Consider after prolonged arrest that does not respond to other therapy

Intravenous (IV) drugs are given via umbilical venous catheter or intraosseous route. Endotracheal (ET) delivery of epinephrine is easier but less reliable as absorption is variable and evidence of its effectiveness in the newborn is lacking. Consider ET route while IV access is obtained.

Special cases

Management of meconium

• If vigorous – no resuscitation needed.
• If not breathing and hypotonic, consider: rapid inspection of oropharynx and suction clearance any obstruction; intubation and suction of the trachea.
• Monitor for subsequent respiratory distress.

Ethical decisions

International guidelines (2010) have been published for:
• non-initiation of resuscitation
  – infants less than 23 weeks of gestation (confirmed) or birthweight less than 400 g
  – anencephaly or trisomy 13 or 18 (confirmed)
• discontinuation of resuscitation
  – if the heart rate is undetectable at birth and remains so for 10 minutes.

Decisions need to be made about comfort care with parents and obstetric team.

This does not address the difficult ethical decisions concerning infants born at 23–25 weeks because of their:
• high mortality
• prolonged neonatal intensive care and hospitalization
• high risk of short-term morbidity and long-term disabilities
• high cost.

Parents will need information about mortality and morbidity, both national and local. Views will be affected by culture, religion and legal framework and may be limited by resources available. A center or country may have a birthweight or gestation cut-off below which respiratory support is not provided.

Neonatal team will need to assess the situation at birth – whether gestation is correct, what is the infant's birthweight and condition. If in doubt, rather than hasty decisions in delivery room, often best to transfer to neonatal unit for detailed assessment. Disadvantage is that once intensive care initiated it may be more difficult to withdraw treatment.

Failure to respond to resuscitation (Fig. 12.9)

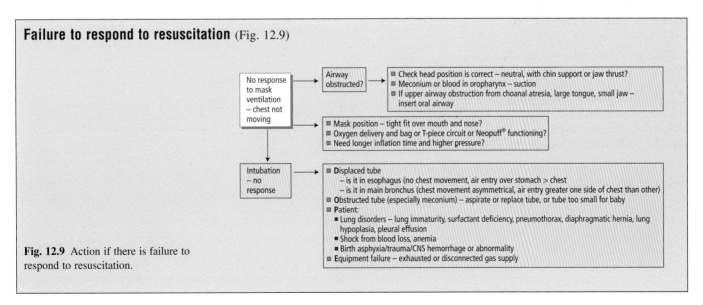

Fig. 12.9 Action if there is failure to respond to resuscitation.

Asphyxia, from the Greek word meaning pulseless, is now used to mean a state in which gas exchange – placental or pulmonary – is compromised or ceases altogether, resulting in cardiorespiratory depression. Hypoxia, hypercarbia and metabolic acidosis follow. Compromised cardiac output diminishes tissue perfusion, causing hypoxic–ischemic injury to the brain and other organs. The neonatal condition is called hypoxic–ischemic encephalopathy (HIE). In developed countries, approximately 0.5–1/1000 liveborn term infants develop HIE and 0.3/1000 have significant neurologic disability.

Hypoxic–ischemic injury is the commonest cause of neonatal encephalopathy, where there is disordered neurologic function. Other causes of neonatal encephalopathy include maternal anesthetic agents, cerebral malformations, metabolic disorders (hypoglycemia, hypocalcemia, hyponatremia, inborn errors of metabolism), infection (septicemia and meningitis), hyperbilirubinemia, neonatal withdrawal (abstinence) syndrome and intracranial hemorrhage. The origin may be antepartum, during labor and delivery or postnatally (Fig. 13.1). As the term 'birth asphyxia' is imprecise and implies that the baby's encephalopathy is a consequence of birth, which may have medicolegal implications, it has been recommended that the term is best avoided.

In hypoxic–ischemic encephalopathy (HIE), there is:
• a significant hypoxic event immediately before or during labor or delivery
• profound acidemia (pH <7 and base deficit >12 mmol/L) on an umbilical cord artery sample, if obtained
• Apgar score 0–3 for longer than 5 minutes
• neonatal neurologic manifestations, e.g. seizures, coma or hypotonia
• multisystem organ dysfunction.

Pathogenic mechanisms

These include:
• failure of gas exchange across the placenta – excessive or prolonged uterine contractions, placental abruption, ruptured uterus
• interruption of umbilical blood flow – cord compression including shoulder dystocia, cord prolapse
• inadequate maternal placental perfusion, maternal hypotension or hypertension – often with intrauterine growth restriction (IUGR)
• compromised fetus – anemia, IUGR
• failure of cardiorespiratory adaptation at birth – failure to breathe (see Chapter 12).

Compensatory mechanisms

These include:
• "diving reflex" – redistribution of blood flow to vital organs (brain, heart and adrenals)
• sympathetic drive – increase in catecholamines, cortisol, antidiuretic hormone (ADH, vasopressin)
• utilization of lactate, pyruvate and ketones as an alternative energy source to glucose.

Neuronal death

Following a severe ischemic insult, some neuronal cells die rapidly (primary neuronal death due to necrosis). When the circulation is re-established, a sequence of biologic reactions may extend the zone of injury (secondary neuronal death due to apoptosis). There is the potential to ameliorate this secondary damage (Fig. 13.2).

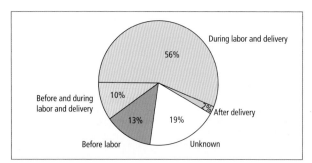

Fig. 13.1 Time of origin of neonatal encephalopathy. (Pierrat V. Prevalence, causes and outcome at 2 years of age of newborn encephalopathy: population based study. *Arch Dis Child Fetal Neonatal Ed* 2005, **90**: F257–261.)

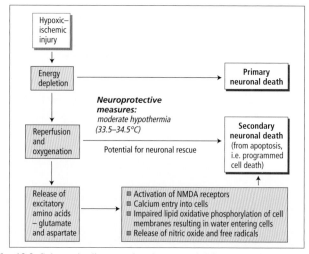

Fig. 13.2 Schematic diagram showing potential for prevention of secondary neuronal death.

Clinical manifestations

The clinical manifestations, investigations and management are summarized in Fig. 13.3.

Clinical staging of hypoxic–ischemic encephalopathy

This is done using a staging system, a sequential, systemic evaluation of the severity of brain injury. The most common is Sarnat (Table 13.1) although the simpler Thomson score is increasingly used.

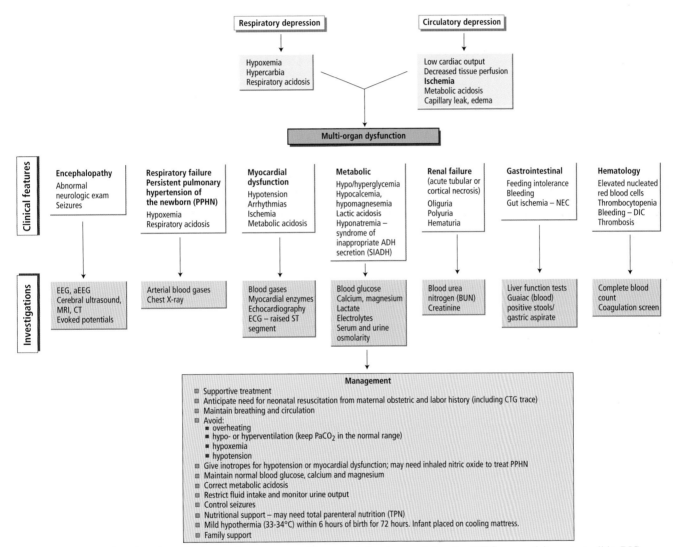

Fig. 13.3 Clinical manifestations, investigations and management of hypoxic–ischemic encephalopathy. (NEC – necrotizing enterocolitis; DIC – disseminated intravascular coagulation; EEG – electroencephalogram; aEEG – amplitude integrated EEG, cerebral function monitor; CTG – cardiotochography.)

Table 13.1 Sarnat staging of hypoxic–ischemic encephalopathy.

	Grade 1 (mild)	Grade 2 (moderate)	Grade 3 (severe)
Level of consciousness	Irritable/hyperalert	Lethargy	Coma
Muscle tone	Normal or hypertonia	Hypotonia	Flaccid
Tendon reflexes	Increased	Increased	Depressed or absent
Myoclonus	Present	Present	Absent
Seizures	Absent	Frequent	Frequent
Complex reflexes			
Suck	Active	Weak	Absent
Moro	Exaggerated	Incomplete	Absent
Grasp	Normal to exaggerated	Exaggerated	Absent
Oculocephalic (doll's eye)	Normal	Overactive	Reduced or absent
Autonomic function			
Pupils	Dilated, reactive	Constricted, reactive	Variable or fixed
Respirations	Regular	Periodic	Ataxic, apneic
Heart rate	Normal or tachycardia	Bradycardia	Bradycardia
EEG	Normal	Low-voltage periodic or paroxysmal	Periodic or isoelectric
Prognosis	Good	Variable	High mortality and neurologic disability

Neuroimaging and functional studies (Table 13.2)

Table 13.2 Neuroimaging and functional studies and their indications and interpretation.

Procedure/test	Indication and interpretation
Standard	
EEG (electroencephalogram) or cerebral function monitor (aEEG) (Fig. 13.4) – best done as soon after birth as possible	aEEG within 6 hours of birth – presence of encephalopathy and prognosis Monitoring of seizures and background activity. If normalizes in first 24 hours – good prognosis
Cranial ultrasound	Easy to perform at bedside. Useful for defining normal anatomy and for evidence of prenatal injury on initial scan on admission or findings suggestive of congenital infection or intracranial hematoma or metabolic disorder. May detect cerebral edema, hyperechogenic basal ganglia, and abnormal blood flow velocity in middle and anterior cerebral arteries Useful for following sequence and timing of any changes. Subsequent scans may show ventriculomegaly and cortical atrophy
MRI scan	Imaging of choice in combination with ultrasound. Allows early recognition of bilateral basal ganglia injury, internal capsule, white matter and cortical injury, focal cerebral infarction, hemorrhage and malformations (Figs 13.5 and 13.6). However, an early scan on day 1–2 may appear normal
Not routinely performed/available	
CT scan	For major malformation, hemorrhage, calcification, edema. Poor for posterior fossa, focal injury and myelin
Magnetic resonance proton spectroscopy (Lactate: N-aspartate acetate ratio)	After 5 days, used to predict later disability
BAER (brainstem auditory evoked responses)	Auditory nerve brainstem conduction
VEP (cortical visual evoked potentials)	Optic nerve – visual cortex pathway
Somatosensory evoked potentials	Median nerve – cortical responses, for prognosis

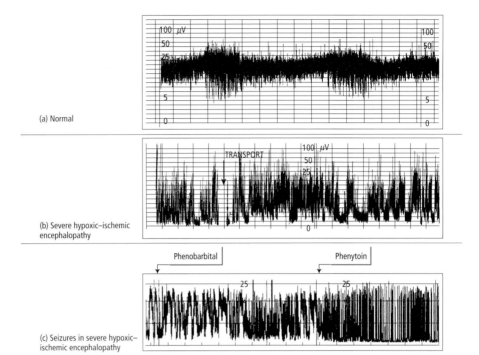

(a) Normal

(b) Severe hypoxic–ischemic encephalopathy

TRANSPORT

Phenobarbital   Phenytoin

(c) Seizures in severe hypoxic–ischemic encephalopathy

Fig. 13.4 Amplitude-integrated EEG (aEEG) trace from cerebral function monitor showing (a) normal term newborn – normal baseline (>5 microV); (b) severe hypoxic–ischemic encephalopathy – low baseline amplitude; (c) seizures in severe hypoxic–ischemic encephalopathy unresponsive to phenobarbital but responsive to phenytoin, although the trace remains abnormal. (Courtesy of Prof. Andrew Wilkinson.)

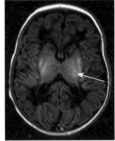

Fig. 13.5 MRI (axial TW1) at the level of the basal ganglia showing abnormal high signal in the posterolateral lentiform nuclei and thalami, loss of the normal high signal from myelin in the posterior limb of the internal capsule (arrow), abnormal signal in the head of the caudate nuclei and low signal throughout the white matter. These are typical of acute perinatal asphyxia in the first week after the insult. (Courtesy of Dr Frances Cowan.)

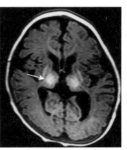

Fig. 13.6 MRI scan showing cerebral atrophy. Axial TW1 MRI at the level of the basal ganglia showing severe atrophy of the basal ganglia (arrow), thalami and white matter with enlarged ventricles and extracerebral space. There is also plagiocephaly. This degree of atrophy takes several weeks to develop. (Courtesy of Dr Frances Cowan.)

Outcome

In general:
- a normal neurologic exam and feeding well by 2 weeks of age suggest good prognosis
- mild HIE – usually normal outcome
- moderate HIE – increased risk for motor and cognitive abnormalities, including cerebral palsy (15–20%)
- severe HIE – mortality rate 75%, 80% of survivors will have neurologic sequelae.

The postnatal markers of poor prognosis are shown in Table 13.3.

Table 13.3 Postnatal markers of poor prognosis.

Persistence of clinical seizures

Persistently abnormal neurologic exam

Not feeding orally by 2 weeks of age

EEG with burst suppression or isoelectric pattern on any day or amplitude-integrated EEG (aEEG) with a low baseline amplitude

Abnormal EEG after several days

Abnormal basal ganglia or marked brain atrophy on MRI

Persistent tissue lactate and low N-aspartate acetate on MR proton spectroscopy, if available

Poor postnatal head growth

14 Birth injuries

The incidence of severe birth injuries has fallen dramatically over the last 50 years. This is because prolonged, obstructed labor and difficult instrumental deliveries are avoided by cesarean section. However, birth injuries still occur, especially in infants who have had instrumental deliveries, shoulder dystocia, malpresentation (e.g. breech deliveries) or are preterm. They are usually classified according to their anatomic location.

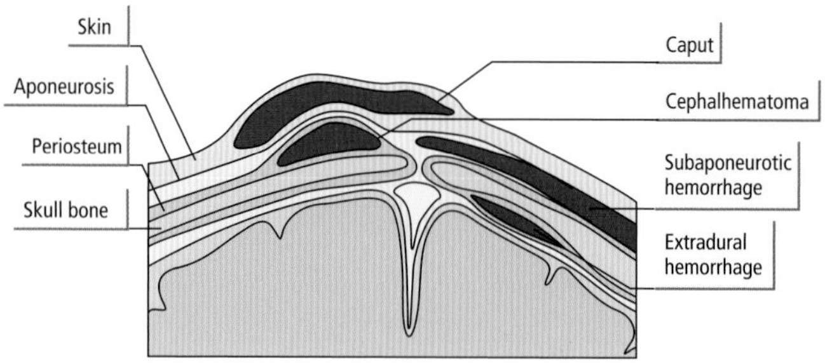

Common or important birth injuries

See Figure 14.1 and Table 14.1.

Fig. 14.1 Anatomic location of injuries to the head.

Table 14.1 Common or important birth injuries.

Lesion	Anatomic location	Comments	Clinical description and management
Injuries to the head			
Caput	Edema of the soft tissue of presenting part Crosses suture lines	Common and benign	Edema, bruising of scalp No treatment necessary; resolves in a few days Good prognosis
Chignon 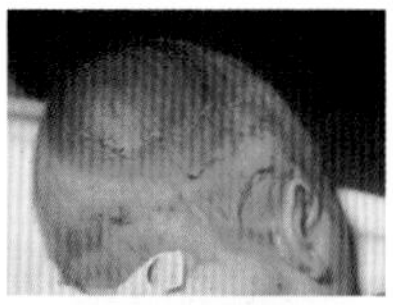	Over site of vacuum extraction	Less common since soft, flexible cups introduced	Edema, sometimes bruising, skin damage Resolves over several days
Cephalhematoma 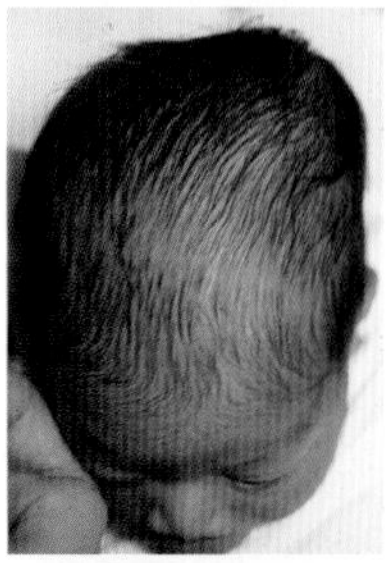	Subperiosteal Usually parietal Does not cross suture lines May be bilateral	Relatively common Associated with prolonged or instrumental labor	Hematoma maximal on second day May be associated with skull fracture May calcify Exacerbates jaundice Resolves in days to months
Subgaleal (subaponeurotic) hemorrhage 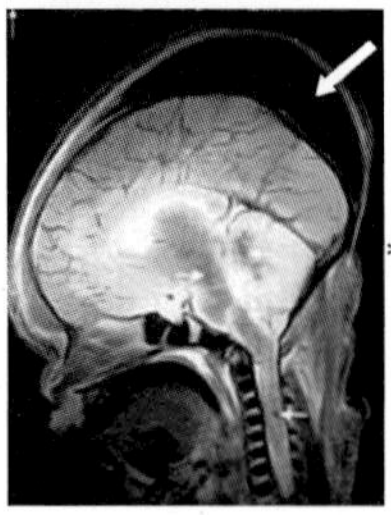	Between galea aponeurosis and periosteum (arrow)	Rare Risk factors: • prematurity • vacuum extraction May have underlying coagulopathy	Boggy appearance and pitting edema of scalp Anterior displacement of the ears Prompt recognition is crucial as may rapidly progress to hypovolemic shock Transfusion of blood, fresh frozen plasma, coagulation factors
Skull fractures	Usually parietal bone; occipital in breech deliveries	Uncommon Usually forceps delivery, but also normal delivery	Soft tissue edema and cephalhematoma Fractures may be linear or depressed Prognosis good
Minor injuries			
Forceps marks	From pressure of blades, especially rotational forceps	Less common as rotational forceps now seldom used	Bruising and/or skin abrasion Heals rapidly

Neonatology at a Glance, 2nd edition. Edited by Tom Lissauer & Avroy A. Fanaroff. © 2011 Blackwell Publishing Ltd.

Lesion	Anatomic location	Comments	Clinical description and management
Scalpel lacerations	Head or face	Scalpel incision at cesarean section	Usually small Depending on size and site, may need tapes to oppose edges, suturing, plastic surgical referral
Injuries to the face			
Facial palsy	Usually unilateral (right side in figure). If bilateral, suspect congenital cause	Pressure on maternal ischial spine or forceps delivery	Unilateral facial weakness on crying Eye remains open Resolves in 1–2 weeks If eye permanently open, use methylcellulose eye drops
Asymmetric crying facies	Unilateral absence of orbicularis oris	More common than facial palsy	In contrast to facial palsy, eye can close
Injuries to the neck and shoulders			
Fractured clavicle	Midclavicular area	Shoulder dystocia, breech Snap may be heard during delivery	Edema, bruising, crepitation at the site; decreased active movement of arm Clavicular lump from callus formation during healing phase Confirm on X-ray Heals spontaneously
Brachial palsy Erb Nerves involved: C5, C6, ±C7		Shoulder dystocia, abnormal presentation, obstructed labor, macrosomia Phrenic nerve palsy – rare, diaphragm is elevated	Decreased shoulder abduction and external rotation, supination of wrist and finger extension (waiter's tip posture) Hand movement is preserved In 5% diaphragm palsy 90% resolve by 4 months To avoid contractures, perform passive range of motion ± splints Surgical referral if not recovered by 2–3 months
Other injuries			
Extremities	Fracture of the humerus/femur	Breech, shoulder dystocia. May have underlying bone/muscle disorder	Deformity, reduced movement of limb, pain on movement Orthopedic referral Splint to reduce pain. Rarely, hypovolemia from blood loss requires treatment Bones rapidly remodel
Spinal cord	Cervical, thoracic, lumbar spine	Rare Instrumental delivery, may occur prenatally	Lack of movement below level of lesion Absent respiratory effort in high lesions Supportive care, steroids for spinal shock
Intra-abdominal organs	Ruptured liver, spleen Renal injury Adrenal hemorrhage	Macrosomia, breech, dystocia Pre-existing hydronephrosis Prematurity, neuroblastoma	Abdomen – distension, mass, discoloration, tenderness. Shock, pallor Hematuria Hypoglycemia, abdominal mass, coma, shock Intravascular volume support Abdominal ultrasound. Surgery unless bleed is contained (subcapsular hematoma)
Genitalia	Scrotum and labia majora	Breech	Bruising, hematoma Resolves

*Photograph of subgaleal hemorrhage with permission from Cheong, JLY *et al. Arch Dis Child Fetal Neonatal Ed* 2006; **91**: F202–F203.

15 Routine care of the newborn infant

Most term infants start to breathe several seconds after birth and rapidly become pink and active. If breathing normally, the baby can be rapidly dried and handed directly to his/her mother. This will allow direct skin-to-skin contact, the baby being kept warm with a towel. Alternatively the baby can first be wrapped in warm towels. It is at this time that most babies are alert and are ready to begin to establish nursing at the breast.

Shortly after birth, the midwife, or pediatrician if attending the delivery, will examine the baby briefly to check there are no abnormalities. A more detailed examination, the routine examination of the newborn, will be performed later, but within 24 hours of birth (see Chapter 16). Name tags will be attached to the baby and a record made to confirm that the baby passes urine and meconium within 24 hours of birth.

Routine care

Vitamin K

The administration of vitamin K as prophylaxis against hemorrhagic disease of the newborn should have been discussed with parents antenatally. It can be given either as a single, large dose by intramuscular injection, which provides reliable prevention but is an injection, or orally, which requires several doses to overcome its variable absorption, and protection is less reliable. Infants are at increased risk if they are breast-fed, as breast milk is low in vitamin K, if they have liver disease and if their mother is on anticonvulsant therapy.

Consent should be obtained before vitamin K is given.

Eye prophylaxis

In the US, all newborn infants are given erythromycin eye drops as prophylaxis against gonococcal and chlamydia eye infection. Silver nitrate eye drops were used, but can cause chemical conjunctivitis and do not prevent chlamydial infection.

In the UK eye prophylaxis is not practiced, but gonococcal or chlamydia eye infection is extremely rare.

Circumcision

Widely performed in the US; only for religious reasons in the UK.

Appropriate analgesia should be provided for the procedure and postoperatively. May disrupt feeding and unsettle the infant for several days (see Chapter 51).

Meeting the family

Siblings, grandparents and other close family should be encouraged to visit in order to be introduced to the new member of the family.

Breast-feeding

Mothers may need assistance and support to establish breast-feeding.

Umbilical cord care

Always wash hands before handling.
Keep dry and exposed to air.
Clean with water, avoid alcohol as it delays cord separation.
Fold diaper (nappy) below umbilicus.
In US, topical antibacterial agents (e.g. triple dye) widely used.

Emotions

Some mothers are emotionally labile during the first few days after birth. Even minor problems can cause considerable upset. Explanation and reassurance are required.

Mothers who develop postnatal depression or who are unable to care for their baby or have no suitable accommodation may be identified during this postnatal period. Liaison with mental health or social services, voluntary services or health visitors and other community health professionals may be required.

Infants with disabilities or complex medical needs may require a multidisciplinary planning meeting before discharge. This is considered further in Chapter 70.

Screening

The use of a screening test depends on:
- prevalence of the disease
- ease with which the test can be performed
- false-positive and false-negative screening rate
- whether it significantly improves the prognosis
- cost.

Availability of screening tests varies with judgment as to whether these criteria are satisfied.

Biochemical screening (called the Guthrie test in the UK)

This is performed on all infants. Blood spots, usually from a heel prick, are placed on a card which is sent to a reference laboratory.

In most centers in the US, tandem mass spectrometry is used to screen a wide range of disorders including:
- phenylketonuria (frequency 1 : 12 000)
- hypothyroidism (1 : 4000)
- sickle cell disease
- thalassemia
- MCAD (medium chain acyl-CoA dehydrogenase) deficiency (1 : 10 000).

In the UK, screening is confined to the disorders listed above as well as cystic fibrosis.

Neonatology at a Glance, 2nd edition. Edited by Tom Lissauer & Avroy A. Fanaroff. © 2011 Blackwell Publishing Ltd.

Audiology (see Chapter 61)

Neonatal hearing screening for all infants is being increasingly introduced. In some centers it is provided only for infants with risk factors, e.g. family history, hyperbilirubinemia requiring treatment or given potentially ototoxic drugs. All infants with preauricular tags or pits should have their hearing checked.

Transcutaneous bilirubin at discharge

Introduced because of recent increase in kernicterus. Can identify infants at increased risk who require close monitoring.

Other possible screening tests

Pulse oximetry on all infants
Lower limb pulse oximetry to detect cyanotic congenital heart disease. However, low yield as prevalence is low. Performed at some centers.

Ultrasound for DDH (developmental dysplasia of the hips)
Performed on all babies in some countries in Europe. Used selectively in UK and US.

Routine hematocrit for polycythemia
Not recommended as not proven that treatment improves prognosis.

Health promotion

Parents should be provided with verbal and written advice about:
- feeding
- the importance of immunizations
- how to reduce the risk of SIDS (sudden infant death syndrome) (Fig. 15.1)
- the need for a car seat to take the baby home and whenever traveling in a car
- when to seek medical attention.

Discharge

Before discharge check that:
- feeding is being established successfully
- the nursing staff do not have concerns about the mother's handling of the baby
- the baby is well and not significantly jaundiced.

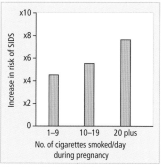

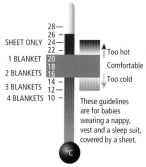

Fig. 15.1 Advice for parents to reduce the risk of SIDS. (Adapted from *Reduce the Risk of SIDS*. Department of Health, UK, 2009 and American Academy of Pediatrics, 2005.)

(a) Back to basics
Always put babies to sleep on their back (not prone or side)

(b) Avoid smoking in your baby's presence

(c) Don't let your baby get too hot or cold

All babies are examined shortly after birth to check that transition to extrauterine life has proceeded smoothly and there are no major abnormalities. A comprehensive medical examination within 24 hours of birth, the 'routine examination of the newborn infant', should be performed.

The purpose is to:
• detect any abnormalities – a significant congenital anomaly is present at birth in 10–20 per 1000 live births
• confirm and/or consider the further management of any abnormalities detected antenatally
• consider potential problems related to maternal pregnancy history or familial disorders
• allow the parents to ask any questions and raise any concerns about their baby
• determine whether there is concern by caregivers about the care of the baby following discharge.
• provide health promotion, especially prevention of sudden infant death syndrome (SIDS) (see Chapter 15).

Preparation

Maternal charts (records):
• Check maternal antenatal, labor and delivery charts.

Equipment:
• Tape measure.
• Stethoscope.
• Ophthalmoscope.
Environment:
• Warm room free from drafts.
• Privacy, suitably lit.
• Examine on firm mattress in crib.
• Both parents present if possible.
• Always wash hands and clean stethoscope before each examination.

The infant

• The baby must be completely undressed during the course of the examination so that all the body is observed.
• Need a content, relaxed infant for successful examination.
• Examination is performed opportunistically, i.e. eyes when open, heart when quiet, hips left until last. However, the examination must be complete.

Routine examination of newborn infants (Table 16.1, Figs 16.2 and 16.3)

Developmental dysplasia of the hip, DDH (congenital dislocation of the hip, CDH)

Clinical examination:
• Performed on all infants – part of routine neonatal examination.
• Infant must be relaxed – if crying or kicking there is tightening of the muscles around the hip.
• There may be asymmetry of skin folds around an affected hip and shortening of the affected leg.
• Pelvis is stabilized with one hand; with the other, the examiner's middle finger is placed round the greater trochanter and the thumb around the distal medial femur.
• Both hips are fully abducted; full abduction may not be possible if the hip is dislocated.
• Check if dislocatable posteriorly (Barlow maneuver) (Fig. 16.1a).
• Check if hip is dislocated and can be relocated into acetabulum (Ortolani maneuver) (Fig. 16.1b).

Risk increased:
• in female infants (9 : 1)
• if positive family history (20% of affected infants)
• if breech presentation (30% of affected infants)
• in infants with a neuromuscular disorder.

If abnormal or questionable clinical examination, arrange hip ultrasound at 4–6 weeks of age. Follow-up ultrasound and re-examination is recommended for breech presentation; similarly in some centers if family history. Role of routine ultrasound screening of all infants still being assessed – can identify some missed on clinical examination and some with shallow acetabular shelf not detectable on clinical examination, but has appreciable false-positive rate (7%) and is expensive. Not recommended for all infants in US or UK.

For management see Chapter 60.

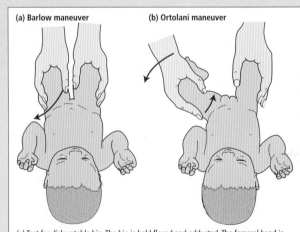

(a) Test for dislocatable hip. The hip is held flexed and adducted. The femoral head is pushed downwards. If dislocatable, the femoral head will be pushed posteriorly out of the acetabulum
(b) Test for dislocated hip. Abduct hip with upward leverage of femur. A dislocated hip will return with a palpable **clunk** into the acetabulum

Fig. 16.1 Barlow and Ortolani maneuvers.

Neonatology at a Glance, 2nd edition. Edited by Tom Lissauer & Avroy A. Fanaroff. © 2011 Blackwell Publishing Ltd.

Table 16.1 Significant congenital abnormalities which may be identified on routine examination.

Dysmorphic infant (see Chapter 8)
Cataracts (see Chapter 61)
Cleft lip and palate (see Chapter 39)
Heart murmurs (see Chapter 48)
Urogenital – hypospadias, undescended testes (see Chapter 51)
DDH (developmental dysplasia of the hip)
Imperforate anus (see Chapter 47)
Spinal anomalies (see Chapter 58)

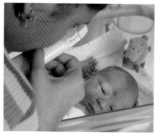

Fig. 16.2 Checking for red reflex. If absent, i.e. the pupil is white (cataracts, glaucoma, retinoblastoma), refer directly to an ophthalmologist. Also check eye looks normal, e.g. for a coloboma, a key-shaped defect in the iris.

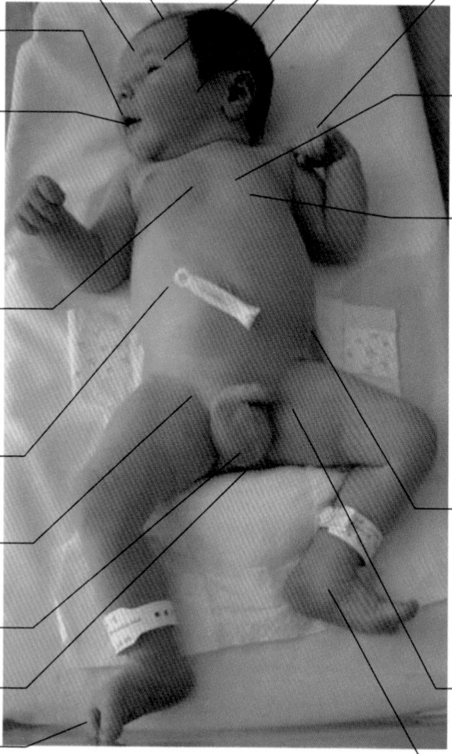

Eyes – check with ophthalmoscope for red reflex

General appearance, posture, movements – are they normal?

Fontanel and skull structures feel normal

Facies – any dysmorphic features e.g. trisomy 21 (Down syndrome)

Palate – inspect and palpate to identify cleft palate

Cyanosis of tongue – if in doubt check oxygen saturation with pulse oximeter

Breathing and chest wall movement – observe for respiratory distress:
■ increased respiratory rate
■ flaring of nostrils
■ grunting
■ chest retractions (sternal and intercostal)

Abdomen:
■ normal liver 1–2 cm below costal margin, spleen tip and left kidney may be palpable
■ any masses – investigate with ultrasound

Hips – check for developmental dysplasia of the hips (see opposite)

Genitalia – check testes in scrotum and normal penis in boys and normal anatomy in girls

Anus – observe patency

Feet – check for talipes

Plethora or pale? If suspected, check hematocrit

Ears – low-set, malformed or preauricular tags/pits?

Hands – check for extra digits, palmar creases

Jaundice – if present in first 24 hours, needs investigation

Heart – auscultate. Normal heart rate 110–160 beats/min but may drop to 80 beats/min during sleep
Heart murmur – see Chapter 48

Back and spine: check from top to bottom. Sacral dimples below the line of the natal cleft – common and benign. If proximal to natal cleft, ultrasound to identify if there is a track to the spinal cord, though rare. Check the back for a tuft of hair, swelling, nevus or other lesion over the spine, which may indicate vertebral or spinal cord abnormality, e.g. spina bifida occulta or tethered cord. If present, arrange ultrasound, but MRI scan may be required

Femoral pulses:
■ reduced in coarctation of the aorta. If suspected, check by measuring blood pressure in all four limbs. Difference >15 mmHg is significant
■ bounding in patent ductus arteriosus

Muscle tone:
■ observe for normal movements of limbs
■ feel when handling the baby (support the head when picking up baby)
■ on holding prone, term babies will lift their head to horizontal position

Measurements (at 40 weeks):	50th centile	(10th–90th centile)	Comments
Birth weight	3.5 kg	(2.8–4.5 kg)	
Head circumference	35 cm	(33.5–37 cm)	Maximal occipito-frontal diameter
Length	51 cm	(48–53.5 cm)	Routinely measured in US, not in UK
			Inaccurate unless hips and knees are straightened

Fig. 16.3 Routine examination of newborn infants.

17 Neurologic examination

The newborn infant's neurologic development progresses markedly with gestational age. This needs to be taken into account when performing a neurologic examination, and accounts for many of the components of the neurologic examination used in the clinical assessment of gestational age (Ballard or Dubowitz score; see Chapter 80).

A detailed neurologic examination is performed if there are any concerns about neurologic abnormality. A normal neurologic exam is helpful prognostically, e.g. following hypoxic–ischemic encephalopathy, a normal neurologic examination and normal feeding by 2 weeks of age are associated with a good prognosis. Very low birthweight infants with a normal neurologic examination and intracranial ultrasound at 40 weeks are highly unlikely to develop significant motor disability and the predictive value of combined assessment is better than ultrasound alone.

The neurologic development described here is adapted from that described by Amiel-Tison, who has also devised a standardized examination with 10 components.

States of alertness

An infant's state of alertness can be classified (Prechtl scale):
- state 1: eyes closed, regular respiration, no movements
- state 2: eyes closed, irregular respiration, no gross movements
- state 3: eyes open, no gross movements
- state 4: eyes open, gross movements, no crying
- state 5: eyes open or closed, crying.

For satisfactory neurologic assessment infants need to be in state 3, when they are quiet but alert, i.e. able to fix and follow. However, the clinician may have to bring the baby to this state. Inability to do this may occur because the infant is abnormally lethargic or hyperexcitable (or deeply asleep or hungry!). An abnormal cry may also indicate abnormal neurology.

Visual fixing and following

A normal term infant should fix and follow a face or target of concentric black and white circles or a red ball moving from side to side. This starts at about 32 weeks' gestation. The infant should make eye-to-eye contact when held about 30 cm from the observer.

Hearing

Infants respond to noise with a facial grimace, turning of the head or startle.

Consolability

This is the response of the crying infant to a voice or soothing movements, such as rocking from side to side. It indicates communication between the infant and caregiver.

Head circumference

This is a surrogate measure of brain volume and subsequently of brain growth.

Face (cranial nerves)

There should be normal facial movements, blinking of the eyes and ability to suck strongly.

Posture and spontaneous motor activity

Posture

Posture at term is flexed (Fig. 17.1). Movements are smooth, symmetric and varied. The infant can move the fingers and can abduct the thumbs.

Passive tone in limbs and trunk

Develops from hypotonia at 24 weeks of gestation to strong flexor tone at 40 weeks, initially in the lower then upper limbs (Fig. 17.2).

Active tone in limbs and trunk

See Fig. 17.3.

32 weeks	40 weeks
Arms extended Some flexion of the legs	Full flexion of all four limbs

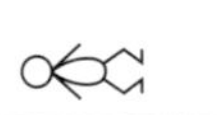

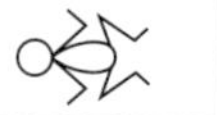

Fig. 17.1 Posture.

Popliteal angle		Foot dorsiflexion		Scarf sign	
With thigh beside abdomen, extend knee as far as possible		With knee flexed, ankle is dorsiflexed Measure angle between dorsum of foot and anterior of leg		Hand pulled across chest towards opposite shoulder Position of elbow noted	
32 weeks	Term	32 weeks	Term	32 weeks	Term
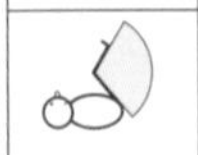	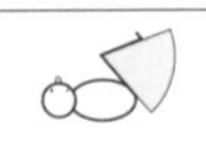	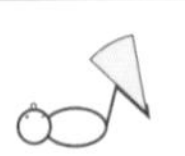	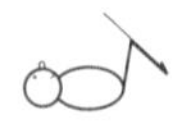	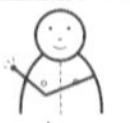 Largely passes midline	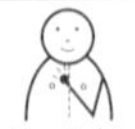 Very tight
120°–110°	90° or less	40°–30°	0°	Very weak resistance	Does not reach midline

Fig. 17.2 Passive tone in limbs and trunk.

Neonatology at a Glance, 2nd edition. Edited by Tom Lissauer & Avroy A. Fanaroff. © 2011 Blackwell Publishing Ltd.

Righting reaction		Neck flexor tone (raise to sit)		Ventral suspension	
Holding infant upright under axillae		Holding infant's shoulders, pull from lying to sitting			
32 weeks	40 weeks	32 weeks	40 weeks	32 weeks	40 weeks
Brief support of lower limbs only	Upright and takes weight for few secs	No movement of head forwards	Minimal head lag. Similarly for neck extensor tone (back to lying)	Some extension of head and back	Head extended above body, back extended and limbs fully flexed

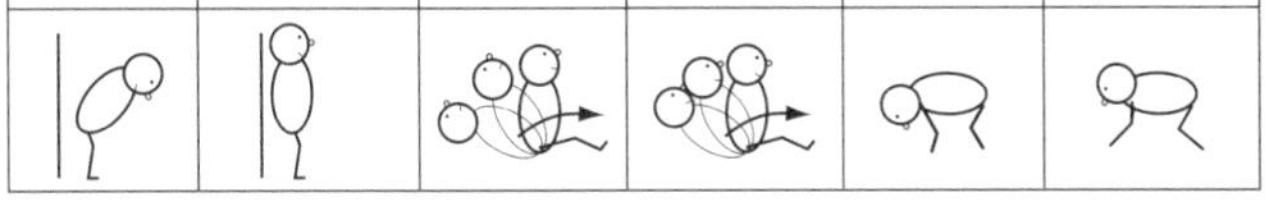

Fig. 17.3 Active tone in limbs and trunk.

Primary reflexes

Primary or primitive reflexes reflect brainstem activity (Fig. 17.4). They are a manifestation of central nervous system programming with later suppression by higher cortical function. If they cannot be elicited, suggests central nervous system depression. More important, their persistence suggests damage to upper cortical control (Table 17.1).

Table 17.1 Primary reflexes.

Reflex	Disappearance (corrected age)
Placing	3 months
Palmar grasp	3 months
Plantar grasp	3 months
Moro	4 months
Asymmetric tonic neck reflex (ATNR)	6 months

Deep tendon reflexes

May be depressed with lower motor neuron lesions, occasionally increased with upper motor neuron lesions. May reveal asymmetry. Ankle clonus is common and usually of no pathologic significance.

Plantar responses

Elicited by stroking the lateral part of the foot from heel to toe. Unhelpful at this age as normal response may be flexor (toe down) or extensor (toe up).

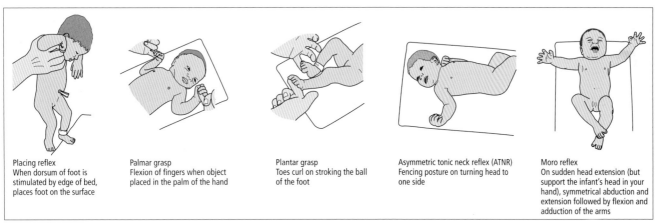

Placing reflex
When dorsum of foot is stimulated by edge of bed, places foot on the surface

Palmar grasp
Flexion of fingers when object placed in the palm of the hand

Plantar grasp
Toes curl on stroking the ball of the foot

Asymmetric tonic neck reflex (ATNR)
Fencing posture on turning head to one side

Moro reflex
On sudden head extension (but support the infant's head in your hand), symmetrical abduction and extension followed by flexion and adduction of the arms

Fig. 17.4 Primary reflexes.

The family must, of course, be included in the care of all newborn infants, whether well or critically ill. The birth of a healthy newborn infant is usually a joyous occasion fulfilling the dreams and hopes of the parents. If the baby is extremely premature, sick, has malformations or dies, these dreams will be shattered and the family will experience considerable distress. The family will need sensitive assessment, discussion and support. How this is done will influence their ability to cope and recover in the short and long term. Family centered care encourages parents to be partners in their infants' care and in decisions about treatment. The way parents see themselves as parents, respond to their baby and react to stressful situations is very individual and will be influenced by personal views and standards, family background and culture. Psychological support from an appropriately trained professional helps parents deal with their distress and anxiety. This may also be needed to help with psychological problems that commonly occur after the infant leaves hospital.

Attachment

What is maternal attachment?

It is the intense relationship which develops between a mother and her child, providing protection and nurturing for the child (Fig. 18.1).

In many animals, e.g. ducks or penguins, there is a critical, sensitive period for mother–infant bonding immediately after birth, when the mother and her offspring must be in direct contact. If this does not happen the mother fails to recognize that the newborn is hers. Attachment in humans does not necessarily happen instantly, but develops over time. Although touching and nursing the baby shortly after birth is helpful in promoting attachment, and should be encouraged, humans can still become attached to their infants where this does not occur, for example if the infant is admitted directly to the neonatal unit.

Fathers and other family members also develop attachment with the newborn baby. Attachment is the foundation of healthy emotional development. In childhood secure attachment gives the child the confidence to explore and learn.

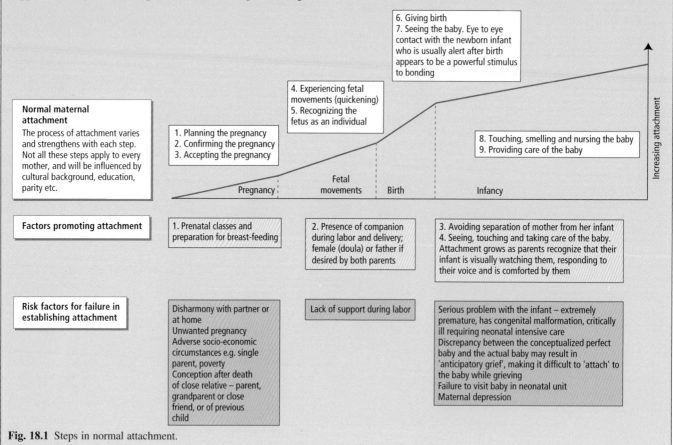

Fig. 18.1 Steps in normal attachment.

Neonatology at a Glance, 2nd edition. Edited by Tom Lissauer & Avroy A. Fanaroff. © 2011 Blackwell Publishing Ltd.

Communicating with parents

Parents and family want open communication about their baby. Professionals need to not only provide accurate and realistic information about the baby's problems but also listen to and address the family's anxieties and feelings. The needs of each of the family members should be elicited, as they may differ. Fathers, who may be at work much of the time, particularly value opportunities for communication.

Some specific circumstances regarding communicating with parents related to perinatal care are considered below.

Antenatal identification of fetal abnormality or potential abnormality

• Many problems, including major malformations and preterm delivery, are now identified before birth. The recognition of many minor malformations or the possibility of an abnormal finding in the fetus has become a common cause of additional anxiety for parents.
• The neonatal team should be involved and present a realistic picture. First discuss the positive aspects and present facts in a positive light – describe a glass as half full rather than half empty. Facts should be disclosed but unsubstantiated fears not shared with the family.
• Problems should be anticipated and their consequences and management discussed with the family. If appropriate, a tour of the neonatal intensive care unit (NICU) before delivery should be conducted.

Admission of the infant to the neonatal unit

See Chapter 22.

Infants with serious congenital malformations

The crisis of the birth of a child with a serious malformation can result in emotional turmoil, the parents mourning the loss of the normal child they expected whilst also needing to become attached to their living but abnormal child. Doctors and other health professionals will need to explain the nature and implications of the disorder to the parents and family and may need to provide considerable emotional support to help families in this difficult situation (Table 18.1).

Table 18.1 How parents wish to be told about a serious problem or life-threatening illness.

Setting	**Explain long-term prognosis**
In private and comfort	If child is likely to die, listen to concerns about time, place and nature
Uninterrupted	of death
Unhurried	Outline the support/treatment available
Both parents (or friend/relative) present if possible	
Senior doctor	**Address feelings**
Nurse or social worker present	Be prepared to tolerate reactions of shock, especially anger or weeping
Translator if necessary	Acknowledge uncertainty
Some families find it helpful to have a tape recording of the interview or	How is it likely to affect the family?
to take notes	What and how to tell other children, relatives and friends?
Establish contact	**Concluding the interview**
Find out what the family knows or suspects	Elicit what parents have understood
Respect family's vulnerability	Clarify and repeat, particularly highlighting immediate situation and
Use the child's name	next steps
Do not avoid looking at them	Acknowledge that it may be difficult for parents to absorb all the
Be direct, open, sympathetic	information
	Mention sources of support
Provide information	Give parents a contact telephone number or e-mail
Flexibility is essential	Give web-site or address of self-help group
Pace rather than protect from bad news. Some families want a lot of	
information at once, others prefer shorter interviews more often	**Follow-up**
Name the illness or condition	Offer early follow-up and arrange date
Describe symptoms relevant to child's condition	Suggest to families that they write down questions in preparation for
Discuss etiology – parents will usually want to know	next appointment
Anticipate and answer questions. Don't avoid difficult issues because	Ensure adequate communication of content of interview to other
parents have not thought to ask	members of staff, family practitioner and health visitor and other
	professionals, e.g. a referring pediatrician

Human milk is recommended as the exclusive food for all term infants for the first 6 months of life. Human milk is also recommended for preterm infants but may need fortification. All mothers should be encouraged and supported to breast-feed. Counseling should commence early in pregnancy and mothers should be assisted by nursing or lactation specialists.

The choice to breast- or bottle-feed is personal and formula feeding should not be criticized.

Nutritional characteristics of human milk compared with unmodified cow's milk

Protein

- Low protein content (whey:casein, 60:40) – more easily digestible.
- High free amino acids and urea; glutamine, the predominant amino acid, stimulates enterotropic hormones, enhancing feeding tolerance.

Fat

- Unsaturated.
- Contains long-chain polyunsaturated fatty acids (LCPUFAs) – needed for nervous system development (now incorporated into formula, as is arachidonic acid, ARA).

Carbohydrate

- High lactose.

Minerals

- Low renal solute load.
- Reduced phosphate:calcium ratio.

Vitamins

Supplementation required to breast milk to meet daily requirements.

Formula

Formula is humanized, i.e. manipulated to resemble human milk. However, there are still differences in amino acid and fatty acid composition and it does not contain the anti-infective properties of human milk. In developing countries, infection from reconstituting milk powder with contaminated water is a major health problem.

Unmodified cow's, goat's and sheep's milks are unsuitable for infants. Soy formula is sometimes used to prevent allergic disorders such as eczema and asthma, although evidence for this is lacking. About 10–30% of infants with cow's milk protein intolerance become sensitive to soy.

Steps to successful breast-feeding

- Place the infant on the breast either immediately or soon after birth.
- Provide quiet, supportive environment with comfortable positioning (Fig. 19.1).
- Demand feeding is preferable to a fixed schedule. This stimulates milk production and reduces feeling of fullness and discomfort. May be put to the breast 8–12 or more times per 24 hours.
- Put to both breasts at each feeding. Switch sides when baby pauses and lets go of breast. Allow unrestricted duration of feeds. Begin each feeding with the breast last nursed from.
- Emptying the breast adequately avoids engorgement.

- Initial milk is colostrum – low in volume, high in protein and immunoglobulin content. Takes 24–72 hours for breast milk to come in.
- Warn mothers that babies initially lose weight (up to 7–10% of birthweight) and only put on weight after day 4 of life. They should be back to birthweight by 10–14 days.
- Do not give supplementary water or formula unless medically indicated.
- Allow mothers and infants to stay together (rooming-in) 24 hours a day.
- Inform mothers of breast-feeding support groups.

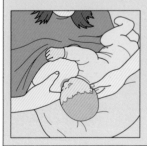
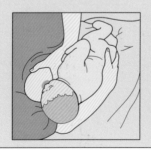
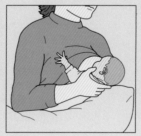

Fig. 19.1 Positioning for breast-feeding. (Adapted from UNICEF UK Baby Friendly Initiative.)

Neonatology at a Glance, 2nd edition. Edited by Tom Lissauer & Avroy A. Fanaroff. © 2011 Blackwell Publishing Ltd.

Breast-feeding

Advantages of breast-feeding for the infant
Immediate:
- Promotes mother–infant bonding.
- Ideal nutritional composition (see below).
- Contains immune factors (e.g. secretory IgA).
- Reduces gastroenteritis, possibly other infections.
- Less feeding intolerance.
- Reduces incidence of necrotizing enterocolitis in preterm infants.
- Promotes ketone production as an alternative energy substrate to glucose in first few days of life.

Long term:
- May reduce risk of SIDS (sudden infant death syndrome).
- May decrease incidence and severity of eczema and asthma.
- Less obesity, insulin-dependent diabetes mellitus (type 1) and inflammatory bowel diseases (Crohn disease and ulcerative colitis).

Advantages of breast-feeding for the mother
- Enhances mother–infant bonding.
- More rapid postpartum weight loss.
- Decreased risk of osteoporosis.
- Decreased risk of breast and ovarian cancer.
- Increases time between pregnancies, which is important in developing countries.

Potential complications of breast-feeding for the infant
- Cannot tell how much milk the baby has taken. This is monitored by checking baby's weight.
- Dehydration may occur if:
  - inadequate milk supply/poor feeding technique
  - hot weather.
- Jaundice associated with breast milk:
  - common
  - exacerbated by dehydration
  - even if requiring phototherapy, breast-feeding should be continued
  - is prolonged (>2 weeks of age) in 15% – will require investigations to be performed.
- Multiple births:
  - twins can often be breast-fed (Fig. 19.2), but rarely higher-order births.
- Vitamin K:
  - low level in breast milk may predispose to hemorrhagic disease of the newborn
  - prophylaxis is required.

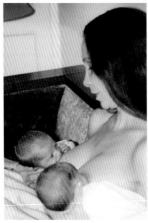

Fig. 19.2 Successful breast-feeding of twins.

Potential complications of breast-feeding for the mother
- Maternal feeling of inadequacy/upset if unsuccessful.
- Breast engorgement, cracked nipples – may be helped by manual expression or breast pump.
- Mastitis – requires maternal treatment and may disrupt feeding.

Contraindications to breast-feeding
- **Maternal HIV** – breast-feeding contraindicated in developed countries. In resource-poor environment, breast-feeding is advised unless formula feeds can be given safely. Low risk with breast-feeding if antiretroviral therapy given to mother or infant. Mixed formula and breast-feeding should be avoided,
- **Maternal TB** infection (active).
- **Inborn errors of metabolism** – galactosemia, phenylketonuria.

Drugs in breast milk
- Most drugs are excreted in breast milk in such small quantities they do not affect the infant.
- Where possible, all drugs, including self-medication, should be avoided during breast-feeding. Most mothers who need medications can continue breast-feeding, but a few drugs preclude breast-feeding. Some examples are listed in Table 63.1.

Check a formulary.

Key point

'Breast is best' for feeding newborn infants.

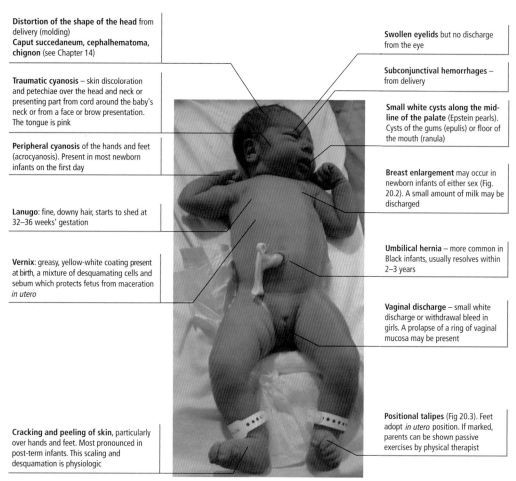

Distortion of the shape of the head from delivery (molding)
Caput succedaneum, cephalhematoma, chignon (see Chapter 14)

Traumatic cyanosis – skin discoloration and petechiae over the head and neck or presenting part from cord around the baby's neck or from a face or brow presentation. The tongue is pink

Peripheral cyanosis of the hands and feet (acrocyanosis). Present in most newborn infants on the first day

Lanugo: fine, downy hair, starts to shed at 32–36 weeks' gestation

Vernix: greasy, yellow-white coating present at birth, a mixture of desquamating cells and sebum which protects fetus from maceration *in utero*

Cracking and peeling of skin, particularly over hands and feet. Most pronounced in post-term infants. This scaling and desquamation is physiologic

Swollen eyelids but no discharge from the eye

Subconjunctival hemorrhages – from delivery

Small white cysts along the mid-line of the palate (Epstein pearls). Cysts of the gums (epulis) or floor of the mouth (ranula)

Breast enlargement may occur in newborn infants of either sex (Fig. 20.2). A small amount of milk may be discharged

Umbilical hernia – more common in Black infants, usually resolves within 2–3 years

Vaginal discharge – small white discharge or withdrawal bleed in girls. A prolapse of a ring of vaginal mucosa may be present

Positional talipes (Fig 20.3). Feet adopt *in utero* position. If marked, parents can be shown passive exercises by physical therapist

Fig. 20.1 Minor abnormalities noted in the first few days of life.

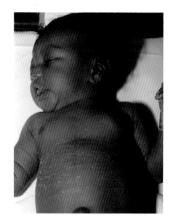

Fig. 20.2 Breast enlargement.

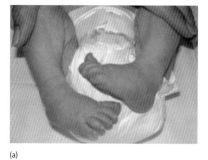
(a)

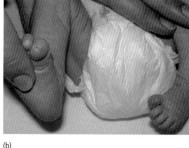
(b)

Fig. 20.3 Positional talipes. (a) Position of the feet. (b) The foot can be fully dorsiflexed to touch the front of the lower leg. In true talipes equinovarus this is not possible.

Neonatology at a Glance, 2nd edition. Edited by Tom Lissauer & Avroy A. Fanaroff. © 2011 Blackwell Publishing Ltd.

Skin lesions

Stork bites
Pink macules on upper eyelids, mid-forehead (also called salmon patch) and nape of the neck (Fig. 20.4). Common. Dilated superficial capillaries. Those on the eyelids and forehead fade over the first year. Those on the neck persist but are covered with hair.

Milia
White, pinhead-sized pimples on the nose and cheeks and forehead. Resolve during first month of life. Are from retention of keratin and sebaceous material in the pilosebaceous follicles.

Miliaria
Pin-sized vesicles, particularly over the neck and chest. Usually develop at 2–3 weeks. Caused by sweat that is retained due to obstructed eccrine glands. Avoid excessive clothing and heating.

Erythema toxicum
Small, firm, white or yellow pustules on erythematous base (Fig. 20.5). It is the most common transient lesion, usually appears at 1–3 days but up to 2 weeks of age; primarily on trunk, extremities and perineum. Moves to different sites within hours. Contains eosinophils. May be present at birth.

Mongolian blue spots
Blue–black macular discoloration at base of the spine and on the buttocks (Fig. 20.6). Usually but not invariably in black or Asian infants. Sometimes also on the legs and other parts of the body. Fade slowly over the first few years. Of no significance unless misdiagnosed as bruises.

Transient pustular melanosis
(transient neonatal pustulosis)
Resembles miliaria, but present at birth and may continue to appear for several weeks. Superficial vesiculo-pustular lesions rupture within 48 hours to leave small pigmented macules with white surround. More common in black infants, in whom the lesions are often hyperpigmented.

Harlequin color change
Sharply demarcated blanching down one half of the body – one side of the body red while the other is pale. Lasts a few minutes. Thought to be due to vasomotor instability. It is benign.

Sucking blisters
Vesicles on hand, fingers or lips, from vigorous sucking *in utero*.

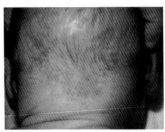

Fig. 20.4 Stork bite (salmon patch).

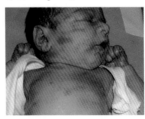

Fig. 20.5 Erythema toxicum. (Courtesy of Dr Nim Subhedar.)

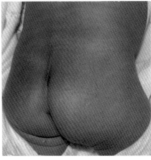

Fig. 20.6 Mongolian blue spot.

Other minor abnormalities (Figs 20.7–20.9)

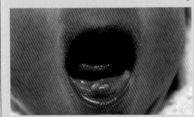

Fig. 20.7 Natal teeth. Front lower incisors present at birth. Remove if loose to avoid the risk of aspiration.

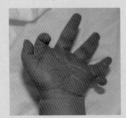

Fig. 20.8 Extra digits. Usually connected by a skin tag but may contain bone. Common anomaly – often hereditary. Consult plastic surgeon. If thin skin tags are tied off with silk thread, need to take care to avoid residual neuroma.

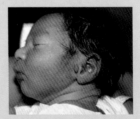

Fig. 20.9 Ear tags. Consult plastic surgeon. Check that the ear and hearing is normal. If there is an ear anomaly, some centers ultrasound the kidneys as slight increased risk of renal abnormalities.

Anticipation

Many neonatal problems can be anticipated or prevented by awareness of conditions that are detected antenatally (Tables 21.1 and 21.2) or which develop during labor or delivery (Table 21.3). This necessitates close liaison between the health professionals caring for the mother and fetus and the pediatricians. Some common examples which may be anticipated developing in the neonatal period are listed below. They are described in more detail in the relevant chapters.

Maternal or antenatal conditions (Table 21.1)

Table 21.1 Neonatal problems associated with maternal conditions.

Maternal medical condition	Neonatal problem
Diabetes mellitus	Neonatal hypoglycemia Polycythemia Jaundice Congenital malformations
Maternal hyperthyroidism	Neonatal hyperthyroidism or hypothyroidism from maternal drug treatment
Autoimmune thrombocytopenia	Neonatal thrombocytopenia
SLE (systemic lupus erythematosus)	Heart block, rash
Red blood cell isoimmunization Rhesus and other red cell antibodies. ABO incompatibility (mother group O, infant A or B)	Jaundice, anemia
Blood tests Hepatitis B positive HIV infection Syphilis serology positive	Immunization ± prophylaxis Preventative therapy, advice about breast-feeding Treatment if necessary
Chlamydia screening (in US) *Chlamydia trachomatis* identified	Check for conjunctivitis
Maternal drugs Drug abuse Alcohol	Neonatal drug withdrawal Fetal alcohol syndrome
Prolonged rupture of membranes **Chorioamnionitis** **Maternal fever >38°C** **Maternal group B streptococcal bacteriuria or colonization**	Neonatal infection

Fetal conditions (Table 21.2)

Table 21.2 Neonatal problems associated with fetal conditions.

Fetal condition	Neonatal problem
Abnormal ultrasound	
Renal (commonest), e.g. hydronephrosis	May need prophylactic antibiotics, ultrasound and VCUG (vesicocystourethrogram)
Cardiac	Echocardiography – liaise with pediatric cardiologist involved antenatally
Other abnormalities	Management as planned antenatally
Intrauterine growth restriction (IUGR) or large for gestational age	Hypoglycemia Polycythemia
Multiple births	Anemia/polycythemia Twin–twin transfusion syndrome Congenital malformations Intrauterine growth restriction (IUGR)

Labor and delivery (Table 21.3)

Table 21.3 Neonatal problems associated with abnormal labor and delivery.

Labor and delivery	Neonatal problem
Antepartum hemorrhage	Hypoxic–ischemic encephalopathy, anemia
Markedly abnormal CTG trace	Hypoxic–ischemic encephalopathy
Cesarean section	TTNB (transient tachypnea of the newborn)
Vacuum extraction	Chignon, jaundice Subgaleal (subaponeurotic) hemorrhage – anemia, shock
Forceps	Localized bruising Facial palsy
Breech position	DDH (developmental dysplasia of the hip) Birth injuries Hypoxic–ischemic encephalopathy
Shoulder dystocia	Hypoxic–ischemic encephalopathy Erb palsy Fractured clavicle or humerus
Meconium	Meconium aspiration
Need for prolonged resuscitation at delivery	Hypoxic–ischemic encephalopathy

Neonatology at a Glance, 2nd edition. Edited by Tom Lissauer & Avroy A. Fanaroff. © 2011 Blackwell Publishing Ltd.

Overview of common medical problems

Most newborn infants are healthy, but may develop some of the clinical features described below. Differentiating the clinically significant from the transient and benign can be difficult. An approach to these problems is given in Fig. 21.1. For details see specific chapters.

Conjunctivitis
Sticky eyes – common
Clean with sterile (boiled) water
If conjunctivitis purulent or eyelids red and swollen, exclude bacterial cause including gonococcus and chlamydia

Vomiting
Babies often vomit milk. If persistent or bile stained may be from intestinal obstruction. If it contains blood, malrotation must be excluded, but is usually swallowed maternal blood from delivery or maternal breast
Abdominal distension may be from lower intestinal obstruction

Poor feeding
Usually related to problems in establishing breast-feeding
However, can be presentation of:
▪ Infection
▪ Hypoglycemia
▪ Electrolyte disturbance
▪ Inborn error of metabolism

Cyanotic/dusky spells
Normal infants sometimes become dusky or cyanosed around the mouth, often during feeds, in the first few days.
Conditions which need to be excluded are:
▪ Cyanotic congenital heart disease
▪ Polycythemia
▪ Infection

Mucus
Many babies produce a considerable amount of mucus on the first day. This needs to be differentiated from the infant with esophageal atresia who is unable to swallow saliva, which pools in the mouth

Jaundice
Check bilirubin on blood sample if:
▪ Jaundice at < 24 hours of age
▪ Looks significantly jaundiced clinically
▪ Significant level on transcutaneous monitor

Skin lesions
White spots – erythema toxicum or milia are common and harmless
Septic lesions – contain pus
Bullous impetigo – serious (staphylococcal or streptococcal) infection. Sacs of serous fluid; their roof is easily broken leaving denuded skin (Fig. 42.4)

Pallor/plethora
▪ Check hematocrit for anemia or polycythemia
▪ Check breathing and circulation

Jitteriness/seizures/lethargy
Jittery movements are common. They stop on holding the limb, in contrast to seizures. If pronounced check blood glucose and consider other causes, e.g. drug withdrawal
Seizures can be subtle, but are rhythmic jerky movements of the limbs
Seizures require prompt treatment and investigation – admit to the neonatal unit
Lethargy may be a sign of sepsis, hypoglycemia or inborn error of metabolism

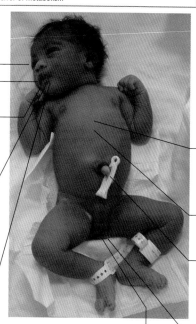

Delay in passing meconium (> 24 hours)
Check for intestinal obstruction

Delay in voiding urine (> 24 hours)
Voiding may be unobserved – often void immediately after birth
Consider urinary outflow obstruction (palpable bladder, ultrasound) or renal failure (serum creatinine, ultrasound)

Weight loss
Babies initially lose weight (1–2% of birth weight per day up to 7–10% of birth weight). They may take up to 10–14 days to regain their birth weight

Collapse (rare but important)
Maintain Airway, Breathing, Circulation
Causes:
▪ Sepsis – bacterial or viral
▪ Duct-dependent heart disease – closure of ductus arteriosus
▪ Inborn error of metabolism

Hypoglycemia
Blood glucose < 40 mg/dL (< 2.6 mmol/L) and asymptomatic – feed infant and recheck
If symptomatic, blood glucose levels are very low < 20 mg/dL (1.1 mmol/L) or persistently < 40 mg/dL (< 2.6 mmol/L) despite adequate feeding – give intravenous glucose

Respiratory distress
Most common cause – TTNB (transient tachypnea of the newborn), but need to exclude infection and other causes
Check Airway, Breathing, Circulation
Give oxygen, respiratory and circulatory support as required
Admit to neonatal unit
Check – complete blood count, blood culture, C-reactive protein and chest X-ray
Start antibiotics

Apneic attacks
The pauses in normal periodic breathing are sometimes misinterpreted as apnea by parents
True apnea with desaturation is uncommon in term infants and is a serious symptom; infection must be excluded

Umbilical cord
Red flare in skin around umbilicus – usually staphylococcal or streptococcal. Give intravenous antibiotics

The septic baby
A combination of some of these clinical features:
▪ Apnea and bradycardia
▪ Slow feeding or vomiting or abdominal distension
▪ Fever, hypothermia or temperature instability
▪ Respiratory distress
▪ Irritability, lethargy or seizures
▪ Jaundice
▪ Petechiae or bruising
▪ Reduced limb movement (bone or joint infection)
▪ Collapse or shock
▪ Hypoglycemia
In meningitis (late signs):
▪ Tense or bulging fontanelle
▪ Head retraction (opisthotonus)
Admit to neonatal unit
Check – complete blood count, blood and other cultures, C-reactive protein/procalcitonin and chest X-ray
Consider lumbar puncture
Start antibiotics
Provide supportive care

Fig. 21.1 Common medical problems of term infants.

Newborn infants should not be separated from their mothers unless it is essential for their well-being. Additional nursing and medical care can be provided on postpartum (postnatal) wards or by providing transitional care facilities beside their mother. However, 6–10% of newborn infants are admitted to a neonatal unit and 1–2% require intensive care.

Families often find neonatal units daunting and frightening. The environment is unfamiliar and their small and fragile baby is surrounded by high-tech equipment. There are large numbers of highly skilled nurses, doctors and other health professionals caring for their baby, and parents and families often feel superfluous as they are unable to help and care for their baby. Much can be done for parents and families to avoid these difficulties or help them cope with them.

If premature delivery can be anticipated arrangements should be made for the parents to visit the neonatal unit and meet the neonatal team before the birth.

Welcoming parents and families

- Parents and families should always be made welcome by staff (however busy they are).
- Parents should be shown around to make sure they know what facilities are available for them, e.g. where they can rest, prepare food and drink, make phone calls, use the internet.
- Ask them how they would like to be addressed and call them by name.
- Always make sure you use the correct gender when talking about the baby.

Open access

- Open visiting policy for parents (Fig. 22.1) and ability to exchange information 24 hours per day. Mothers should be transported to be near their baby.
- Visits by grandparents (Fig. 22.2) and close family members who are part of the parents' support network, as well as supervised sibling visits (Fig. 22.3) should be encouraged.

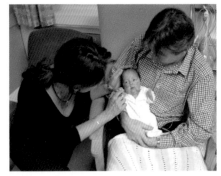

Fig. 22.1 Encourage parents to visit at any time.

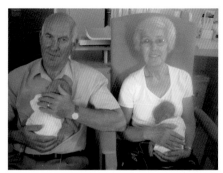

Fig. 22.2 Grandparents on the neonatal unit visiting the latest additions to their family.

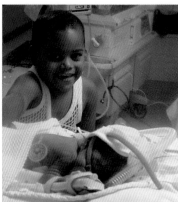

Fig. 22.3 Supervised sibling visits should be encouraged.

Explanation and facilitating communication

- Explain the infant's medical condition and equipment. Provide written information.
- Check with parents how they think their baby is doing and determine their level of understanding about their infant's condition and care. Correct misconceptions. Listen to the parents. Use interpreters if necessary.
- Arrange privacy for more detailed discussions. Parents appreciate respect for personal values and being involved in decision-making as appropriate.
- Assist the family to experience their new baby as a little person by visualizing the infant beyond the tubes and devices.
- Utilize other professionals, e.g. counselors, social workers. They may also provide helpful liaison between the neonatal intensive care unit (NICU) team and family as they may be perceived by the family as being less threatening than health-care professionals.
- The primary nurse, who is responsible for that baby, can facilitate identification of areas of concern and organize discharge.
- Arrange care conferences with the family, including all subspecialists involved in the care of infants with complex problems. These meetings are invaluable in keeping the family up-to-date and planning for discharge and subsequent care.
- Make sure that fathers do not miss out on communications.
- Listen to parents when they express concerns about changes in their baby's behavior.

Neonatology at a Glance, 2nd edition. Edited by Tom Lissauer & Avroy A. Fanaroff. © 2011 Blackwell Publishing Ltd.

Assisting attachment

• Give the mother the opportunity to touch and hold her baby in delivery room, if at all possible.

• Explain the value of breast milk and encourage the mother to express breast milk if the baby cannot be breast-fed. This enables her to make a unique contribution to her baby's care. Success depends on support and encouragement by staff.

• Promote loving touch of infant (Fig. 22.4); even if on a ventilator the parents can soothe their baby. Like all new parents the parents of premature infants need time to watch their baby to learn their ways of responding.

• Encourage parents to actively participate in their infant's care (Fig. 22.5). From the beginning parents can provide comfort and begin to take part in caregiving, e.g. with mouth care and tube feeds. When the baby is stable enough, parents may hold their baby during feeding (Fig. 22.6) and provide kangaroo care (Fig. 22.7a and b). Individualized nursing plans address the baby's behavioral and environmental needs and may reduce morbidity and length of stay (see Chapter 23).

• Encourage parents to keep a diary or journal and to collect mementos. Refer to the baby by name. Ensure the family has or is provided with good quality photos of their baby. Enable parents to personalize the isolette (incubator) with family pictures, religious texts etc. (Fig. 22.8).

Providing a family-friendly environment

• Make appearance of the unit as family-friendly as possible.

• Provide space and facilities for parents and families to have some privacy with their baby.

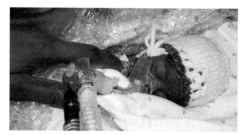

Fig. 22.4 Ventilated baby grasping her mother's finger.

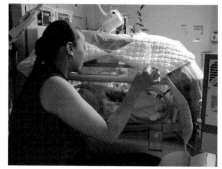

Fig. 22.5 Mother gavage (tube) feeding her ill baby. Parents also need to feel comfortable to watch their baby for as long as they like.

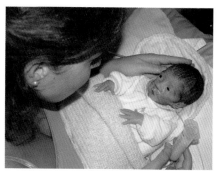

Fig. 22.6 Mother gavage (tube) feeding her baby. One of many activities that give mother and baby an opportunity to get to know each other.

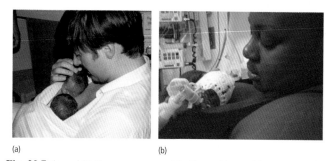

(a)   (b)

Fig. 22.7 (a and b) Kangaroo care, with direct skin-to-skin contact with parent. In some developing countries where isolettes (incubators) are not available, prolonged use has been shown to reduce mortality.

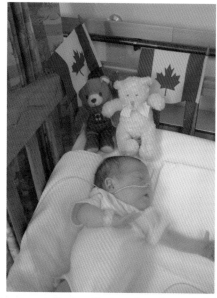

Fig. 22.8 Parents may like to add personal touches to their baby's bed, with toys and in this case flags to represent the baby's home country.

• Try to create a quiet calm environment with soft lighting

• Provide facilities for families to relax near but separate from the unit, with play area for siblings.

• Provide rooms for parents to stay overnight. This is particularly important if their infant is critically ill or prior to discharge.

Developmental care complements high-tech medical and nursing care with strategies that reduce stress and promote the development of infants in NICU. Some of these strategies are of general benefit to all infants, e.g. adapting the nursery environment, and require understanding and commitment rather than skill. Others are individualized to suit the condition, stage of development and characteristics of the infant; these depend on professionals and parents understanding infant behavioral cues.

Observing newborn behavior

Babies tell us how they are coping by their behavioral cues. These include physiological signs (e.g. color changes, breathing pattern, heart rate and blood oxygen); motor signs (e.g. muscle tone, smoothness of movements, pattern of movement and posture); signs of state organization (e.g. level of arousal, quality of sleep and alertness); and capacity to pay attention. There are many different behavioral patterns that are helpful in understanding when a baby is comfortable and ready to interact (approach cues), or uncomfortable and needing rest or support (avoidance cues) (Table 23.1).

Table 23.1 Behavioral observation.

	Approach behavior	Avoidance behavior
Autonomic	Regular, gentle breathing	Breathing irregular, fast, labored
	Healthy pink coloring	Pale, dusky, flushed or mottled
	Comfortable digestion	Straining, gagging, vomiting
Motor	Smooth varied movement	Jerky, disorganized movement
	Softly flexed posture	Extended (Fig. 23.1b) or flat posture
	Modulated muscle tone	Flaccid or stiff tone
State	Restful sleep	Restless sleep
Attention	Sustained, focused alertness (Fig. 23.1a)	Glazed, strained, hyperalert look
Self-regulation	Self-calming	Inconsolable
	Socially responsive	Shut down

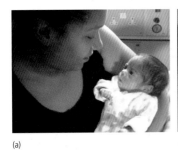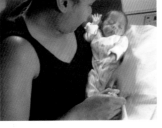

(a)   (b)

Fig. 23.1 (a) This baby's controlled posture and focused expression show successful self-regulation and readiness for interaction, i.e. approach behavior. (b) Extended limbs and turning away suggest avoidance behavior.

These observations take into account the context in which patterns of behavior occur, helping us to adjust the infant's experience and challenges to fit current developmental needs.

Parent participation

Developmental care can help parents to tune into their baby's behavior, laying the foundations for a secure attachment relationship, the basis of healthy emotional and social development. Parents are the baby's most consistent and dedicated carers and even in intensive care they can be involved, e.g. by placing a finger in the palm of the baby's hand or comforting their baby by cradling with still hands, Wherever possible plan the baby's day with parents to make opportunities to participate (Fig. 23.2). Share with parents observations about how their baby reacts to sounds, touch and movement, to build up a picture of each infant's individual characteristics and preferences (Fig. 23.3). Close physical contact, including skin to skin 'kangaroo care', helps parents to enjoy loving contact with their baby and grow in confidence.

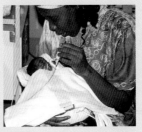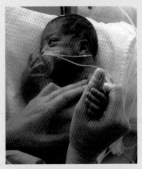

Fig. 23.2 Promotion of parental attachment by involvement with their baby's care.

Fig. 23.3 Promotion of parental attachment through touch.

The nursery environment

Preterm infants are not ready to deal with bright light, loud mechanical noises, hard surfaces, drafts, being moved through space and frequent sleep disruption. These experiences can be modified, e.g. ambient lighting can often be safely reduced and shade can be provided with isolette (incubator) covers and crib (cot) canopies (Fig. 23.4); noise can be reduced with acoustic engineering, by lowering the volume of alarms and encouraging staff to work and talk quietly; nesting and soft bedding can be used to support the baby in a comfortable position (Fig. 23.5).

Adapting care

All caregiving activities and procedures can be adapted to make them go smoothly and provide opportunities for communication (Fig. 23.6). Infants in intensive care are frequently disturbed for

Neonatology at a Glance, 2nd edition. Edited by Tom Lissauer & Avroy A. Fanaroff. © 2011 Blackwell Publishing Ltd.

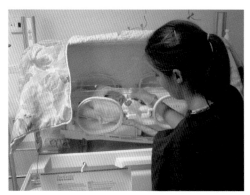

Fig. 23.4 Isolette (incubator) covered to shade the baby. A flap always folded back so that the baby can be observed.

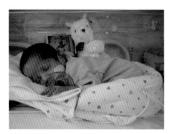

Fig. 23.5 Soft bedding with supportive nesting can contain disorganized movement and provide the baby with comforting boundaries.

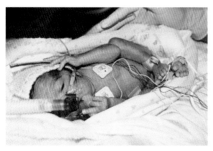

Fig. 23.6 Many activities can be done with the baby lying on one side to give more control of movement – lying quietly and calmly with legs folded in, one hand holding onto his head and the other grasping the pacifier which he is sucking.

nursing observations, examinations, diaper (nappy) changes, blood and other tests, giving medications, etc. Procedures can often be performed together to minimize disturbing a sleeping baby, even if this means being flexible about timing routine observations and care, or when to perform tests and therapy. Very sensitive babies may find this too challenging and will need periods of rest between procedures. A soft spoken greeting with gentle touch helps the baby to adjust at the start. Timing and pacing of procedures can

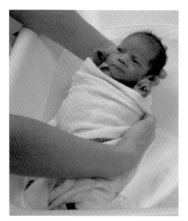

Fig. 23.7 Help sensitive infants to find bathing pleasurable by loosely wrapping in a towel.

be adjusted according to the behavioral cues that show when the baby needs time out to rest and recover. Ask parents or a colleague to soothe a sensitive or agitated baby. Wrap the baby when moving through space, e.g. for weighing or bathing (Fig. 23.7). Try positioning the baby on the side for procedures and diaper (nappy) change. Give the baby opportunities to steady him or herself by grasping your finger, sucking a pacifier or pressing feet against the nest wall.

Questions

What is the Newborn Behavioral Assessment Scale (NBAS)?

A neurobehavioral assessment suitable for infants from term to 2 months. It reveals infant maturity and individuality with a series of maneuvers designed to test habituation, orientation to visual and auditory stimuli, state regulation, motor maturity and reflex responses. The baby's reactions to increasingly demanding activities are noted. The examiner must be skillful in eliciting the baby's best response as well as in scoring the assessment. It enables parents and professionals to enhance the parent–infant relationship and promote the baby's capacity for self-regulation. The Newborn Behavioral Observation is a recent shorter version.

What is NIDCAP®?

This is the Newborn Individualized Developmental Care and Assessment Program. Practitioners have formal training in systematic, behavioral observation, analysis and care planning. Has promoted developmental care in many countries. It involves observations before, during and after caregiving which are reported in a narrative style suitable for parents and professionals. Recommendations are made about the infant's environment and caregiving.

Seriously ill or extremely preterm infants may require resuscitation. Thereafter, they all need to be promptly stabilized and therapy should be initiated for organ-specific dysfunction (Fig. 24.1).

Airway, Breathing
Examination
■ Respiratory distress—respiratory rate, chest retractions, nasal flaring, grunting
Treatment as required with:
■ Clearing the airway
■ Oxygen
■ CPAP
■ Mechanical ventilation

Give surfactant therapy as indicated

Circulation
Examination
■ Heart rate, pulses, capillary refill time, skin color and temperature
■ Blood pressure
Treat shock—see facing page

Central nervous system
Examination
■ Response to handling
■ Posture
■ Movements
■ Tone
■ Reflexes

Monitoring
■ Oxygen saturation
■ Heart rate
■ Respiratory rate
■ Apnea >20 seconds
■ Temperature – central and peripheral if ill
■ Blood pressure
■ Blood glucose
■ Blood gases
■ Weight
■ Transcutaneous O_2 and CO_2 —used in some centers

X-rays
Chest X-ray +/– abdominal X-ray assist in identifying cause of respiratory distress, position of tracheal tube and central lines

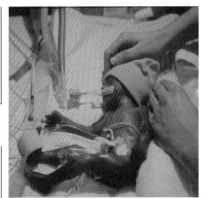

Venous and arterial lines
Peripheral intravenous line
■ Required for intravenous fluids, antibiotics, other drugs and parenteral nutrition
Umbilical venous catheter
■ Sometimes used for immediate intravenous access or for CVP (central venous pressure) monitoring or obtaining blood samples or administration of fluid or medications.
Some centers use multilumen catheters to avoid the need for peripheral IV lines
Arterial line
■ Inserted if frequent blood gas analysis, blood tests and continuous blood pressure monitoring is required. Usually umbilical artery catheter (UAC), sometimes peripheral cannula if for short period or no umbilical artery catheter possible
Central venous line for parenteral nutrition
■ Inserted peripherally when infant is stable

Antibiotics
Usually given before results of cultures and other investigations are available (although most infants are not septic)

Temperature control
To keep the infant warm, stabilization is performed under a radiant warmer or in an isolette (incubator)

Investigations
■ Hemoglobin/hematocrit
■ Neutrophil count
■ Platelets
■ Blood urea nitrogen (urea)/creatinine
■ Electrolytes
■ Culture—blood, CSF, urine
■ Blood glucose
■ CRP/acute phase reactant
■ Surface cultures
■ Coagulation screen if indicated

Pain/sedation
Analgesia and sedation given according to assessment of need, e.g. painful procedures, artificial ventilation
Muscle relaxants may sometimes be required during mechanical ventilation

Parents
Time needs to be found to explain to parents and immediate relatives what is happening. If the mother cannot see the baby, e.g. following cesarean section or severe hypertension, photographs or videolinks are reassuring

Vitamin K
Routine prophylaxis against hemorrhagic disease of the newborn

Fig. 24.1 Stabilizing the newborn infant requiring intensive care.

Oxygen saturation

What arterial oxygen saturation should one aim for?

This depends on the infant's maturity and underlying clinical condition.
• Healthy term infants have an oxygen saturation >95%.
• Term infants with cyanotic congenital heart disease tolerate saturations of around 80%.
• Preterm infants – oxygen saturation between 90 and 95% is compatible with adequate oxygen tension and this range is widely adopted. Lower saturations appear to be associated with lower incidence of ROP (retinopathy of prematurity) but higher mortality.
• Preterm infants receiving supplemental oxygen must be monitored with arterial oxygen tension measurements to detect hypoxemia and because high saturations may represent extremely high tissue oxygen tensions (Fig. 24.2), which are potentially dangerous to the eyes (retinopathy of prematurity) and lungs (bronchopulmonary dysplasia, chronic lung disease).

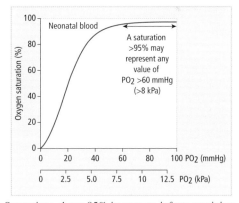

Neonatal blood

A saturation >95% may represent any value of PO_2 >60 mmHg (>8 kPa)

Fig. 24.2 Saturations above 95% in preterm infants receiving supplemental oxygen may represent dangerously high oxygen tensions.

Heart rate

What information can be obtained by monitoring heart rate? (Table 24.1)

Interpreting the heart rate is best done in conjunction with respiratory rate and oxygen saturation. Episodes of apparent desaturation

---

Neonatology at a Glance, 2nd edition. Edited by Tom Lissauer & Avroy A. Fanaroff. © 2011 Blackwell Publishing Ltd.

Table 24.1 Some causes of isolated changes in heart rate.

Increased heart rate (>160 beats/minute)
Movement/crying
Respiratory distress
Hypovolemia
Fever, infection
Pain
Fluid overload, e.g. heart failure, patent ductus arteriosus
Supraventricular tachycardia
Anemia
Thyrotoxicosis

Decreased heart rate (<100 beats/minute)
Apnea, hypoxia
Seizures
Shock (uncompensated)
Heart block, arrhythmia
Raised intracranial pressure
Hypothermia
Artifact

are mostly transient. They may be caused by movement artifact, but if more severe and prolonged will be accompanied by bradycardia and require prompt attention.

Circulation

How is the need for circulatory support determined?

The causes of shock are shown in Fig. 24.3. The clinical signs of shock are difficult to interpret.

The circulation is assessed by:
• Heart rate – usually tachycardia in shock; bradycardia is a late sign.
• Temperature gap: central–peripheral, i.e. tummy–toe, difference >2°C. Also caused by a cold environment. Capillary refill time is prolonged if >3 seconds in neonates.
• Blood pressure measurement – hypotension. But central blood pressure correlates poorly with circulating blood volume.
• Metabolic acidosis (increased lactate levels).
• Oliguria.
• Echocardiography – used increasingly to help identify low cardiac output from cardiac underfilling suggesting hypovolemia and/or poor contractility from myocardial dysfunction.
• Chest X-ray – excludes pneumothorax, diaphragmatic hernia.

Cardiovascular function may be compromised by overinflation of lungs or high mean airway pressure on mechanical ventilation obstructing venous return to both the right and left atrium.

A management regimen is shown in Fig. 24.4.

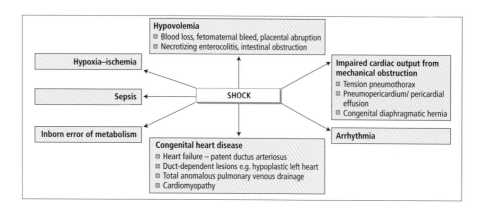

Fig. 24.3 Causes of shock.

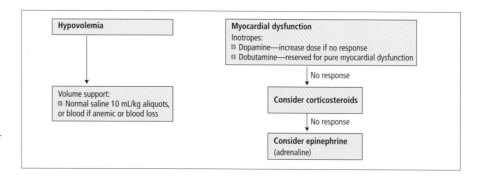

Fig. 24.4 Example of management regimen for circulatory support. This differs between centers.

Forms of respiratory support

These are:
- supplemental oxygen
- CPAP – continuous positive airway pressure
- positive pressure ventilation
- HFOV – high-frequency oscillatory ventilation
- NO – nitric oxide
- ECMO – extracorporeal membrane oxygenation.

Although many new forms of respiratory support are becoming available, teams of professionals fully familiar with a limited range of modes of ventilation and equipment are likely to have better outcomes than those using an array of ventilation modes and sophisticated new equipment with which they are not fully conversant.

The increase in use of nasal CPAP and surfactant for very low birthweight (VLBW) infants during the last two decades is shown in Fig. 25.1. It also shows the use of HFOV has stabilized and that of postnatal corticosteroids has declined (see Chapter 36).

Supplemental oxygen therapy

- Oxygen is given to avoid hypoxemia (Fig. 25.2), which may cause ischemic damage to the brain and other organs, apnea and pulmonary hypertension. Hyperoxemia should also be avoided as it may increase the risk of ROP (retinopathy of prematurity) in preterm infants and of tissue damage from release of free radicals. The optimal values for arterial oxygen tension and saturation have not been established, but in practice:
- In preterm infants, arterial oxygen tension is maintained at 45–80 mmHg (6.0–10.5 kPa) and oxygen saturation at 90–95%. There is some evidence that lower saturations are associated with a reduced incidence of ROP but an increase in mortality.
- Term infants – maintain oxygen saturation at >95%.

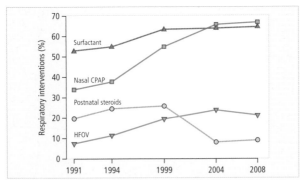

Fig. 25.1 Changes in use of respiratory interventions in VLBW (very low birthweight) infants with time. (Vermont–Oxford Network; courtesy of Dr Jeff Horbar.)

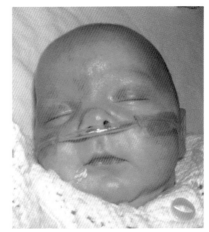

Fig. 25.2 Oxygen delivered via nasal cannula.

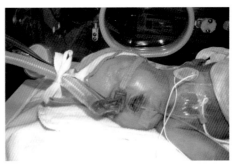

Fig. 25.3 Nasal CPAP (continuous positive airway pressure).

Continuous positive airway pressure (CPAP)

Distending pressure is usually applied via nasal prongs (Fig. 25.3) in the nasal airway. CPAP aims to prevent alveolar collapse at end expiration and stabilize the chest wall. It also allows supplemental oxygen to be delivered continuously. It is used for infants with moderate respiratory distress and for recurrent apnea. There is increasing use of early CPAP as respiratory support immediately after birth even for very preterm infants, with mechanical ventilation used only as required. CPAP may also facilitate weaning from mechanical ventilation.

CPAP may be delivered as:
- bubble CPAP – the pressure is determined using a water manometer
- flow-driver CPAP – the flow driver provides a constant stream of oxygen; special nasal prongs maintain a constant pressure throughout the infant's respiratory cycle by changing the direction of flow during expiration (fluidic flip).

Complications of CPAP are:
- pneumothorax
- feeding difficulties due to gaseous distension of the stomach
- often poorly tolerated by term infants.

Neonatology at a Glance, 2nd edition. Edited by Tom Lissauer & Avroy A. Fanaroff. © 2011 Blackwell Publishing Ltd.

If respiratory failure develops, mechanical ventilation is required.

Some infants with bronchopulmonary dysplasia (chronic lung disease) require nasal CPAP for many weeks. Prolonged use of nasal prongs may cause nasal trauma, long-term damage to the nasal septum and deformity of the nose. Correct fixation will minimize this.

Question

Is it better to commence nasal CPAP or intubate and give surfactant in extremely preterm infants at birth?

Trials (SUPPORT and COIN) have shown no significant difference in BPD (bronchopulmonary dysplasia) or mortality but nasal CPAP infants need fewer days of ventilation.

Nasal CPAP has the attraction of being less invasive though many subsequently require mechanical ventilation.

Positive pressure ventilation

Indications

- Increasing oxygen requirement or work of breathing or increasing $PaCO_2$ while on nasal CPAP.
- Respiratory failure – defect in oxygenation (hypoxemia) and/or carbon dioxide elimination (hypercarbia).
- Respiratory support of the extremely preterm infant for first few days of life to prevent respiratory failure – depends on unit policy
- Apnea – prolonged/recurrent.
- Upper airway obstruction.
- Congenital diaphragmatic hernia.
- Circulatory failure.

Intermittent positive pressure ventilation (IPPV)

Ventilatory support is administered using a mechanical ventilator through a tracheal tube. With conventional ventilation, intermittent positive pressure ventilator breaths are given on a background of continuous distending pressure (positive end expiratory pressure, PEEP) (Fig. 25.4). Alveolar ventilation is determined by the difference between peak inspiratory pressure (PIP) and PEEP, the inspiratory time and respiratory rate.

Most conventional neonatal ventilators are pressure-limited and time-cycled. They are used as tracheal tubes are not cuffed and so there is an air leak.

Key points

In the presence of marked chest retractions, provide respiratory support, including mechanical ventilation if necessary, even if the blood gases are normal.

Evidence of respiratory failure on blood gases is a late feature.

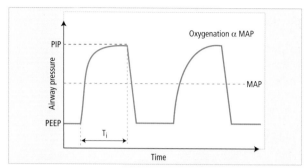

Fig. 25.4 Intermittent positive pressure ventilation (IPPV). Diagram of change in airway pressure with time. (PIP – peak inspiratory pressure; PEEP – positive end-expiratory pressure; Ti – inspiratory time; MAP – mean airway pressure.)

Patient-triggered (assist/control) ventilation and synchronous intermittent mandatory ventilation

Two forms of synchronized mechanical ventilation are available to promote synchrony between the ventilator and a baby's own respiratory efforts – patient-triggered ventilation (PTV) and synchronous intermittent mandatory ventilation (SIMV). Both methods use a baby's own spontaneous respiration to trigger the ventilator to deliver a breath, usually from the change in airway pressure or flow measured in the ventilator circuit; or from a recording of the infant's respiration. In PTV each breath triggers the ventilator; in SIMV only a preset number of breaths in a given time are triggered. In both, there is a backup ventilation rate if the infant does not breathe.

Multicenter studies have failed to show any advantages of PTV or SIMV over conventional ventilation for preterm infants with respiratory distress syndrome, although these forms of ventilation may decrease the need for sedation.

There is also increasing use of combining nasal CPAP with IMV (intermittent mandatory ventilation), i.e. additional positive pressure ventilation or SIMV.

Question

What are the causes of deterioration of a ventilated infant?
Sudden deterioration:
- Tracheal tube blocked/displaced.
- Ventilator/circuit disconnected or malfunction.
- Air leak – tension pneumothorax or pneumomediastinum.
- Pulmonary hemorrhage.
- Hemorrhage – intraventricular or other sites.

Slow deterioration:
- Increased lung secretions.
- Infection.
- Patent ductus arteriosus.
- Anemia.
- Developing bronchopulmonary dysplasia (chronic lung disease).

Question

How are the settings of conventional ventilators adjusted?

Monitoring

Continuous oxygen saturation, vital signs, regular blood gases, transcutaneous PaO_2 and $PaCO_2$ if available – to identify acute changes in infant's condition.

Target arterial blood gases
- PaO_2: 45–75 mmHg (6–10 kPa).
- $PaCO_2$: 35–55 mmHg (4.5–7 kPa).
- pH: 7.20–7.4.

Abnormal blood gases

Check:
- infant – for satisfactory chest wall movement, bilateral air entry, no pneumothorax (transilluminate chest if necessary), airway is clear, and ventilator functioning correctly
- breathing and circulation – adjust ventilator settings if necessary
Recheck blood gases 20 mins after changing settings.

Oxygen

To increase oxygen, options are:
- increase inspired oxygen concentration
- increase mean airway pressure – increase PIP, PEEP, tidal volume or inspiratory time (Fig. 25.5).

Consider surfactant therapy or HFOV (high frequency oscillation).

Carbon dioxide
- Keep $PaCO_2$ in normal range during first 72 hours – to keep cerebral blood flow in normal range during time of maximum risk of intraventricular hemorrhage. Thereafter, allow somewhat higher levels of $PaCO_2$ (permissive hypercapnia) to minimize ventilator-induced lung injury, but keep pH above 7.20.
- Avoid low $PaCO_2$ (<30 mmHg, 4 kPa) – lowers cerebral blood flow and is associated with ischemic brain injury (periventricular leukomalacia).

To reduce $PaCO_2$:
- increase ventilator rate (but allow sufficient expiratory time for carbon dioxide removal)
- increase breath size – increase PIP, or reduce PEEP or increase inspiratory time

Consider if tracheal tube is blocked (suction or replace if necessary), or if excessive dead space in circuit.

Metabolic acidosis

In extremely preterm infants it may be due to:
- circulatory hypoperfusion
- hypoxemia
- urinary loss of bicarbonate (alkaline urine)
- anemia
- parenteral nutrition.

When adjusting ventilator, aim to minimize ventilator-induced lung injury (inflammation, air leaks) by:
- optimal lung expansion – avoid lung overexpansion from too high mean airway pressure (volutrauma) or ventilating underexpanded atelectatic lung from using too low mean pressure (sometimes called atelectotrauma). Aim to synchronize ventilator with the infant's breathing – can use patient-triggered (PTV) or synchronous intermittent mandatory ventilation (SIMV). Sedation, analgesia and occasionally muscle relaxants are given as indicated.

High-frequency oscillatory ventilation (HFOV)

High-frequency ventilators operate at frequencies approximately 10 times greater than conventional ventilators and can achieve good gas exchange despite using tidal volumes smaller than dead space (Fig. 25.5). The rationale for using high-frequency ventilation is to recruit collapsed alveoli and minimize ventilator-induced lung damage. Rescue treatment with high-frequency ventilation in term and preterm infants with severe respiratory failure is associated with short-term improvement in gas exchange, especially when used in combination with inhaled nitric oxide. Some units choose to ventilate all their extremely preterm infants by HFOV to minimize barotrauma. Studies have failed to show a decrease in duration of ventilation, incidence of bronchopulmonary dysplasia (chronic lung disease), mortality or need for extracorporeal membrane oxygenation (ECMO) compared with conventional ventilation.

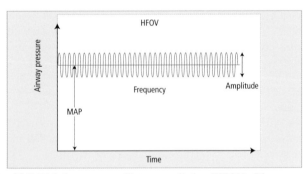

Fig. 25.5 High-frequency oscillatory ventilation (HFOV). Diagram showing changes in airway pressure with time. (MAP – mean airway pressure.)

Volume-limited ventilation

Used in some neonatal units. The tidal volume is set at a predetermined level and the ventilator adjusts the peak inspiratory pressure to achieve this.

Respiratory failure

The severity of hypoxemic respiratory failure is assessed by calculating the oxygenation index (OI):

$$OI = \frac{\text{mean airway pressure (cm } H_2O) \times FiO_2 \times 100}{PaO_2 \text{ (mmHg)}}$$

In term infants OI ≥ 40 is associated with a 40% risk of mortality.

In preterm infants OI ≥ 20 is associated with a 50% risk of mortality.

Therapeutic options for respiratory failure if on conventional mechanical ventilation with high pressures and high concentration of oxygen are:

- extra rescue doses of surfactant
- high-frequency ventilation
- nitric oxide or sildenafil (Viagra) therapy
- ECMO for infants of ≥ 34 weeks' gestation.

Inhaled nitric oxide (iNO)

Inhaled nitric oxide causes selective pulmonary vasodilation. It is used in infants with hypoxemic respiratory failure with or without persistent pulmonary hypertension of the newborn (PPHN) to improve oxygenation (Fig. 25.6). It reduces the need for ECMO in term and near-term infants with severe respiratory failure. There is increasing evidence that sildenafil (Viagra) is as effective with reduced expense and complexity. The efficacy of inhaled nitric oxide in preterm infants remains to be established.

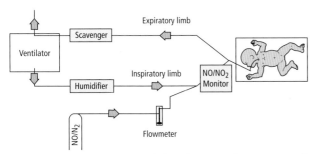

Fig. 25.6 Circuit for delivering nitric oxide. There is a scavenger for removing nitric oxide released into the atmosphere. The blood concentration of methemoglobin, a potentially toxic byproduct, is checked periodically. Inspired nitrogen dioxide (NO_2) levels (a byproduct of mixing nitric oxide and oxygen) are monitored continuously.

Extracorporeal membrane oxygenation (ECMO)

Infants are placed on heart–lung bypass for up to several days to allow the lungs to recover (Fig. 25.7). It is performed in relatively few specialized centers. Because of the need for anticoagulation, there is a risk of intraventricular hemorrhage in preterm infants and it is therefore reserved for infants ≥ 34 weeks' gestation and birthweight $>2\,$kg. Conditions that cause recoverable respiratory failure that may respond to ECMO are listed in Table 25.1. Indication is an oxygenation index of ≥ 40 in spite of optimal mechanical ventilation and circulatory support. Other requirements are <10 days' mechanical ventilation, no lethal congenital abnormalities and no significant intracranial hemorrhage. The need for ECMO has declined markedly since the introduction of nitric oxide and sildenafil and HFOV and the reduced incidence of severe meconium aspiration syndrome.

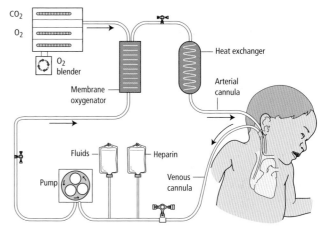

Fig. 25.7 ECMO (extracorporeal membrane oxygenation) circuit. The infant's venous blood is pumped through a membrane oxygenator (an artificial lung), which extracts carbon dioxide and adds oxygen. The blood is returned to the baby into the right carotid artery (veno-arterial ECMO, as shown in the diagram). In veno-venous ECMO blood is removed and returned into the superior vena cava. The lungs continue to be ventilated but at a low resting level.

Table 25.1 Conditions that may require ECMO.

Severe respiratory failure from:
- meconium aspiration syndrome
- persistent pulmonary hypertension of the newborn (PPHN)
- sepsis
- respiratory distress syndrome (RDS)
- congenital diaphragmatic hernia
- heart disease – congenital or cardiomyopathy
- severe airway obstruction/malformation

Key point

Trials have shown that for every three infants with severe respiratory failure treated with ECMO rather than conventional ventilation, one more will survive (Cochrane Review, 2008).

The preterm infant differs markedly from the term infant in size, appearance and development. Some of these differences are shown schematically in Figs 26.1–26.4.

Gestation	23–25 weeks	29–31 weeks	37–42 weeks (term)
Birthweight (50th centile)	At 24 weeks – Female: 620 g; Male: 700 g	At 30 weeks – Female: 1.4 kg; Male: 1.5 kg	At 40 weeks – Female: 3.4 kg; Male: 3.55 kg
Skin	Very thin, gelatinous Dark red all over body	Medium thickness Pink	Thick skin with cracking on hands and feet. Pale pink: pink all over ears, lips, palms and soles
Ears	Pinna soft, no recoil	Cartilage to edge of pinna in places, recoils readily	Firm pinna cartilage to edge of pinna, recoils immediately
Breast	No breast tissue palpable	One or both breast nodules 0.5–1.0 cm	One or both nodules > 1.0 cm
Genitalia	Male: scrotum smooth, testes impalpable Female: prominent clitoris. Labia majora widely separated, labia minora protruding	Male: scrotum – few rugae, testes – in inguinal canal Female: labia minora and clitoris partially covered	Male: scrotum – rugae, testes in scrotum Female: labia minora and clitoris covered
Posture	Extended, jerky, uncoordinated	Some flexion of legs	Flexed, smooth limb movements
Vision	Eyelids may be fused or partially open Absent or infrequent eye movements	Pupils react to light	Looks at faces. Follows faces, curvy lines and light/dark contrast in all directions
Hearing	Startles to loud noise		Turns head and eyes to sound Prefers speech and mother's voice
Breathing	Needs respiratory support. Apnea common	Sometimes needs respiratory support. Apnea common	Need for respiratory support uncommon. Apnea rare
Sucking and swallowing	No coordinated sucking	Coordinated at 34–35 weeks' gestation	
Feeding	Usually need TPN (total parenteral nutrition)	Gavage (nasogastric) feeds Sometimes need TPN (total parenteral nutrition)	At term, cries when hungry. Takes full feeds on demand Coordinates breathing, sucking and swallowing
Taste		Reacts to bitter taste	Differentiates between sweet, sour, bitter. Prefers sweet
Interaction	Seldom available for interaction Easily overloaded by sensory stimulation		Makes eye contact and alert wakefulness
Cry	Very faint		Loud
Sleep/wake cycle	Intermediate sleep state		Clearly defined sleeping and waking states

Fig. 26.1 Maturational changes in appearance and development with age.

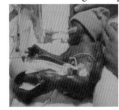
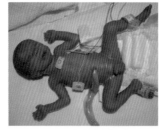
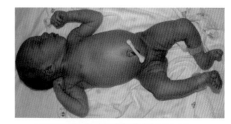
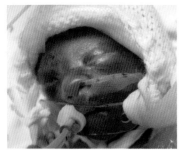
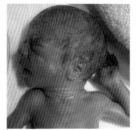
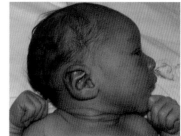

Fig. 26.2 Preterm infant at 23 weeks' gestation, showing extended posture, thin, gelatinous skin and fused eyelids.

Fig. 26.3 Preterm infant at 30 weeks' gestation, showing medium-thickness skin and ear with cartilage to edge of pinna.

Fig. 26.4 Term infant showing flexed posture and thick skin, and well-formed ear.

Neonatology at a Glance, 2nd edition. Edited by Tom Lissauer & Avroy A. Fanaroff. © 2011 Blackwell Publishing Ltd.

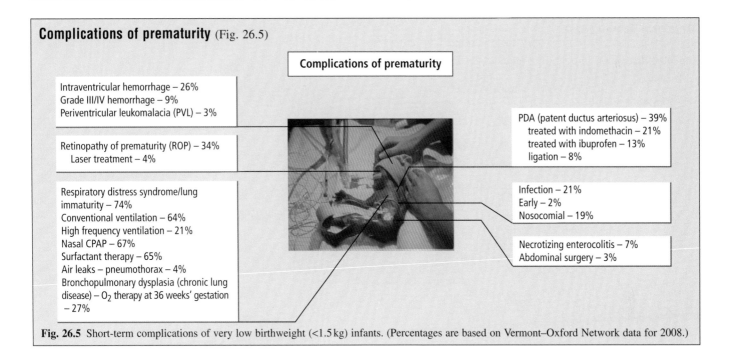

Complications of prematurity (Fig. 26.5)

Complications of prematurity

Intraventricular hemorrhage – 26%
Grade III/IV hemorrhage – 9%
Periventricular leukomalacia (PVL) – 3%

Retinopathy of prematurity (ROP) – 34%
  Laser treatment – 4%

Respiratory distress syndrome/lung
immaturity – 74%
Conventional ventilation – 64%
High frequency ventilation – 21%
Nasal CPAP – 67%
Surfactant therapy – 65%
Air leaks – pneumothorax – 4%
Bronchopulmonary dysplasia (chronic lung
disease) – O_2 therapy at 36 weeks' gestation
– 27%

PDA (patent ductus arteriosus) – 39%
  treated with indomethacin – 21%
  treated with ibuprofen – 13%
  ligation – 8%

Infection – 21%
Early – 2%
Nosocomial – 19%

Necrotizing enterocolitis – 7%
Abdominal surgery – 3%

Fig. 26.5 Short-term complications of very low birthweight (<1.5 kg) infants. (Percentages are based on Vermont–Oxford Network data for 2008.)

Morbidity

Being born preterm has many disadvantages, including stress for the parents and family, prolonged hospitalization and is extremely expensive. After 30 weeks of gestation, most preterm infants in developed countries survive without neurologic or other impairment. However, at lower gestational age there is a considerable complication rate (Fig. 26.5). The rate is highly dependent on gestational age (Fig. 26.6).

Mortality

Mortality is mainly determined by gestational age (see Figs 2.3a and 37.1) and birthweight (Fig. 26.7). They interact with each other as well as with other risk factors:

• gender (males have higher mortality)
• ethnicity
• multiple birth (increases mortality).

There has been a marked improvement in survival in infants born at the limit of viability, i.e. 23–25 weeks of gestational age. However, mortality, morbidity and adverse neurodevelopmental outcome are highest in these infants. This is considered further in Chapters 2 and 71.

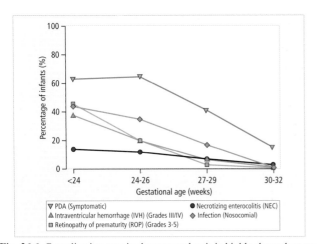

Fig. 26.6 Complication rate in the neonatal unit is highly dependent on gestational age. (Vermont–Oxford Network for very low birthweight infants for 2008.)

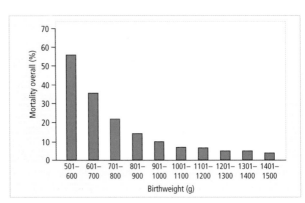

Fig. 26.7 Mortality by birthweight in very low birthweight (VLBW) infants. (Vermont–Oxford Network for 2008.)

27 Lung development and surfactant

Structural development

The fetal lung passes through four main stages of lung development during gestation (Fig. 27.1).

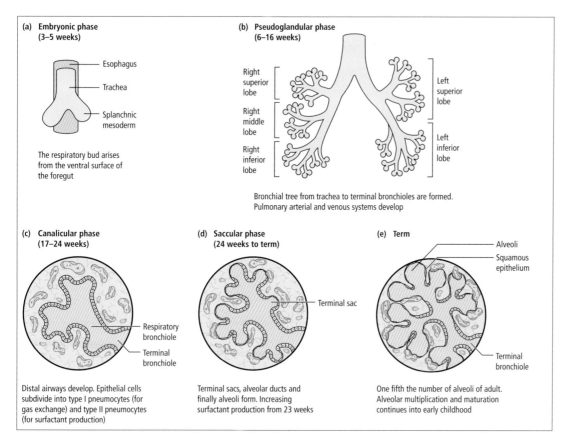

(a) Embryonic phase (3–5 weeks)

- Esophagus
- Trachea
- Splanchnic mesoderm

The respiratory bud arises from the ventral surface of the foregut

(b) Pseudoglandular phase (6–16 weeks)

- Right superior lobe
- Right middle lobe
- Right inferior lobe
- Left superior lobe
- Left inferior lobe

Bronchial tree from trachea to terminal bronchioles are formed. Pulmonary arterial and venous systems develop

(c) Canalicular phase (17–24 weeks)

- Respiratory bronchiole
- Terminal bronchiole

Distal airways develop. Epithelial cells subdivide into type I pneumocytes (for gas exchange) and type II pneumocytes (for surfactant production)

(d) Saccular phase (24 weeks to term)

- Terminal sac

Terminal sacs, alveolar ducts and finally alveoli form. Increasing surfactant production from 23 weeks

(e) Term

- Alveoli
- Squamous epithelium
- Terminal bronchiole

One fifth the number of alveoli of adult. Alveolar multiplication and maturation continues into early childhood

Fig. 27.1 Phases of lung development.

Physiology and composition of surfactant (Figs 27.2–27.4)

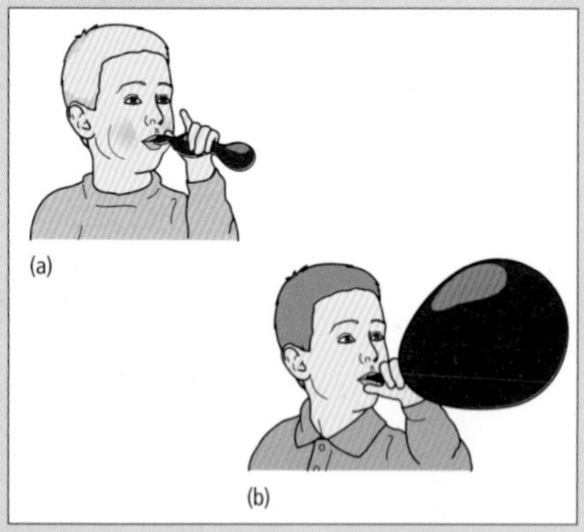

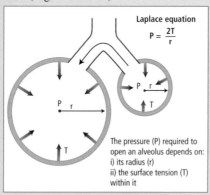

Fig. 27.2 (a) It is hard to blow up a balloon that is collapsed, i.e. has a small radius. Surfactant-deficient lungs are like this. (b) It is easier to blow up once the balloon is partially filled with air, i.e. has a larger radius. Lungs with surfactant are like this.

Laplace equation

$$P = \frac{2T}{r}$$

The pressure (P) required to open an alveolus depends on:
i) its radius (r)
ii) the surface tension (T) within it

Fig. 27.3 In the absence of surfactant, the pressure at the surface of the alveolus is greater in the smaller than the larger alveolus, so the small alveoli collapse and the large ones expand. Surfactant lowers the surface tension (T) and prevents alveolar collapse.

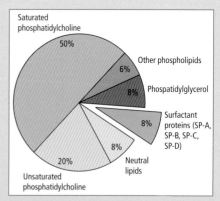

- Saturated phosphatidylcholine 50%
- Other phospholipids 6%
- Phospatidylglycerol 8%
- Surfactant proteins (SP-A, SP-B, SP-C, SP-D) 8%
- Neutral lipids 8%
- Unsaturated phosphatidylcholine 20%

Fig. 27.4 Composition of surfactant.

Neonatology at a Glance, 2nd edition. Edited by Tom Lissauer & Avroy A. Fanaroff. © 2011 Blackwell Publishing Ltd.

Surfactant

Surfactant:
- is a naturally occurring substance containing lipids (90%) and proteins (10%)
- is synthesized in type II pneumocytes in the lung and released onto the alveolar surface
- lowers surface tension at the air–water interface in the alveolus through the action of its lipid components (mainly dipalmitoyl phosphatidylcholine, DPPC). This effect helps to prevent alveolar collapse (atelectasis) and improves lung compliance (lung stiffness), reducing the work of breathing
- is only produced late in the second trimester and early third trimester
- deficiency causes respiratory distress syndrome (RDS).

Clinical implications of surfactant deficiency

In surfactant deficiency, as the lung has low compliance (i.e. it is stiff), the change in lung volume for a given change in airway pressure is much less than in the normal healthy newborn lung (Fig. 27.5). The pressure required to initiate lung inflation ('opening pressure') is also higher. Without surfactant the lung alveoli collapse to zero volume during expiration and the next breath starts from a low lung volume. These changes result in increased work of breathing and hypoxemia (Fig. 27.6).

Antenatal corticosteroids

Promote surfactant synthesis and lung maturation. The original studies showed they reduced the incidence of RDS by 60% and mortality by 40%. There is no increase in infection rate or maternal adverse side effects. The maximum benefit is when given more than 24 hours before delivery. It is uncertain whether it needs to be repeated. Generally advised for deliveries at 24–34 weeks.

Surfactant therapy

Surfactant therapy is given directly down a tracheal tube.
   There are two types of surfactant:
- natural surfactants – made from animal lung extracts, porcine – poractant alfa (Curosurf), calf – beractant (Survanta)

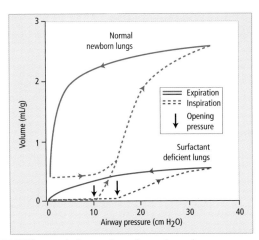

Fig. 27.5 Difference in lung volume for a given airway pressure between normal and surfactant-deficient lungs. If surfactant is present (a) there is a large change in volume for small changes in pressure once the opening pressure is exceeded, and (b) the lungs do not collapse on expiration.

- artificial surfactants – manufactured synthetically, but not currently available as the original preparation was less effective than natural. New preparations are under investigation.
   Preterm babies are given surfactant to either prevent or treat RDS. The strategies used are:
- prophylactic surfactant – elective intubation and surfactant given in the first few minutes after birth
- early selective surfactant – intubation and surfactant if infant needs artificial ventilation after birth
- rescue surfactant therapy – once the baby develops RDS.
   Systematic reviews have shown that prophylactic therapy is more effective than rescue treatment. It is usually given to infants of 29 weeks' gestation or less in the delivery room. If early nasal CPAP is used, some units intubate just to give surfactant, others delay and give as rescue therapy.
   Surfactant may also be beneficial in infants with meconium aspiration and pneumonia who may develop secondary surfactant deficiency.

Key point

- Surfactant therapy – a major advance in neonatal care.

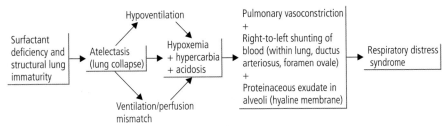

Fig. 27.6 Effect of surfactant deficiency and lung immaturity in preterm infants.

28 Respiratory distress syndrome

Respiratory distress syndrome (RDS) is:
- also called hyaline membrane disease (HMD) or surfactant deficient lung disease (SDLD)
- the commonest respiratory disorder affecting preterm infants
- a major cause of morbidity and mortality in preterm infants, although this has decreased markedly in recent years.

Risk factors

The predominant risk factor is:
- prematurity (Fig. 28.1), as surfactant is only produced towards the end of the second trimester and early third trimester.
  Other risk factors are:
- maternal diabetes mellitus
- sepsis
- hypoxemia and acidemia
- hypothermia.

Pathology

Characteristic histopathologic features include:
- collapsed terminal air saccules
- overdistended terminal airways
- influx of inflammatory cells into the airway lumen
- interstitial edema and protein leak onto the surface of the airways and air saccules
- hyaline membrane formation in distal and terminal airways (Fig. 28.2)
- necrotic damage to airway epithelial cells.

Pathogenesis

Caused by a deficiency in surfactant production or function. This results in poor lung compliance (i.e. stiff lungs), which in turn

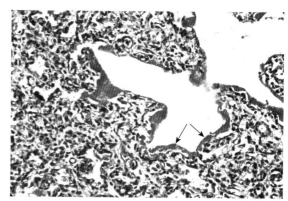

Fig. 28.2 Histology showing characteristic features. The hyaline membrane is shown (arrows).

leads to alveolar collapse and impaired gas exchange. Lung immaturity may also contribute (see Chapter 27).

Key point

Antenatal corticosteroids markedly reduce:
- incidence of respiratory distress syndrome
- mortality.

Clinical features

Onset within 4 hours of birth of respiratory distress:
- tachypnea (>60 breaths/minute)
- chest retractions (sternal and intercostal retractions) (Fig. 28.3)
- nasal flaring
- expiratory grunting
- cyanosis (if severe).
  Diagnosis is based on history, physical signs, characteristic chest X-ray (Fig. 28.4) and clinical course.

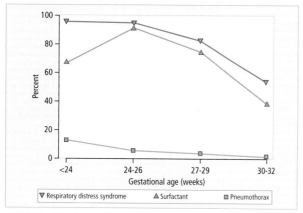

Fig. 28.1 Decline in incidence of RDS with gestation in very low birthweight infants. The use of surfactant and incidence of pneumothorax is also shown. (Vermont Oxford Network data for 2008.)

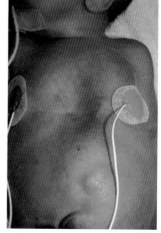

Fig. 28.3 Chest retraction in a preterm infant with respiratory distress.

Neonatology at a Glance, 2nd edition. Edited by Tom Lissauer & Avroy A. Fanaroff. © 2011 Blackwell Publishing Ltd.

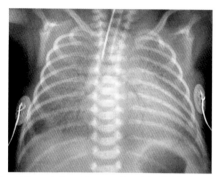

Fig. 28.4 Chest X-ray (after 4 hours of age) in RDS showing:
• diffuse, uniform granular (ground glass) appearance of the lungs from atelectasis
• air bronchogram – outline of air-filled large airways against opaque lungs
• reduced lung volume
• indistinct heart border as the lung fields are opaque ('white-out'). A tracheal tube is in place.

Table 28.1 Causes of respiratory distress in preterm infants.

Common
Respiratory distress syndrome (surfactant deficiency)
Pneumonia/sepsis
Transient tachypnea of the newborn
Uncommon
Pulmonary hypoplasia
Pneumothorax
Congenital heart disease
Rare
Diaphragmatic hernia
Non-respiratory – anemia, hypothermia, metabolic acidosis
Other causes
These are listed in Chapter 38

Causes of respiratory distress in preterm infants are listed in Table 28.1.

Natural course

The natural course is for the illness to become worse over the first 24–72 hours and then improve over the next few days. There is initially tissue edema from transudation of fluid into alveoli and subcutaneous tissues, which resolves with improvement of lung disease. These clinical features are markedly ameliorated by antenatal corticosteroids and postnatal surfactant therapy.

Management

This includes:
• antenatal corticosteroids
• surfactant therapy – prophylaxis/rescue via tracheal tube
• oxygen therapy

• prevention of lung collapse – by applying CPAP (continuous positive airway pressure) or PEEP (positive end-expiratory pressure) on a mechanical ventilator
• lung expansion – by applying a peak inspiratory pressure with a mechanical ventilator, if necessary
• provision of intensive care (see Chapter 24).

Complications

The main complications are:
• infection/lung collapse
• air leaks
• patent ductus arteriosus
• pulmonary hemorrhage
• intraventricular hemorrhage
• bronchopulmonary dysplasia (chronic lung disease).

Air leaks

Pulmonary interstitial emphysema (PIE)
There is tracking of air from the overdistended terminal airways into the interstitium. Increases risk of pneumothorax and bronchopulmonary dysplasia (chronic lung disease).

Pneumothorax
Occurs in about 10% of infants ventilated for RDS. Presents with:
• increased oxygen requirement
• reduced breath sounds and chest movement on the affected side
• hypoxemia, hypercarbia and acidosis on blood gases
• shock.
Confirmed by transillumination of the chest or chest X-ray (see Chapter 25).
A tension pneumothorax is treated by urgent aspiration followed by insertion of a chest tube.
May occur spontaneously, but is less likely if high airway pressure and asynchrony of the infant's breathing and lung expansion by the ventilator are avoided.

Pulmonary hemorrhage

This is hemorrhagic pulmonary edema. In preterm infants it is usually associated with left heart failure from a patent ductus arteriosus (left-to-right shunting) with respiratory distress syndrome requiring mechanical ventilation.
Causes blood staining of tracheal aspirate with or without shock.
Incidence is about 3% of infants with respiratory distress syndrome requiring mechanical ventilation. Most of these infants will have received surfactant, but this is no longer considered to be a risk factor. Coagulation may be deranged.
Treatment:
• increase ventilation
• surfactant
• if necessary, replace blood/volume and clotting factors, but avoid fluid overload
• close patent ductus arteriosus.
Massive pulmonary hemorrhage has a high mortality.

Hypothermia

Temperature regulation is fundamental to neonatal care.
    Hypothermia can cause:
- increased oxygen and energy consumption, resulting in hypoxia, metabolic acidosis and hypoglycemia
- apnea
- neonatal cold injury – redness of the skin from dissociation of hemoglobin
- reduced blood coagulability
- failure to gain weight
- increased mortality.
    Newborn babies are particularly liable to hypothermia as:
- they have a large surface area relative to their mass, so there is an imbalance between heat generation (related to mass) and heat loss (surface area)
- their skin is thin and permeable to heat
- they have little subcutaneous fat for insulation
- they have a limited capacity to generate heat as they mainly rely on non-shivering thermogenesis using a special form of adipose tissue, brown fat, which is distributed in the neck, between the scapulae and surrounding the kidneys and adrenals
- their ability to produce heat from sympathetic responses is poor – shivering occurs only at an ambient temperature of <16°C in term infants and does not occur in preterm infants until 2 weeks of age
- preterm infants are unable to curl up to reduce skin exposure.

Evaporative heat loss in preterm infants

Transepidermal water loss:
- is markedly increased in very premature infants (Fig. 29.2a)
- is increased by radiant warmers, phototherapy (unless cold light source) and if the skin is denuded
- declines with increasing postnatal age, as the skin thickens
- is reduced by humidity (Fig. 29.2b).

Neutral thermal environment

Infants should be nursed in the neutral thermal environment (Fig. 29.3), and have a core body temperature of 37°C.

Keeping neonates warm

If extremely premature or ill and needs to be naked for observation/procedures:
- place in isolette (incubator) or under radiant warmer
- intensive care unit kept warm and draft-free
- use warm, humidified ventilator gases
- clothe with boots and hat (important as the surface area of babies' heads are large relative to their bodies).

How newborn infants lose heat

Convection (Fig. 29.1a)
Determined by:
- temperature difference between skin and air
- area of skin exposed to the air
- movement of surrounding air.
    Is an important cause of heat loss, minimized by:
- clothing the infant
- raising temperature of ambient air
- avoiding drafts.

Radiation (Fig. 29.1b)
Depends on temperature difference between skin and surrounding surfaces, i.e. walls of isolette (incubator) or, if under radiant warmer, windows and walls of room; is independent of the air temperature.

Reduced in isolettes (incubators) by having a double wall.

Evaporation (Fig. 29.1c)
Important:
- at birth, when skin is wet
- in preterm infants, as their skin is very thin and water-permeable
- from the respiratory tree with artificial ventilation/nasal CPAP unless air/oxygen is warm and humidified.
    Minimized at birth by drying the infant and wrapping in a warm towel; extremely preterm infants placed directly in plastic wrapping with only the face exposed.

Conduction (Fig. 29.1d)
Loss is small as babies are on mattresses.

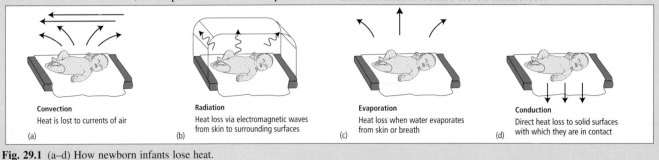

Convection
Heat is lost to currents of air
(a)

Radiation
Heat loss via electromagnetic waves from skin to surrounding surfaces
(b)

Evaporation
Heat loss when water evaporates from skin or breath
(c)

Conduction
Direct heat loss to solid surfaces with which they are in contact
(d)

Fig. 29.1 (a–d) How newborn infants lose heat.

Neonatology at a Glance, 2nd edition. Edited by Tom Lissauer & Avroy A. Fanaroff. © 2011 Blackwell Publishing Ltd.

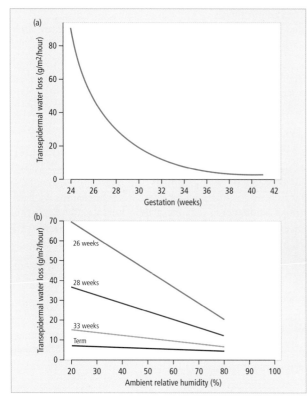

Fig. 29.2 (a) Transepidermal water loss increases with decreasing gestation. (b) Transepidermal water loss is reduced by humidity. (From Hammerlund *et al.* Transepidermal water loss in newborn infants. *Acta Paediatr Scand* 1983; **72**: 721–728.)

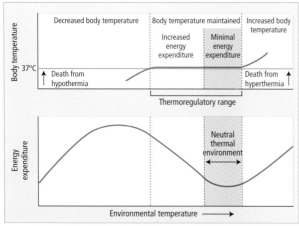

Fig. 29.3 The neutral thermal environment is the temperature range where the heat production is at the minimum needed to maintain normal body temperature. It depends on birthweight and postnatal age and whether the infant is clothed or naked.

If premature but stable:
- clothe
- place in isolette (incubator) or heated mattress in crib/cot
- wrap, keep in a warm, draft-free room.

Isolettes (incubators)

Advantages
- Provide constant, warm environment, even when doors are open.
- Can minimize transepidermal water loss – with high relative humidity.
- Can reduce radiant heat loss if the baby is covered and the isolette has double walls.

Disadvantages
- Reduced access for procedures, but improved in modern isolettes (incubators).
- May inhibit parental interaction.
- Noise from isolette's motor and doors.

Radiant warmers

Advantages
- Ease of access for observation and procedures.
- Rapid increase in temperature.

Disadvantages
- High transepidermal water loss makes fluid balance problematical.
- Difficult to provide extra humidity – partially achieved by covering the infant with cling film, insulating material, etc., and giving extra humidity.
- High convective heat losses.

Combined isolettes (incubators) with inbuilt radiant warmers

Now widely used for infants requiring intensive care. Radiant heat is used only when access is required, e.g. for procedures.

Key point

A normal core temperature does not mean a neutral thermal environment – it may be achieved by thermal stress.

Question

When are heated mattresses useful?
They allow some stable preterm infants to be nursed in a crib (cot) instead of an isolette (incubator). Also to warm infants who have become cold, or in the operating room, during imaging studies or transport.

30 Growth and nutrition

Growth

Between 24 and 36 weeks' gestation, a fetus growing along the 50th centile gains 15 g/kg/day. Infants who are fed enterally require 120–140 kcal/kg/day to maintain this rate of growth. As these high energy requirements often cannot be met, the weight of extremely preterm infants is often initially static or may decline, and the infant may take up to 21 days to regain birthweight. Thereafter, their growth improves but is often suboptimal. The reason for this growth failure includes:

- the infant is unable to tolerate high volumes of nutrients
- fluids may be restricted, e.g. patent ductus arteriosus
- intercurrent illness, e.g. infection.

Nutrition

Which milk?

Breast milk
Is the milk of choice. Advantages over formula feeds (also see Chapter 19) are:

- better tolerated
- associated with a lower incidence of necrotizing enterocolitis and provides some protection against infection
- contains hormones and growth factors
- has better absorption of fats and improved bioavailability of trace minerals
- promotes mother–infant bonding
- it is associated with improved cognitive development later in childhood.

  Disadvantages are:
- depends on the mother being able to express sufficient milk over a prolonged period
- growth of the preterm infant may be suboptimal. Breast milk may need to be enhanced with human milk fortifier to increase its energy, protein and mineral content. Human milk fortifiers contain cow's milk protein. Fortification is usually stopped once the infant is entirely breast-fed or weighs more than 2 kg.

Donor human milk
In the UK some neonatal units give donor breast milk to extremely preterm infants or infants at increased risk of NEC (necrotizing enterocolitis) when maternal breast milk is not available. Donors are screened by questionnaire and serological testing for infection, the milk is pasteurized and screened for bacteria. The efficacy of donor human milk in improving outcome has not been determined.

Low birthweight infant formulas
These have been developed to supply the increased energy (24 kcal/oz, 80 kcal/100 mL), protein, sodium, calcium and phosphate required by low birthweight infants (Table 30.1). They are increasingly further modified to be more like breast milk, with the addition of long-chain polyunsaturated fatty acids which are used as structural fats in nervous tissue, and oligosaccharides which act as probiotics to encourage a more breast-fed-like gut bacterial flora.

Supplements

- **Iron** is given to all preterm infants once they are on full enteral feeds and are not receiving blood transfusions. Supplementation is usually continued for six months to one year.
- **Multivitamins** (A, B_{12}, C, D and E) are given routinely. Folic acid is given in some centers.
- **Vitamin K** is given to all infants, including the preterm, as prophylaxis against hemorrhagic disease of the newborn.

Feeding

Whereas the healthy newborn term infant can be put to the breast shortly after birth, extremely preterm infants cannot feed for themselves as they:

- are unable to suck and swallow until about 34–35 weeks of gestation (Figs 30.1–30.3)
- are initially unable to tolerate milk in sufficient quantity to meet their nutritional requirements.

  A number of strategies are adopted to overcome these problems.

Table 30.1 Composition of various milks.

	Mature term breast milk	Preterm breast milk	Fortified preterm breast	Low birthweight formula	Term formula
Energy (kcal/100 mL)	70	67	74	80	66
Carbohydrate (g/100 mL)	7	6	8	8.5	6.9
Fat (g/100 mL)	4.2	4	4	4.4	3.6
Protein (g/100 mL)	1.3	1.8–2.4	2.9	2.2	1.5
Na (mmol/L)	7	13	18	13–20	8
K (mmol/L)	15	15	17	18	17
Ca (mmol/L)	9	6	22	30	12–20
Phosphate (mmol/L)	5	5	18	21	12–18

Question

What is the daily nutritional requirement of a well preterm infant?

It is:

Energy	120–140 kcal
Protein	3.0–3.8 g
Carbohydrate	8–12 g
Fat	10–20% of calorie intake
Sodium	2–3 mmol
Potassium	2–3 mmol
Calcium	2–3 mmol
Phosphate	1.9–4.5 mmol

Neonatology at a Glance, 2nd edition. Edited by Tom Lissauer & Avroy A. Fanaroff. © 2011 Blackwell Publishing Ltd.

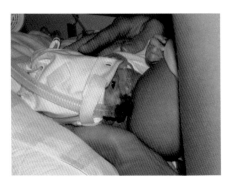

Fig. 30.1 Preterm infant learning to suck at the breast whilst still on continuous positive airway pressure (CPAP).

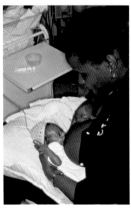

Fig. 30.2 Preterm infant learning to breast-feed whilst still receiving nasogastric gavage (tube) feeds.

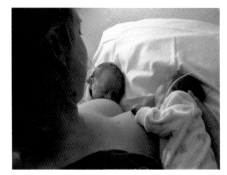

Fig. 30.3 Preterm twins successfully learning to feed at the breast.

Minimal enteral (non-nutritive) feeding

A small volume (e.g. 10–20 mL/kg/day), preferably with expressed breast milk, is given during the first few days to stimulate gut hormone production even when the infant is too unwell or unstable to tolerate the expected volume of feeds. This helps intestinal maturation, motility and gallbladder function, decreasing the time taken to establish full enteral feeding; it also lowers serum bilirubin concentrations. Feeding is introduced particularly slowly in infants who are growth-restricted and have reversed end-diastolic blood flow velocity on antenatal Doppler ultrasound because of their increased risk of necrotizing enterocolitis.

Gavage (tube) feeding

Used when infants are too immature (<34 weeks' gestational age) or ill to feed for themselves but are able to tolerate enteral feeds. The volume of milk is gradually increased. Feeds are withheld if aspirates are more than half the volume given or if bilious with abdominal distension, blood in the stool or other features suggesting necrotizing enterocolitis. Reduced gut motility in very low birthweight infants may necessitate suppositories for constipation.

The tube may be orogastric or nasogastric. As nasogastric tubes lie in the narrowest part of the upper airway, just behind the nose, a size 5 French gauge tube increases airway resistance by 30–50% in preterm infants. This increases the work of breathing and may increase the frequency of apnea. Some units avoid nasogastric tubes if less than 35 weeks' gestation, but orogastric tubes are more difficult to fix securely.

There is conflicting evidence regarding continuous versus bolus feeding in relation to weight gain and the incidence of apnea and bradycardia. The infant's oxygen tension falls with feeds in both preterm and term infants. It has been argued that continuous feeding is more physiologic for preterm infants because it is a closer approximation to the way a fetus is fed *in utero*. However, bolus feeds are preferred as the response of gut hormones is more physiologic.

Total parenteral nutrition (TPN)

A mixture of carbohydrate, protein, fat, vitamins and trace elements allows nutrition to be provided whilst oral feeding is established. It is usually given via a central venous line but may be given peripherally. It is associated with a number of complications:

- line-related infection
- conjugated hyperbilirubinemia
- electrolyte disorders
- hyperglycemia
- chemical burns from extravasation
- pleural or pericardial effusion – if tip of the central line becomes displaced and lies in the heart.

Volume of fluids

A guide to average total fluid intake is shown in Table 30.2. It is adjusted according to plasma electrolytes, creatinine, acid–base status and the infant's weight, all of which are measured regularly over the first few days. It is markedly affected by:

- gestational age
- thermal environment (radiant warmer or isolette)
- evaporative water loss (reduced by humidity, etc.).

Once the preterm infant is stable and on full enteral feeds, electrolytes, creatinine and phosphate, calcium and alkaline phosphatase can be checked weekly.

Table 30.2 Typical fluid intake according to postnatal age.

Postnatal age	Fluid intake (mL/kg/24 h)	
	<2.5 kg	>2.5 kg
Birth	60–100	40–80
Day 1	90–120	60–100
Day 2	120–150	90–120
Day 3	150	120–150
Days 4 and over	150–180	150

These are the most common causes of acquired brain injury in premature infants. Their incidence is inversely related to gestational age.

- **Hemorrhage** – occurs in 25–30% of VLBW (very low birthweight) infants. Involves the germinal matrix, an immature capillary network, which overlies the head of the caudate nucleus. The hemorrhage may be confined to the germinal matrix (GMH-IVH), may extend into the ventricle (IVH) or involve the parenchyma. Hemorrhagic parenchymal lesions are thought to be mainly venous infarcts from impaired venous drainage. Hemorrhage usually occurs within 72 hours of birth. The germinal matrix disappears at about 32 weeks' gestation, so hemorrhage is uncommon beyond this gestation.
- **Periventricular leukomalacia (PVL)** – loss of periventricular white matter in watershed areas around the lateral ventricles from hypoxia–ischemia. Probably most occur before birth, but some occur postnatally. Only becomes evident as cystic lesions on ultrasound three or more weeks after the insult. Cystic PVL is detectable on ultrasound in 3% of VLBW infants; less severe damage is represented by a persistent flare (echodensity) in the periventricular white matter.

The appearance of these lesions on cranial ultrasound is shown in Chapter 78.

Diagnosis

This is by cranial ultrasound at the bedside (Table 31.2). In very low birthweight (VLBW) infants, it is performed shortly after birth to identify antenatal lesions, during the first week of life to identify hemorrhages and repeated periodically to identify and monitor hydrocephalus and appearance of periventricular leukomalacia (PVL).

Ultrasound is excellent for detecting hemorrhage and ventricular dilatation, but is relatively insensitive in detecting white matter damage. MRI when the baby is older is more sensitive than ultrasound for white matter injury.

Pathogenesis (Figs 31.1 and 31.2) and incidence (Table 31.1)

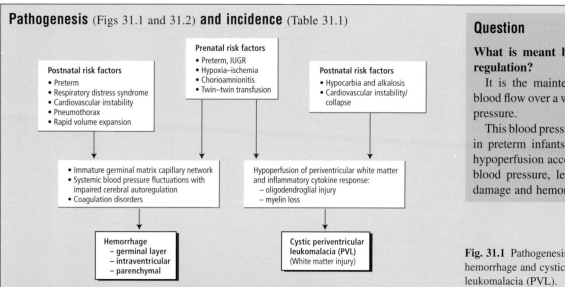

Postnatal risk factors
- Preterm
- Respiratory distress syndrome
- Cardiovascular instability
- Pneumothorax
- Rapid volume expansion

Prenatal risk factors
- Preterm, IUGR
- Hypoxia–ischemia
- Chorioamnionitis
- Twin–twin transfusion

Postnatal risk factors
- Hypocarbia and alkalosis
- Cardiovascular instability/collapse

- Immature germinal matrix capillary network
- Systemic blood pressure fluctuations with impaired cerebral autoregulation
- Coagulation disorders

Hypoperfusion of periventricular white matter and inflammatory cytokine response:
- oligodendroglial injury
- myelin loss

Hemorrhage
- germinal layer
- intraventricular
- parenchymal

Cystic periventricular leukomalacia (PVL) (White matter injury)

Fig. 31.1 Pathogenesis of cerebral hemorrhage and cystic periventricular leukomalacia (PVL).

Question

What is meant by cerebral autoregulation?

It is the maintenance of cerebral blood flow over a wide range in blood pressure.

This blood pressure range is narrow in preterm infants; there is cerebral hypoperfusion accompanying falls in blood pressure, leading to ischemic damage and hemorrhagic infarction.

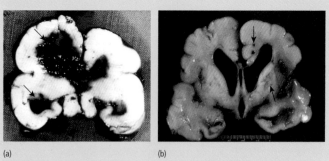

(a)   (b)

Fig. 31.2 Autopsy specimen showing (a) large parenchymal and intraventricular hemorrhage and (b) ventricular dilatation and cystic periventricular leukomalacia (PVL).

Table 31.1 Incidence of intraventricular hemorrhage (IVH) or periventricular leukomalacia (PVL) by gestational age (Vermont–Oxford Network data for 2008).

Gestational age (weeks)	IVH (all grades)	IVH (Grades III/IV)	PVL
<24	62	38	7
24–26	43	20	5
27–29	23	6	3
30–32	13	2	2

Key point

There has been a marked reduction in the incidence of posthemorrhagic hydrocephalus requiring shunts.

Neonatology at a Glance, 2nd edition. Edited by Tom Lissauer & Avroy A. Fanaroff. © 2011 Blackwell Publishing Ltd.

Table 31.2 A classification of lesions identified on intracranial ultrasound.

Hemorrhage
Grade I – isolated germinal matrix hemorrhage (GMH-IVH)
Grade II – intraventricular hemorrhage (IVH) without ventricular dilatation
Grade III – intraventricular hemorrhage with acute ventricular dilatation
Grade IV – parenchymal hemorrhagic infarct (parenchymal lesion)
Periventricular leukomalacia (PVL)
Cysts – localized and small or widespread
Porencephalic cyst – single, large cyst
Post-hemorrhagic ventricular dilatation (PHVD)

Clinical features

Most infants are asymptomatic. Clinical features include:
- increased ventilatory support
- abnormal neurologic signs including seizures
- apnea and bradycardia
- shock.

Laboratory findings

Mostly not specifically attributable to cerebral hemorrhage. May include:
- acute anemia
- hyperglycemia
- unexplained, severe metabolic acidosis
- hyperkalemia
- electrolyte imbalance
- coagulation abnormalities.

Key point

Don't overestimate the long-term significance of minor abnormalities on cranial ultrasound.

Management

- Optimize:
  – airway and breathing – provide oxygenation/ventilation as needed; avoid hypo- or hypercarbia, synchronize infant's breathing and ventilator
  – circulation – maintain adequate intravascular volume and blood pressure
  – comfort – avoid unnecessary or uncomfortable manipulation of infant.
- Treat seizures.
- Correct significant coagulation abnormalities.
- Monitor for complications (Fig. 31.3) – sequential head circumference measurements and serial head ultrasound for ventricular dilatation (PHVD, post-hemorrhagic ventricular dilatation) (see Chapter 78).

Prognosis

- Small germinal matrix or intraventricular hemorrhage – similar to normal ultrasound.
- Large parenchymal hemorrhage/large porencephalic cyst/hydrocephalus needing shunt – appreciable mortality, high risk of cerebral palsy and learning difficulties.
- Localized anterior cysts/transient flares – normal.
- Widespread cysts – all have cerebral palsy, usually spastic diplegia or quadriplegia with or without learning difficulties and visual impairment.

Prevention

- Avoid delivery before 30 weeks of gestation unless essential, and give antenatal corticosteroids.
- Avoid perinatal hypoxia–ischemia.
- Efficient resuscitation.
- Optimize intensive care – especially ventilation and circulation.
  Giving preterm infants indomethacin prophylactically reduces the incidence of severe hemorrhage but does not improve neurodevelopmental outcome.

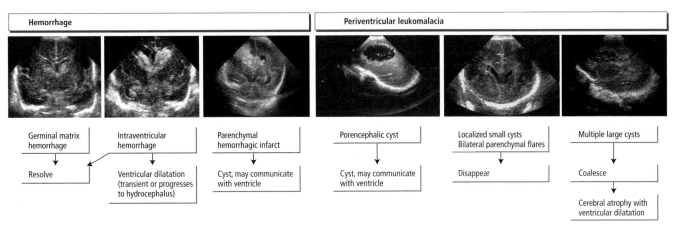

Fig. 31.3 Natural history and complications of cerebral hemorrhage and periventricular leukomalacia.

Ductus arteriosus – connects the pulmonary artery with the descending aorta (Fig. 32.1). Ongoing patency of the ductus arteriosus may be beneficial in patients with pulmonary hypertension or some forms of congenital heart disease.

In utero – ductal patency:
- dependent on low PaO_2 and high concentrations of vasodilating prostaglandins (PGE_2 and PGI_2).

Postnatal – ductal constriction is promoted by:
- the rise in oxygen tension with the first breaths
- the increase in pulmonary blood flow, which enhances clearance of the local vasodilating prostaglandins.

Ductal closure

Ductal closure takes place in two stages:
- functional closure – 24–48 hours after birth
- anatomic closure – may take 2–3 weeks.

In preterm infants, there may be delay in anatomic closure. Blood flows left to right across the patent ductus, from the higher systemic blood pressure to the low pulmonary artery pressure. However, in respiratory distress syndrome, pulmonary artery pressure is increased and the shunt may be bidirectional or right to left. Eventually, the duct will close spontaneously, but intervention is sometimes required to achieve this.

In contrast to preterm infants, in term infants a patent ductus arteriosus is a permanent defect in the muscle wall of the duct and is unlikely to close spontaneously.

Risk factors

- Prematurity – incidence increases with decreasing gestational age; most are less than 32 weeks' gestational age.
- Respiratory distress syndrome.
- Sepsis
- Pulmonary hypertension.

Clinical features

A patent ductus arteriosus becomes significant when the volume of blood flow across it leads to hemodynamic compromise.

The clinical features are attributable (Fig. 32.2) to:
- excessive pulmonary blood flow (pulmonary overcirculation)
- reduced systemic perfusion (systemic hypoperfusion) from shunting of blood across the duct; its magnitude depends on size of the vessel (transductal diameter) and the difference between systemic and pulmonary vascular resistance (transductal pressure differential).

Excessive pulmonary blood flow:
- Tachypnea.
- Increase in oxygen requirement.

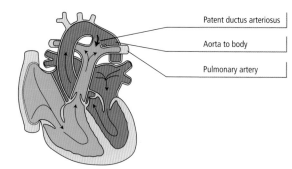

Fig. 32.1 Anatomy of the ductus arteriosus, with left to right flow across it.

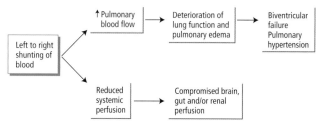

Fig. 32.2 Physiologic consequences of a patent ductus arteriosus.

- Carbon dioxide retention, difficulty weaning from mechanical ventilation.
- Apnea and bradycardia.

Reduced systemic perfusion:
- Tachycardia
- Widened pulse pressure, causing bounding pulses
- Active precordium
- Heart murmur (see below)
- Hepatomegaly (from right-sided heart failure).
- Systemic hypotension; low diastolic arterial pressure in all.

Heart murmur (Fig. 32.3):
- systolic
- best heard at left sternal border.
  If heart failure is present:
- gallop rhythm (extra third heart sound)
- may be loud pulmonic component (P_2) of second heart sound.
  Silent PDA, i.e. no murmur but PDA present – common, usually large shunt.

The classic continuous murmur, systole extending into diastole, heard in older infants is rarely present in preterm infants.

Investigations

Chest X-ray (Fig. 32.4)

Echocardiography with pulsed color Doppler
- Confirms the diagnosis (Fig. 32.5).
- Provides details of size and direction of the shunt and its hemodynamic consequences (Fig. 32.6).

Neonatology at a Glance, 2nd edition. Edited by Tom Lissauer & Avroy A. Fanaroff. © 2011 Blackwell Publishing Ltd.

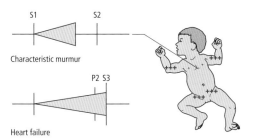

Fig. 32.3 Cardiac murmur and bounding pulses from shunting across a patent ductus arteriosus.

Echocardiographic diagnosis may be from:
- Direct visualization – diameter (>1.5 mm), direction of shunt
- Left atrial enlargement (left atrial:aortic root ratio >1.5:1)
- Increased left atrial pressure
- High cardiac output (> 350 mL/kg/min)
- Absent or retrograde diastolic flow in postductal aorta.
- Absent or retrograde diastolic flow in celiac, renal and middle cerebral arteries,

Management

Medical management

Aim is to control heart failure and for duct to close spontaneously or pharmacologically.

It consists of:
- **Fluid management** – although fluid restriction has been widely practiced, it may be harmful if renal output is normal as systemic blood flow is often compromised. Fluid restriction may though be desirable during treatment with indomethacin or ibuprofen as they cause fluid retention.
- **Diuretics** – used infrequently for heart failure. Furosemide leads to increased renal production of prostaglandins which may promote ductal patency. Only used when medical therapy has failed or is contraindicated and surgery is awaited.
- **Prostaglandin synthase inhibitors**, also called cyclooxygenase inhibitors (COXi):
  - indomethacin
  - ibuprofen.

Table 32.1 Indomethacin and ibuprofen.

Side effects	Contraindications
Decrease platelet aggregation, may worsen bleeding	Abnormal renal function with oliguria
Gastrointestinal bleeding	Thrombocytopenia (platelet count <75 000/mm^3 (<75 × 10^9/L)
	Gastrointestinal bleeding

Indomethacin – used for many years; ibuprofen introduced more recently. It has similar efficacy but less reduction in cerebral, renal and mesenteric blood flow. Other side effects and contraindications are shown in Table 32.1. Indomethacin may be given as a short course in high dosage or a longer course in lower dosage. The duct closes in >60% after a single course, but often remains patent and further courses are required.

Surgical closure

Performed if medical treatment fails.

Video-assisted thoracoscopic surgery (VATS) is now available in some centers, avoiding the need for a thoracotomy.

Complications of surgery are:
- post-ligation cardiac syndrome – low systolic arterial pressure, need for cardiotropes and difficulty with oxygenation secondary to impaired left ventricular function
- recurrent laryngeal nerve damage, common, causing vocal cord paralysis
- chylothorax from damage to thoracic duct
- pneumothorax
- ligation of pulmonary artery by mistake
- mortality (<1%) but surgical closure is associated with worse long-term neurological outcome.

Associated morbidity

- Pulmonary hemorrhage
- Cranial hemorrhage
- Necrotizing enterocolitis
- Bronchopulmonary dysplasia (chronic lung disease).

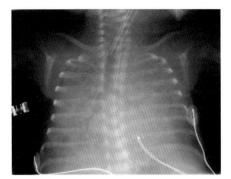

Fig. 32.4 Chest X-ray showing increased pulmonary vasculature markings and cardiomegaly. But often unhelpful diagnostically.

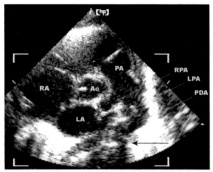

Fig. 32.5 Visualization of a patent ductus arteriosus (arrow).

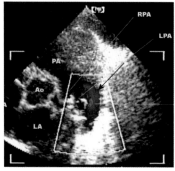

Fig. 32.6 Pulsed color Doppler showing shunting across the ductus arteriosus (arrow).

Infection

In preterm infants, infection is a major cause of morbidity and mortality.

Preterm infants are especially vulnerable because:
• they have reduced cellular and humoral immunity – this is because IgG antibodies are transferred from mother to fetus mainly during the third trimester
• their skin is thin and readily denuded by skin electrodes, catheters and tape, providing a portal of entry and a site of colonization for organisms
• central venous catheters and tracheal tubes are left in place for prolonged periods and are a potential focus for infection
• cross-infection is readily spread from infant to infant in neonatal nurseries on the hands of staff and from contaminated equipment.

Early-onset infection (<72 hours)
Acquired before birth from chorioamnionitis or maternal bacteremia or from the birth canal.

The most common organisms are group B streptococci and coliforms.

Late-onset sepsis (>72 hours)

Mainly due to nosocomial (hospital-acquired) infection, rather than community-acquired infection.. The most common cause is coagulase-negative staphylococcus (CONS). Other organisms are shown in Fig. 33.1.

There is marked variation in nosocomial infection rates among units. This results in wide variation in infection-related morbidity, duration of hospitalization, cost and mortality.

Fungal infections

In very low birthweight infants:
• incidence 1–10%
• mortality (up to 35%).

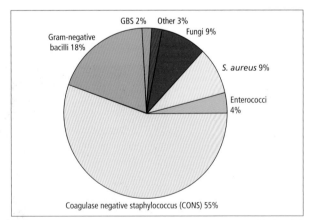

Fig. 33.1 Organisms causing late-onset sepsis in very low birthweight infants. (NICHD Neonatal Network. *J Pediatr* 1996; **129**: 63.)

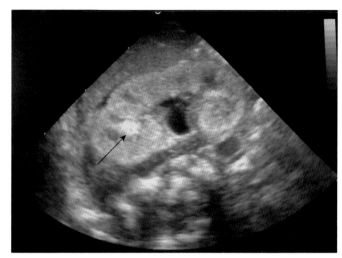

Fig. 33.2 Fungal ball in the kidney from *Candida* sepsis on renal ultrasound.

Candida albicans is the most common organism (Fig. 33.2). The source of infection is colonization of the gastrointestinal tract. Oral and topical antifungal agents are often given as prophylaxis to infants receiving prolonged antibiotic therapy, although this practice is not uniformly accepted. Broad-spectrum antibiotics, parenteral nutrition, central venous catheters are risk factors for fungal infection.

Treatment is with amphotericin B, fluconazole or flucytosine, depending on infection site and fungus species.

Presentation and management

These are described in Chapter 41.

Jaundice

Most preterm infants develop jaundice from unconjugated hyperbilirubinemia in the first week of life. The level of bilirubin that is potentially damaging is lower than in more mature infants. The bilirubin peaks at around day 5 of life and should be closely monitored.

Conjugated hyperbilirubinemia is mainly associated with total parenteral nutrition (TPN), necrotizing enterocolitis and congenital infection. Management is described in Chapter 40.

Anemia

Common in VLBW (very low birthweight) infants, mainly because of:
• blood loss from repeated blood sampling and the preterm infant's small blood volume of only 80 mL/kg

Neonatology at a Glance, 2nd edition. Edited by Tom Lissauer & Avroy A. Fanaroff. © 2011 Blackwell Publishing Ltd.

- physiologic anemia of prematurity. This occurs at 1–3 months of age due to:
  - reduced red cell production
  - shortened red cell survival
  - markedly increased requirements from growth.

Treatment

Blood transfusions

Aim is to restore or maintain adequate tissue oxygen delivery, but as there are no reliable symptoms or signs to determine this, the indications in neonates are controversial and varies between centers (Table 33.1). Kept to a minimum because of potential hazards. Splitting adult donor bags to allow several transfusions from the same donor is recommended to reduce potential risk of blood-borne pathogens by reducing number of donors. Blood transfusions are also associated with an increased risk of retinopathy of prematurity.

Oral iron therapy

Given to prevent anemia of prematurity, unless the infant has received a recent blood transfusion or iron-fortified formula.

Oral folic acid

Given in some centers.

Question

Is erythropoietin therapy used in newborn infants?

Recombinant human erythropoietin (EPO) could potentially reduce the need for red cell transfusions. However, it does not significantly reduce the transfusion requirements in the first 2 weeks of life, when sick neonates are most dependent on transfusion. It is therefore used selectively. It may be useful for treatment of chronic anemia when transfusion is declined (e.g. for religious or cultural reasons). It is not useful for treatment of acute anemia because of the lag of >1 week after starting treatment before the hemoglobin increases significantly.

Osteopenia of prematurity

Metabolic bone disease may occur at several weeks of age, causing:
- reduced bone mineralization with widening and cupping of the wrists, knees and ribs on X-ray, as with rickets (Fig. 33.3)
- failure in linear growth
- pathologic fractures, particularly of ribs and long bones (Fig. 33.4).

Investigations show:
- calcium – normal or raised
- phosphate – low
- alkaline phosphatase (a marker of bone turnover) – markedly raised.

Table 33.1 An example of indications for blood transfusions in preterm infants (College of American Pathologists, 1998).

Acute blood loss with shock
Hb <12 g/dL – if in oxygen with mechanical ventilation, congenital heart disease with cyanosis or heart failure
Hb <10 g/dL – if moderate oxygen requirement via nasal cannula
Hb <8 g/dL – if apnea and bradycardia, sustained tachycardia, failure to gain weight, mild oxygen requirement
Hb <7 g/dL and reticulocyte count <100 000/mL – even if asymptomatic

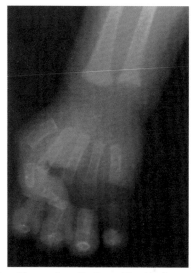

Fig. 33.3 Reduced bone mineralization with widening and cupping of the wrist bones from osteopenia of prematurity.

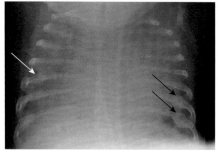

Fig. 33.4 Rib fractures (arrows) and reduced bone mineralization from osteopenia of prematurity. (Courtesy of Dr Richard Nicholl.)

Osteopenia of prematurity is due to phosphorus deficiency from urinary loss and increased requirements.

It can be prevented by providing additional phosphate in total parenteral nutrition, by fortifying expressed breast milk or by giving oral phosphate to maintain age-appropriate plasma phosphate levels. It can be problematic to provide sufficient phosphate for infants requiring total parenteral nutrition for a prolonged period.

Treatment is with sodium or potassium acid phosphate and vitamin D supplements.

Apnea, bradycardia and desaturations

Common in VLBW (very low birthweight) infants.

Definition (Fig. 34.1)

Interrelationship between apnea, bradycardia and desaturation is complex, so monitor not only respiration but also heart rate and oxygen saturation.

Hypoxemia with bradycardia is harmful if prolonged.

Classification

• **Central** – cessation of chest wall motion due to loss of respiratory neural output.
• **Obstructive** – persistence of obstructed inspiratory efforts throughout the apnea with no airflow. Rare, unless associated with neck flexion. Presents with bradycardia with or without desaturation. May not be detected on standard clinical impedance respiratory monitor as they detect chest wall movement as a breath, although there is no airflow.
• **Mixed** – most common for prolonged apnea; a combination of both of above, with obstructed inspiratory efforts intermittently throughout the apnea.

Episodes of desaturation

• May accompany short (5–10 seconds) respiratory pauses, especially if baseline SaO_2 is low.
• During assisted ventilation they are secondary to hypoventilation.
• Variable relationship with bradycardia.

Causes

Usually due to prematurity – must consider or exclude:
• infection (most common)
• necrotizing enterocolitis
• heart failure – patent ductus arteriosus, etc.
• hypoglycemia, electrolyte abnormality
• inborn error of metabolism
• anemia
• seizures.

Treatment

Most apneic spells are brief and self-limiting.
If not:
• Check airway.
• Gentle tactile stimulation.
• Nasal CPAP (continuous positive airway pressure) – very effective, eliminates obstructive apnea. Nasal CPAP may be combined with IMV (intermittent mandatory ventilation) or SIMV (synchronized ventilation).
• Methylxanthines – caffeine or theophylline. Caffeine more widely used as fewer side-effects and drug level monitoring not needed. Caffeine lowers the incidence of bronchopulmonary dysplasia (BPD) and of neurodevelopmental delay.
• Mechanical ventilation.

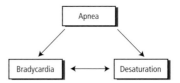

Fig. 34.1 Apnea is absence of breathing for more than 10–15 seconds and may result in bradycardia and/or desaturation.

Prognosis

Apnea and bradycardia continue in some preterm infants beyond 36 weeks of gestational age, particularly in association with bronchopulmonary dysplasia (chronic lung disease), but rarely beyond 43–44 weeks. Continue to hospitalize if symptomatic apnea and bradycardia until absent for several days. Not a risk factor for SIDS (sudden infant death syndrome).

Question

What is the relationship of apnea to feeding?

Hypoventilation, apnea and even cyanosis commonly accompany onset of oral (especially bottle) feeds.

These episodes of hypoventilation typically resolve rapidly without the need for further intervention.

Gastroesophageal reflux and apnea are both common in preterm infants, but rarely temporally related.

Pharmacologic treatment of reflux often fails to abolish apnea and is associated with an increased risk of infection.

Retinopathy of prematurity (ROP)

Eye disease of prematurity. Highest incidence in extremely low birthweight infants.

Hyperoxia restricts retinal vascular growth by inhibiting vascular endothelial growth factor (VEGF). Subsequent hypoxia acts as a stimulus for inappropriate and excessive growth of retinal vessels, mediated by increased VEGF. Keeping preterm infants in inappropriately high oxygen concentrations results in a high incidence of ROP, causing blindness (see Chapter 66). However, in VLBW (very low birthweight) infants, even with oxygenation closely monitored (attempting to keep PaO_2 at 50–80 mmHg, i.e. 6.5–10.5 kPa, oxygen saturation 90–95%), about 30–40% develop ROP, with 4–5% needing treatment and 1% have severe visual impairment.

Visual outcome also depends on associated neurologic injury, myopia and squint.

ROP causes 3–10% of childhood visual impairment in developed countries.

Neonatology at a Glance, 2nd edition. Edited by Tom Lissauer & Avroy A. Fanaroff. © 2011 Blackwell Publishing Ltd.

Screening

Preterm infants are screened selectively (Table 34.1). Findings are classified according to the stage of advancement and the zone affected (Table 34.2 and Fig. 34.2).

Treatment

Stage 1 or 2 disease resolves spontaneously. Stage 3 plus disease requires laser therapy to ablate the peripheral avascular retina (Fig. 34.6).

Table 34.1 Screening guidelines for retinopathy of prematurity.

	US (2006)	UK (2008)
Who?	Birth: <1500 g or <30 weeks Bigger/older infants who are particularly unstable	Birth: <1501 g and <32 weeks
When?	<27 weeks gestational age at 31 weeks	<27 weeks gestational age at 30–31 weeks
	>27 weeks at 4 weeks postnatal age	>27 weeks at 4–5 weeks postnatal age
Follow up?	Until retinopathy shows signs of regression or until 36 weeks' postmenstrual age if no disease Post-discharge follow-up of visual development	

Table 34.2 International classification of retinopathy of prematurity (revised 2005).

Stage 1 – flat demarcation line between normally vascularized and non-vascularized retina (Fig. 34.3)

Stage 2 – demarcation line extends off the retina as a ridge

Stage 3 – new vessels behind the ridge with or without vitreous hemorrhage (extraretinal fibrovascular proliferation) (Fig. 34.4)

Stage 4 – partial retinal detachment

Stage 5 – total retinal detachment (Fig. 34.5)

Plus disease – active progressive disease

Pre-plus disease – abnormal dilatation and tortuosity of posterior pole vessels

Aggressive posterior ROP – rapidly progressing, severe form

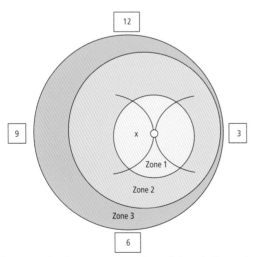

Fig. 34.2 Zones of retina. Numbers at the periphery indicate clock hour.

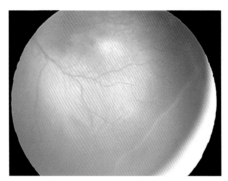

Fig. 34.3 Stage 1 retinopathy of prematurity. (Courtesy of Prof. Alistair Fielder.)

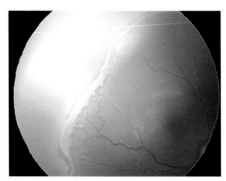

Fig. 34.4 Stage 3 retinopathy of prematurity in a black African infant. (Courtesy of Prof. Alistair Fielder.)

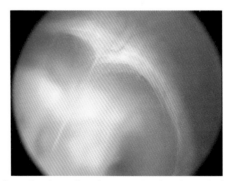

Fig. 34.5 Stage 5 retinopathy of prematurity showing retinal detachment.

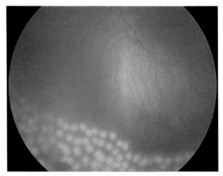

Fig. 34.6 Following laser therapy for retinopathy of prematurity.

Apnea, bradycardia and desaturations, retinopathy of prematurity 85

Necrotizing enterocolitis (NEC) is the most serious abdominal disorder of preterm infants. It occurs in 2–10% of VLBW (very low birthweight) infants and has a mortality of 25–30%.

The incidence increases with decreasing gestational age; it is rare in term infants. It is a syndrome characterized by abdominal distension, bilious aspirates, bloody stools and intramural air (pneumatosis intestinalis) on abdominal X-ray.

There is inflammation of the bowel wall, which may progress to necrosis and perforation. It may involve a localized section of bowel (most often the terminal ileum) or be generalized.

Cases may be sporadic or sometimes occur in epidemics.

Risk factors

Pathogenesis is unknown, but several risk factors have been identified (Fig. 35.1).

Clinical features

Onset is at 1–2 weeks but may be up to several weeks of age, with:
- bilious aspirates/vomiting
- feeding intolerance
- bloody stools
- abdominal distension and tenderness (Fig. 35.2), which may progress to perforation (Table 35.1).
- features of sepsis:
  - temperature instability
  - jaundice
  - apnea and bradycardia
  - lethargy
  - hypoperfusion, shock.

Laboratory findings

These include:
- raised acute-phase reactant (C-reactive protein, CRP or procalcitonin)
- thrombocytopenia

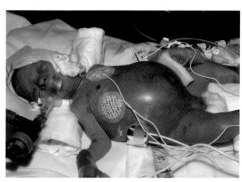

Fig. 35.2 Abdominal distension and shiny abdominal skin in necrotizing enterocolitis.

Table 35.1 Clinical signs of peritonitis/perforation.

Abdominal tenderness
Guarding
Tense, discolored abdominal wall
Abdominal wall edema
Absent bowel sounds
Abdominal mass

- neutropenia, neutrophilia
- anemia
- blood culture positive
- coagulation abnormalities
- metabolic acidosis
- hypoxia, hypercapnia
- hyponatremia, hyperkalemia
- increased BUN (blood urea)
- hyperbilirubinemia.

Radiologic abnormalities

- Dilated loops of bowel.
- Thickened intestinal wall.
- Inspissated stool (mottled appearance).
- Intramural air (*pneumatosis intestinalis*) (Fig. 35.3).
- Air in portal venous system (Fig. 35.4).

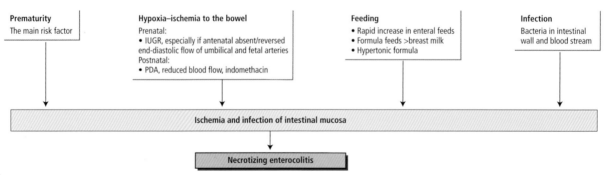

Fig. 35.1 Risk factors in the pathogenesis of necrotizing enterocolitis.

Neonatology at a Glance, 2nd edition. Edited by Tom Lissauer & Avroy A. Fanaroff. © 2011 Blackwell Publishing Ltd.

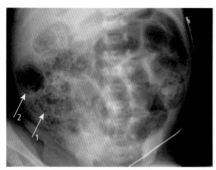

Fig. 35.3 Abdominal X-ray showing dilated loops of bowel, inspissated stool (arrow 1) and intramural air (arrow 2). (Courtesy of Dr Annemarie Jeanes.)

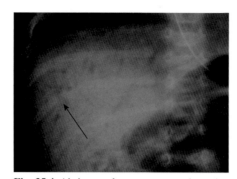

Fig. 35.4 Air in portal venous system (arrow). (Courtesy of Dr Annemarie Jeanes.)

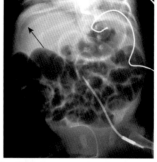

Fig. 35.5 Bowel perforation showing air under the diaphragm (arrow) and outlining the falciform ligament. (Courtesy of Dr Annemarie Jeanes.)

- Bowel perforation:
  - gasless abdomen/ascites
  - pneumoperitoneum
  - air below diaphragm/around the falciform ligament (Fig. 35.5).

Management (Table 35.2)

Table 35.2 Management of necrotizing enterocolitis.

Treatment	Rationale/goals
Secure airway and breathing	Maintain adequate oxygenation and ventilation
	Abdominal distension may compromise breathing
Circulation	
• establish vascular access	Infusion of fluids
• give intravascular volume replacement (saline, blood, fresh frozen plasma)	Treat hypoperfusion/hypovolemic shock
• correct metabolic acidosis	Improve organ and tissue perfusion
Place large-bore naso/orogastric tube	Intestinal decompression, bowel rest
NPO (nil by mouth) – start parenteral nutrition	Support nutritional demands for growth
Broad-spectrum antibiotics	Gram-positive, -negative and anaerobic coverage
	Consider antifungal agents
Treat coagulopathy (fresh frozen plasma, platelets, cryoprecipitate)	Avoid bleeding complications
Monitor regularly – clinical, radiographic and laboratory investigations	Necrotizing enterocolitis can worsen very quickly
Surgery – options are:	Indications – bowel perforation or failure to resolve on medical treatment
• peritoneal drainage at bedside	
• laparotomy – resection of non-viable bowel and anastomosis or ileostomy or colostomy	However, peritoneal drainage alone is associated with worse neurodevelopmental outcome than laparotomy

Sequelae

Short term

These are:
- electrolyte depletion.
- complications of prolonged parenteral nutrition – infection, electrolyte derangement, conjugated hyperbilirubinemia, etc.

Long term

Short bowel syndrome following bowel resection:
- diarrhea (from loss of bowel mucosa and rapid gastrointestinal transit)
- growth failure
- vitamin B_{12} deficiency if terminal ileum resected
- stricture formation – causes intestinal obstruction and/or intestinal hemorrhage.

Prevention

- Use breast milk if possible.
- Avoid hyperosmolar feeds.
- Avoid rapid increase in feed volume in very immature infants, especially if intrauterine growth restriction with absent/reverse end-diastolic Doppler waveform antenatally.
- Use of prebiotics and probiotics with or without lactoferrin to maintain normal gut flora is being investigated.

Key point

NEC is often suspected, although all the classic clinical features are not present. Treatment may need to be started whilst awaiting investigation results and before the clinical course becomes evident. Surgical consultation should be initiated early.

36 Bronchopulmonary dysplasia

Bronchopulmonary dysplasia (BPD, chronic lung disease) is a major cause of morbidity and mortality in preterm infants. It develops in 25–35% of very low birthweight infants. The incidence is highest in the extremely preterm (Fig. 36.1). It is uncommon in infants born after 32 weeks' gestational age.

Definition

A consensus conference (NICHD/NHLB/ORD, 2004) recommended definitions based on severity of illness:
- oxygen requirement at 28 days of age (used in many trials)
- oxygen requirement and characteristic chest X-ray at 28 days
- oxygen requirement at 36 weeks' postmenstrual age. This is usually used as it identifies infants most likely to have long-term complications.

It also recommended that the term 'bronchopulmonary dysplasia' be used rather than 'chronic lung disease'.

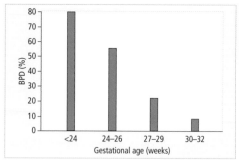

Fig. 36.1 Incidence of bronchopulmonary dysplasia (BPD, chronic lung disease) at 36 weeks with gestational age in VLBW (very low birthweight infants) (Vermont–Oxford Network data for 2008).

Predisposing factors

The cause is unknown. It is a multifactorial disorder.

It most often develops in extremely preterm infants with surfactant deficiency or immature lungs who require mechanical ventilation. The higher the pressures and oxygen concentration required and the longer mechanical ventilation is needed, the more likely the infant is to develop bronchopulmonary dysplasia. However, with current respiratory management of minimal ventilatory support, bronchopulmonary dysplasia is increasingly seen in extremely preterm infants who had minimal lung disease in the first few days of life. There may be a genetic predisposition – it is more common if there is a family history of reactive airway disease. Other risk factors are shown in Fig. 36.2.

Clinical features

In addition to the need for oxygen with or without respiratory support:
- skin pallor
- tachypnea
- hyperexpanded chest
- chest retractions
- auscultation – crackles and wheezes
- fluid retention
- heart failure
- recurrent pneumonia
- growth failure.

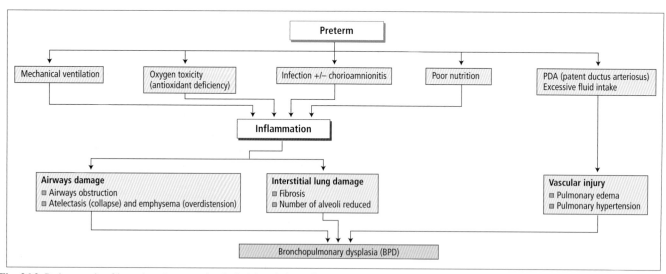

Fig. 36.2 Pathogenesis of bronchopulmonary dysplasia (chronic lung disease).

Neonatology at a Glance, 2nd edition. Edited by Tom Lissauer & Avroy A. Fanaroff. © 2011 Blackwell Publishing Ltd.

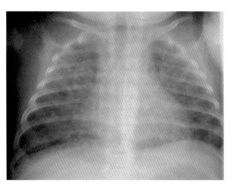

Fig. 36.3 Chest X-ray in bronchopulmonary dysplasia (chronic lung disease) showing generalized opacification of lung fields, lung collapse, fibrosis, cystic changes and overdistension of the lungs.

Investigations – chest X-ray (Fig. 36.3)

Management

This is with:
• oxygen and respiratory support (low flow nasal cannula or nasal CPAP or mechanical ventilation) but kept to a minimum to maintain satisfactory oxygenation (SaO₂ 90–95%) (Fig. 36.4)
• attention to nutritional problems of:
 – increased caloric requirements (130–150 kcal/kg) because of increased work of breathing
 – delay in establishing feeding
 – gastroesophageal reflux (may result in aspiration)
 – prevention of osteopenia of prematurity with phosphate supplements
• drug therapy may be considered:
 – inhaled bronchodilators
 – diuretics (transient improvement only)
 – corticosteroid therapy (see below).

Long-term consequences of severe BPD

• Prolonged oxygen therapy over many months. May need to be given at home.
• Feeding problems requiring prolonged nasogastric/gastrostomy feeding.
• Inguinal hernias (from raised intra-abdominal pressure and muscular weakness associated with failure to thrive).
• Risk of RSV (respiratory syncytial virus) infection causing bronchiolitis (risk of hospitalization reduced by monoclonal antibody palivizumab).
• Rehospitalization because of respiratory infection – needing additional oxygen or nasal CPAP (continuous positive airway pressure)/mechanical ventilation.
• Increased risk of asthma and sleep-disordered breathing including obstructive sleep apnea
• Increased risk of neurodevelopmental problems.

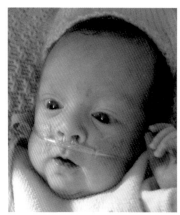

Fig. 36.4 Infant with bronchopulmonary dysplasia receiving low-flow nasal oxygen.

• Rarely, death from acute chest infection or cor pulmonale (pulmonary hypertension).

Strategies for prevention

These include:
• antenatal corticosteroids.
• surfactant therapy.
• possibly synchronized or high-frequency oscillatory ventilation.
• avoidance of fluid overload.
• closure of patent ductus arteriosus.
• vitamin A (given in some centers).

Question

What is the controversy about corticosteroid therapy?

Antenatal corticosteroids (betamethasone) reduce the severity of lung disease and mortality of VLBW infants.

However, when corticosteroids (dexamethasone) were given to VLBW infants in the first few days of life, it was associated with increased incidence of gastrointestinal hemorrhage and bowel perforation.

In infants still requiring oxygen at several weeks of age, a course of dexamethasone sometimes dramatically reduces the oxygen requirement and may allow weaning from mechanical ventilation. However, it is associated with serious side effects:
• short term – high blood pressure, hyperglycemia, increased risk of sepsis
• longer term – Cushingoid facies, hypertrophic cardiomyopathy, osteopenia and failure of growth in length and head circumference, and increase in cerebral palsy.

As a result of the increased incidence of cerebral palsy and other side-effects, it is now used only sparingly and after informing parents of the potential risks (Fig. 25.1).

Inhaled corticosteroids may reduce the need for systemic corticosteroids.

Survival in developed countries of very preterm (<32 weeks) and very low birthweight (VLBW) infants has increased dramatically, and babies from 23–24 weeks of gestation are now expected to survive (Fig. 37.1). However, this increased survival has been achieved at the expense of high rates of neurodisability although recent outcome data suggest the neurodisability rates in early life are falling (Fig 37.2).

The development of VLBW infants is monitored in a follow-up program (see Chapter 71) or in the community. Data from these programs can then be compared with other programs, but such comparisons may be misleading if based on an individual unit as sample size of each individual unit will be small, with wide variations from year to year, and there may be differences in the demography of the mothers and referral patterns.

The most meaningful outcome data are regional or national, provided the data collection is standardized and complete. A follow-up rate greater than 90% is desirable for all cohorts.

Growth

At discharge from hospital, over 90% of VLBW infants are below the 10th centile for weight, length and head circumference. Many show catch-up growth in the first 2–3 years, first of the head circumference, then weight and then length. Energy requirements are increased and

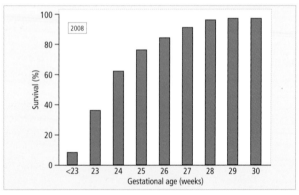

Fig. 37.1 Increase in survival with gestational age. (Vermont–Oxford Network, Birthweight 501–1500, 2009.)

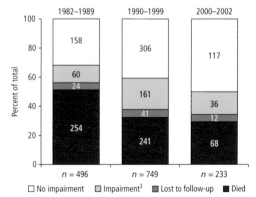

Fig. 37.2 Neurodevelopmental outcome for babies <1000 g birthweight over 20 years in a tertiary perinatal center. The proportion with impairment has decreased. (Wilson Costello *Pediatrics* 2007; **119**: 37–45.)

growth is better if the infant is in good health. Catch-up growth is often less in infants with intrauterine growth restriction.

Medical complications

These include:
- bronchopulmonary dysplasia – may require additional oxygen therapy for many months
- pneumonia/wheezing/asthma often requiring rehospitalization (more common in children with bronchopulmonary dysplasia)
- bronchiolitis from RSV (respiratory syncytial virus) infection (hospitalization reduced by giving RSV monoclonal antibody, palivizumab)
- gastroesophageal reflux – especially with bronchopulmonary dysplasia
- complex nutritional and gastrointestinal disorders – following necrotizing enterocolitis or gastrointestinal surgery
- inguinal hernias – require surgical repair.

The commonest reasons for rehospitalization are respiratory disorders and surgical repair of inguinal hernias.

Neurodisability and behavior problems

Although the rate of neurodisability among very preterm infants has fallen over the past 20 years, they continue to be at high risk of long-term problems (Fig. 37.2). They are at markedly increased risk of developing cerebral palsy (Fig. 37.3). Neurodisability outcomes (see Table 37.1) usually classify children into those with severe disability (unable to walk, very low IQ, blind or profoundly deaf), moderate disability (walk with support, IQ 55–70, hear with aids) and mild disability (less severe impairments, IQ 70–85). The neurodisability outcomes of infants born at <26 weeks' gestation at different ages are shown in Figure 37.4.

The most common impairments are, however, learning difficulties. The prevalence of cognitive impairment and of other associated difficulties increases with decreasing gestational age at birth (Fig. 37.5) and become increasingly evident when the individual child is compared to their peers at nursery or school. In addition, children may have difficulties with:

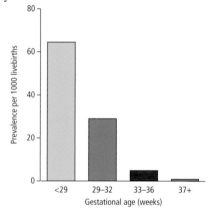

Fig. 37.3 Gestation-specific prevalence of cerebral palsy in 4Child Register 1984–2003. (Data from 4Child annual report 2009.)

Neonatology at a Glance, 2nd edition. Edited by Tom Lissauer & Avroy A. Fanaroff. © 2011 Blackwell Publishing Ltd.

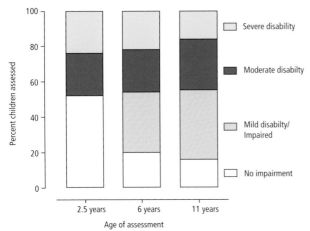

Fig. 37.4 Evolution of disability from birth to 11 years in births 22–25 weeks of gestation in the UK (Johnson *et al. Pediatrics* 2009; **124**: e249–257).

- fine motor skills, e.g. threading beads
- concentration, with short attention span
- behavior problems, especially attention deficit disorders
- abstract reasoning, e.g. mathematics
- processing several tasks simultaneously.

A small proportion also have hearing impairment, with 1–2% requiring amplification, or visual impairment, with 1% blind in both eyes. A greater proportion have refraction errors and squints and therefore require glasses.

Educational outcomes

At school age problems with low IQ, poor executive function and behavior problems are evident in the need for special educational support. These are more prevalent as gestation or weight at birth decreases (Fig. 37.5). Around two-thirds of UK children born <26 weeks of gestation have special needs at 11 years including learning, behavior and physical support needs and 13% require separate

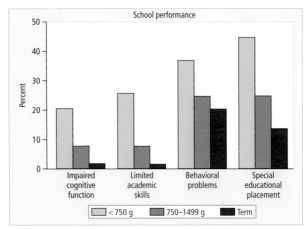

Fig. 37.5 Increased incidence of impaired cognitive function, academic skills, behavioral problems and special education placement in infants with birthweight below 750 g and 750–1499 g compared with term infants. (Adapted from Hack M *et al.*, School-age outcomes in children with birth weights under 750 g. *N Engl J Med* 1994; **331**: 753–759.)

educational provision. When children are permitted to repeat grades, many more very preterm children are either not ready to start school or are kept back one year.

Adulthood

A study of adults, at 20 years of age, comparing those born VLBW with those born at term, showed that:
- fewer had graduated from high school (74% versus 83%)
- fewer men (30% versus 53%) but not women were enrolled in postsecondary study
- they had a lower mean IQ (87 versus 92) and lower academic achievements
- they had a higher rate of neurosensory impairment (10% versus <1%)
- they had less alcohol and drug use and lower pregnancy rate, probably because of closer parental supervision.

Table 37.1 Definitions of disability for use at 18–24 months of corrected age in follow-up of very preterm infants (from Classification of health status at 2 years as a perinatal outcome, BAPM, London, 2008).

Domain	Severe neurodevelopmental disability Any one of below:	Moderate neurodevelopmental disability Any one of below:
Motor	Cerebral palsy with GMFCS level 3, 4 or 5	Cerebral palsy with GMFCS level 2
Cognitive function	Score <3 standard deviations below norm (DQ <55)	Score <2 standard deviations below norm (DQ 55–70)
Hearing	No useful hearing even with aids	Hearing loss corrected with aids (usually moderate 40–70 dBHL) or Some hearing but loss not corrected by aids (usually severe 70–90 dBHL)
Speech and language	No meaningful words/signs	Some but fewer than 5 words or signs
Vision	Blind or can only perceive light	Moderately reduced vision
Other disabilities		
Respiratory	Requires continued respiratory support or oxygen	Limited exercise tolerance
Gastrointestinal	Requires TPN, NG or PEG feeding	On special diet or has stoma
Renal	Requires dialysis or awaiting transplant	Renal impairment requiring treatment or special diet

GMFCS (Gross Motor Function Classification System): level 2 – walks with limitations; level 3 – walks using hand-held mobility device; level 4 – self-mobility with limitations, may use powered wheelchair; level 5 – manual wheelchair.

DQ, developmental quotient; TPN, total parenteral nutrition; NG, nasogastric; PEG, percutaneous endoscopic gastrostomy.

Overview

The clinical features of respiratory distress are shown in Fig. 38.1.

Monitoring

- Oxygen saturation (maintain >95% in term infants).
- Respiratory rate, heart rate, BP, temperature.
- Arterial blood gases if needing oxygen >30%.

Investigations

- Chest X-ray – confirms respiratory disease, excludes pneumothorax, diaphragmatic hernia, lung malformations.
- Complete blood count, blood cultures, C-reactive protein, consider lumbar puncture.

Management

- Airway and breathing – oxygen/CPAP/mechanical ventilation as required.
- Circulatory support if necessary.
- Intravenous fluids or frequent nasogastric feeds.
- Intravenous antibiotics – broad-spectrum coverage.

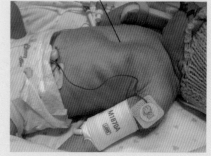

Respiratory distress:
Tachypnea (RR > 60/min)
+
Nasal flaring
+
Grunting (prolonged expiration against closed glottis)
+
Chest retraction
– suprasternal
– intercostal
– subcostal

Cyanosis (if severe)

Fig. 38.1 Clinical features of respiratory distress.

Causes (Fig. 38.2)

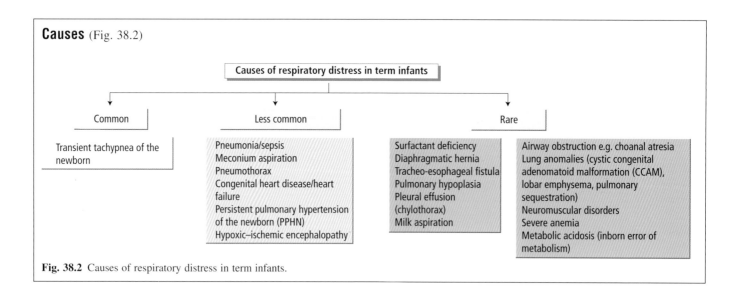

Causes of respiratory distress in term infants

Common

Transient tachypnea of the newborn

Less common

Pneumonia/sepsis
Meconium aspiration
Pneumothorax
Congenital heart disease/heart failure
Persistent pulmonary hypertension of the newborn (PPHN)
Hypoxic–ischemic encephalopathy

Rare

Surfactant deficiency
Diaphragmatic hernia
Tracheo-esophageal fistula
Pulmonary hypoplasia
Pleural effusion (chylothorax)
Milk aspiration

Airway obstruction e.g. choanal atresia
Lung anomalies (cystic congenital adenomatoid malformation (CCAM), lobar emphysema, pulmonary sequestration)
Neuromuscular disorders
Severe anemia
Metabolic acidosis (inborn error of metabolism)

Fig. 38.2 Causes of respiratory distress in term infants.

Neonatology at a Glance, 2nd edition. Edited by Tom Lissauer & Avroy A. Fanaroff. © 2011 Blackwell Publishing Ltd.

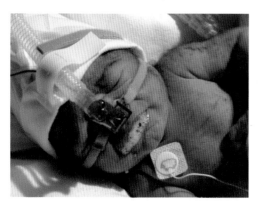

Fig. 38.3 Lung liquid in the mouth of a newborn term infant with transient tachypnea of the newborn requiring nasal CPAP.

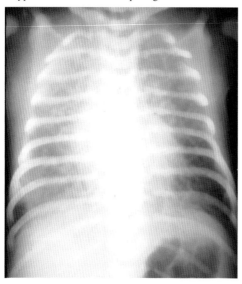

(a)

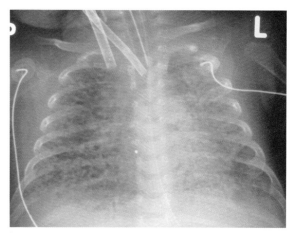

(b)

Fig. 38.4 Chest X-ray in transient tachypnea of the newborn showing fluid in the horizontal fissure and some streaky infiltrates with hyperinflation and perihilar haziness (a). Some hours later, the perihilar haziness has cleared, but there is still fluid in the horizontal fissure and hyperinflation (b).

Common causes

Transient tachypnea of the newborn (TTNB)

This is by far the most common cause of respiratory distress in term infants. Caused by delay in the absorption of lung liquid (Figs 38.3 and 38.4), especially following elective cesarean section. Usually settles within first day or two of life, but may have mild oxygen requirement and take several days to resolve.

Less common causes

Pneumonia

- Risk factors – prolonged rupture of the membranes (PROM), maternal fever, chorioamnionitis, preterm.
- All infants with respiratory distress should be started on broad-spectrum antibiotics until the results of the blood culture, C-reactive protein (CRP), complete blood count (CBC), lumbar puncture (if performed) are known.
- Group B streptococcus is the most common cause.

Meconium aspiration

The proportion of infants who pass meconium at birth increases with gestational age, affecting 20–25% at 42 weeks. Asphyxiated infants may start gasping and aspirate meconium before delivery. At birth infants may inhale thick meconium (see Chapter 12) which results in mechanical obstruction, chemical pneumonitis and inactivation of surfactant (Fig. 38.5). There is a high incidence of air leak. Surfactant therapy may be beneficial. Mechanical ventilation is often required. Accompanying persistent pulmonary hypertension (PPHN) may require nitric oxide or sildenafil and

Fig. 38.5 Chest X-ray in meconium aspiration. There is hyperinflation of the lungs, flattened diaphragm and widespread patchy areas of collapse evident in coarse irregular densities with areas of overinflation. There is a tracheal tube and central lines to deliver extracorporeal membrane oxygenation (ECMO).

Respiratory distress in term infants 93

sometimes ECMO (extracorporeal membrane oxygenation), i.e. cardiopulmonary bypass.

Pneumothorax (see Chapter 28)

May occur spontaneously or more commonly as a complication of mechanical ventilation or CPAP.

Heart failure (see Chapter 48)

Check for evidence of heart failure – including active precordium, enlarged heart, gallop rhythm, heart murmurs and enlarged liver. and that femoral pulses are palpable (reduced in coarctation of the aorta, hypoplastic left heart syndrome).

Persistent pulmonary hypertension of the newborn (PPHN)

Pulmonary hypertension leads to right-to-left shunting of blood (Fig. 38.6):
- across the patent foramen ovale
- across the patent ductus arteriosus
- intrapulmonary.

The condition
Usually secondary to:
- birth asphyxia
- meconium aspiration
- sepsis
- diaphragmatic hernia.
  Occasionally it is the primary disorder.

Presentation
Cyanosis or difficulty in oxygenation.

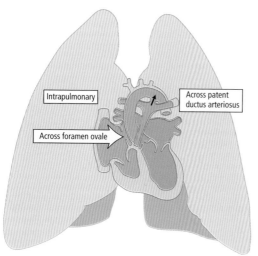

Fig. 38.6 Pulmonary hypertension leads to right-to-left shunting.

Specific investigations
- Chest X-ray – shows underlying cause or may be normal or show pulmonary oligemia (diminished vascularity).
- Echocardiography is needed to exclude congenital heart disease. It can also allow estimation of the magnitude of pulmonary hypertension (see Chapter 79).

Management
- Oxygen.
- Optimize mechanical ventilation.
- Circulatory support as required.
- Consider surfactant therapy.
- Pulmonary vasodilator – nitric oxide (NO). Sildenafil (Viagra) also appears to be effective.
- Consider high-frequency oscillatory ventilation (HFOV).
- Extracorporeal membrane oxygenation (ECMO) as rescue therapy for severe respiratory failure.

Rare causes

Surfactant deficiency

Rare in term infants. May occur in infants of maternal diabetes or with surfactant protein B deficiency, a rare genetic disorder.

Diaphragmatic hernia

Main problems
- Pulmonary hypoplasia, as herniated bowel reduces lung development in the fetus.
- Lung compression by the bowel, which increases in size as air enters it.
- Pulmonary hypertension (PPHN) – pulmonary arterioles reduced in number and size, and smooth muscle is hypertrophied.
- Other anomalies – present in 15–25%.

Incidence
1 in 4000 births.

Most common site
Left-sided hernia of bowel through the posterolateral foramen of the diaphragm (Bochdalek).

Presentation
- **Prenatal** – on ultrasound screening, polyhydramnios. Most identified antenatally. For antenatal management see Chapter 4.
- **Resuscitation** – failure to respond; deteriorates with bag and mask ventilation.
- **Respiratory distress** – but onset may be delayed if underlying lung well developed.

Physical signs
- Respiratory distress.
- Asymmetry of chest.

- Reduced air entry on affected side.
- Apex beat displaced.
- Scaphoid abdomen – from reduced content of bowel.

Diagnosis

X-ray-chest and abdomen (Fig. 38.7).

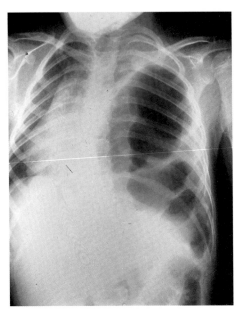

Fig. 38.7 Chest X-ray showing diaphragmatic hernia. There is bowel in the left chest and the heart and trachea are displaced to the right.

Management

- Intubate and ventilate from birth. Gentle ventilation, allowing permissive hypercapnia, i.e. $PaCO_2 > 60\,mmHg$ (8 kPa) but maintaining pH > 7.25. Avoid mask ventilation.
- Pass large nasogastric tube and apply suction.
- Stabilize and support circulation.
- Early TPN (total parenteral nutrition).
- Surgical repair – delay until stable and PPHN is resolving.
- Nitric oxide or sildenafil (Viagra) for PPHN.
- Extracorporeal membrane oxygenation (ECMO) – pre- and post-surgery in selected cases.

Mortality

20–30%.

Milk aspiration

Risk of aspiration if infant has cleft palate, neurologic disorder affecting sucking and swallowing or has respiratory distress. Infants with bronchopulmonary dysplasia (chronic lung disease) often have gastroesophageal reflux, which predisposes to aspiration.

Cleft lip and palate

Incidence – 1 in 1000 live births.

Inheritance – polygenic, but increased risk if family history.

Varies in severity from a mild unilateral cleft to severe bilateral cleft palate (Figs 39.1 and 39.2).

It is increasingly diagnosed on antenatal ultrasound scanning. This allows counseling of the parents and family before birth. Showing parents photographs is often helpful; photos of the lesion may help minimise the shock at birth as the defect is unsightly, photos after surgery are reassuring that the defect can be corrected.

A specialist multidisciplinary team from a tertiary center is required to provide:

• a key worker, usually a specialist nurse, for advice and to act as advocate for the child and family. Will visit the parents shortly after birth and also gives advice about feeding.

• craniofacial surgeon, orthodontist, speech and language therapist and audiologist.

• surgical repair of the lip, usually at 3 months of age for best long-term results, but some centers perform it immediately after birth. The palate is usually repaired at 6–12 months of age. Further surgery may be required when the child is older.

Long-term complications include middle ear infection and otitis media with effusion, difficulties with speech and orthodontic problems.

There are active self-help groups for parents who provide information and practical help. In the US there is Wide Smiles; in the UK it is CLAPA, the Cleft Lip and Palate Association.

Questions

Can babies with a cleft lip and palate breast-feed?

Yes, it is often possible, with expert assistance and encouragement.

What help with feeding can be provided for parents if their infant has a cleft lip and palate?

Special nipples (teats) are available and a dental plate may need to be made to occlude the cleft palate.

Choanal atresia

The condition

A rare bony obstruction between the nasal cavity and the nasopharynx (Fig. 39.3).

Main problem

Bilateral lesions cause respiratory distress and cyanosis immediately after birth due to airways obstruction as newborn infants are

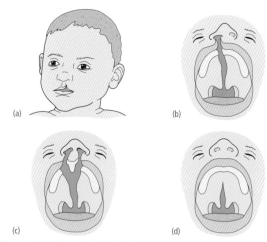

Fig. 39.1 Types of cleft lip and palate. (a) Unilateral cleft lip. (b) Unilateral cleft lip and palate. (c) Bilateral cleft lip and palate. (d) Cleft palate.

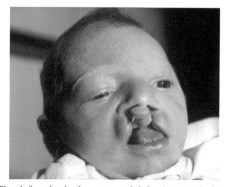

Fig. 39.2 The deformity looks very unsightly. Antenatal ultrasound diagnosis allows preparation before birth. Showing parents photographs before and after surgery is reassuring.

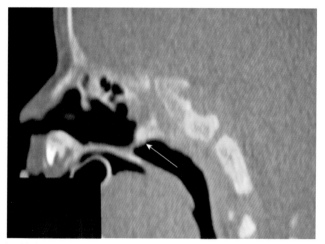

Fig. 39.3 Choanal atresia on MRI scan. There is a bony bar across the posterior nasal space (arrow).

Neonatology at a Glance, 2nd edition. Edited by Tom Lissauer & Avroy A. Fanaroff. © 2011 Blackwell Publishing Ltd.

obligatory nose breathers. The airway obstruction is relieved on crying or opening the mouth.

Treatment

- Initial – insert oral airway or tracheal tube.
- Definitive – surgical correction.

Pierre Robin sequence

This comprises (Fig. 39.4):
- micrognathia (small jaw)
- posteriorly displaced tongue
- posterior palatal defect
- increased incidence of other anomalies, especially of the heart.
  Most serious complication is respiratory obstruction; may lead to hypoxia and cor pulmonale (pulmonary hypertension).

Management

- Avoid obstruction by the tongue:
  – nurse prone
  – may need CPAP (continuous positive airway pressure) via nasopharyngeal tube.

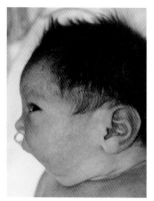

Fig. 39.4 Pierre Robin sequence. (Courtesy of Dr David Clark.)

- Micrognathia and airway obstruction improve over the first 2 years.
- Surgery to the posterior palate is usually performed at about 1 year.
- Feeding can be problematic and initially nasogastric feeding may be required.

40 Jaundice

Visible jaundice occurs in about 75% of term infants and 80% of preterm infants during the first week of life. It is caused by a raised level of bilirubin, a breakdown product of red blood cells. Reasons for elevated bilirubin in newborns are (Fig. 40.1):
• the hemoglobin concentration is high at birth so there is considerable heme degradation
• lifespan of newborn red blood cells is shorter than that of adult red blood cells
• immaturity of liver enzymes impairs bilirubin conjugation and excretion
• absorption of unconjugated bilirubin by intestines (enterohepatic circulation).

Physiologic jaundice peaks at 2–5 days of life and then declines.

Question

What are possible effects of severe hyperbilirubinemia?

Kernicterus describes acute or chronic bilirubin encephalopathy. In acute bilirubin encephalopathy there may be hyptonia, lethargy, poor feeding, irritability, high-pitched cry, fever, apnea, hypertonia with arching of the neck and trunk (opisthotonus, Fig. 40.2), seizures, coma, and death. In chronic bilirubin encephalopathy there is permanent neurologic injury resulting from the deposition of unconjugated bilirubin in the basal ganglia and brainstem nuclei (Fig. 40.3). Long-term consequences include dental dysplasia with yellow staining of the teeth, high-frequency sensorineural hearing loss, paralysis of upward gaze of the eyes, choreoathetoid cerebral palsy, and learning difficulties. Kernicterus is rare in developed countries.

Question

What level of bilirubin is safe?

There is no level of bilirubin that causes kernicterus, but in term infants it is extremely uncommon with bilirubin levels below 26 mg/dL (450 micromol/L). It may occur at lower levels if infants are preterm, or sepsis, hypoxia, seizures, acidosis or hypoalbuminemia are present.

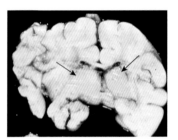

Fig. 40.2 Cross-section of the brain at autopsy showing yellow staining, predominantly in basal ganglia from deposition of unconjugated bilirubin.

Fig. 40.3 Opisthotonus from kernicterus. This is now rarely seen in developed countries.

Causes

Cause is often categorized according to age of onset (Table 40.1).

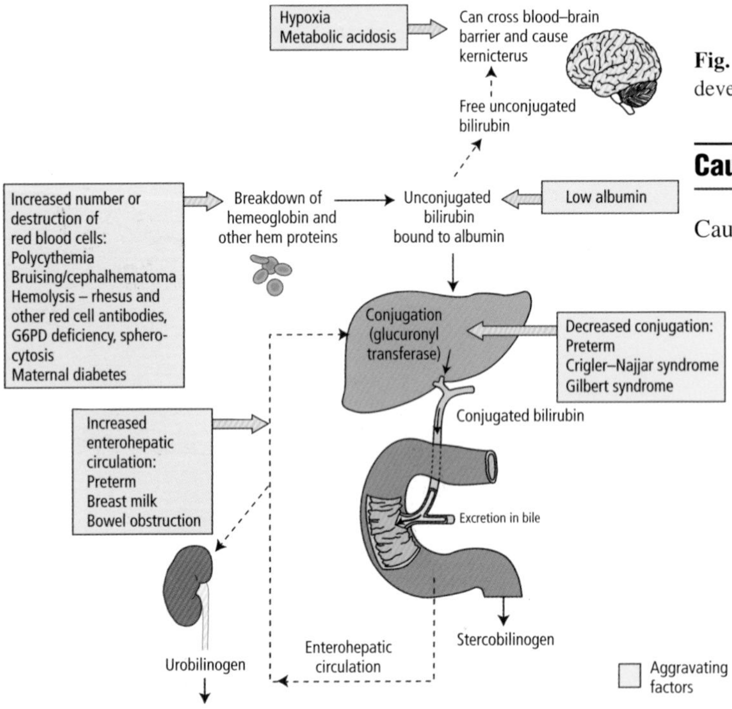

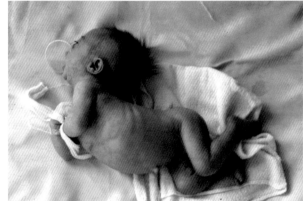

Fig. 40.1 Metabolism of bilirubin. Bilirubin is the product of the metabolism of hemoglobin and other heme proteins. The initial breakdown product is unconjugated bilirubin (indirect bilirubin), which is carried in the blood bound to albumin. When the albumin binding is saturated, free unconjugated bilirubin can cross the blood–brain barrier as it is lipid soluble. Unconjugated bilirubin bound to albumin is conjugated in the liver (direct bilirubin), which is excreted via the biliary tract into the gut. Some bilirubin is reabsorbed from the gut (enterohepatic circulation). Risk factors for jaundice are shown in green.

Neonatology at a Glance, 2nd edition. Edited by Tom Lissauer & Avroy A. Fanaroff. © 2011 Blackwell Publishing Ltd.

<24 hours old

Hemolytic

Jaundice within 24 hours of birth is most likely to be hemolytic. Total bilirubin levels may rise rapidly to very high levels.

RHESUS DISEASE

This is the most severe form of hemolytic disease. Onset *in utero*. At birth, infants may have anemia, hydrops (edema), jaundice and hepatosplenomegaly. Usually identified on antenatal screening tests. Now uncommon because of prophylaxis (see Chapter 5).

ABO INCOMPATIBILITY

- Mother's blood type O.
- Infant's blood type A or B. Maternal anti-A or anti-B IgG crosses the placenta and causes hemolysis in the infant.
- Infant's direct antibody test (DAT or Coombs test) is positive, but positive test is poor predictor that the infant will become significantly jaundiced.
- Generally less severe than rhesus disease, but can still cause significant hemolysis and hyperbilirubinemia. Onset is after birth.
- Hemolysis with anemia may progress during the first few weeks of life, and requires monitoring for anemia.
- Previous sibling may have been affected.

MINOR ANTIGEN INCOMPATIBILITY (KELL, DUFFY, KIDD, ETC.)

- Mother's indirect antibody test is positive.
- Infant's direct antibody test (DAT or Coombs test) is positive.
- Usually moderately severe hemolysis and hyperbilirubinemia.

G6PD (GLUCOSE-6-PHOSPHATE DEHYDROGENASE) DEFICIENCY

- Most common enzyme defect in the world, affecting 200–400 million people.
- Can cause severe hyperbilirubinemia and kernicterus in people originating from central Africa, the Mediterranean or Middle or Far East.
- X-linked disorder, so mostly affects males; can affect females but usually less severe.
- Is accentuated both in males and females who also have Gilbert syndrome (a liver enzyme defect present in about 5% of the population in the US).

- Diagnosed by measuring G6PD activity in red blood cells. However, during hemolytic crises this may be misleadingly elevated due to the increased number of reticulocytes, which have a higher enzyme concentration. A repeat assay in the steady state is required to avoid missing the diagnosis.
- Affected infants should avoid certain medications, i.e. some antimalarials and antibiotics (nalidixic acid, nitrofurantoin and sulfonamides), contact with moth balls (naphthalene) and eating fava beans when older.

HEREDITARY SPHEROCYTOSIS

Uncommon. Red blood cells are spherical with limited deformability causing splenic sequestration and hemolysis.

Autosomal dominant inheritance – family history positive in 75%.

Congenital Infection

Increases hemolysis and may impair conjugation, causing elevated conjugated bilirubin. Other stigmata of congenital infection will be present.

24 hours to 2 weeks

Breast-feeding jaundice

Common. Exacerbated if there is difficulty in establishing breast-feeding. Cause uncertain; may be related to low volume of breast milk, and increased enterohepatic circulation of bilirubin. Breast-feeding should be continued but support with breast-feeding may be needed. Continues beyond 2 weeks of age in 15%.

Infection

Always consider infection, including urinary tract infection. Jaundice occurs because of hemolysis, impaired conjugation, reduced fluid intake and increased enterohepatic circulation.

Other causes

These include:

- hemolysis – may develop after first 24 hours of life
- bruising, cephalhematoma
- polycythemia
- liver enzyme defects, e.g. Crigler–Najjar syndrome; rare but cause severe and protracted hyperbilirubinemia, Gilbert syndrome
- gastrointestinal obstruction, e.g. pyloric stenosis
- metabolic disorders, e.g. galactosemia.

Table 40.1 Causes of jaundice by age of onset.

<24 hours old	24 hours to 2 weeks old	Prolonged jaundice
Hemolytic	Breast-feeding jaundice	Unconjugated:
Rhesus disease	Hemolytic	Breast milk jaundice
ABO incompatibility	Infection	Hypothyroidism
Minor antigen incompatibility	Bruising/cephalhematoma	Gastrointestinal obstruction
G6PD deficiency	Gastrointestinal obstruction	Infection
Hereditary spherocytosis	Polycythemia	Liver enzyme defects
Congenital infection	Metabolic disorders	Conjugated:
	Liver enzyme defects	Neonatal hepatitis syndrome
		Biliary atresia

Clinical examination and assessment

Jaundice is clinically detectable from skin color on blanching the skin with digital pressure or yellow color of the sclerae when bilirubin exceeds 5 mg/dL (85 micromol/L).

It starts on the head, spreads to the abdomen and then to the limbs. It is harder to detect in preterm and dark-skinned infants. The severity of jaundice cannot be reliably assessed by clinical examination. However, an infant who is not jaundiced clinically will not have significant hyperbilirubinemia.

If jaundiced, also check for:
- pallor
- evidence of infection
- bruising, cephalhematoma
- hepatosplenomegaly (hemolysis)
- weight loss, dehydration
- family history of neonatal jaundice.

Investigations

Term infants who become jaundiced should have a transcutaneous bilirubin (TcB) measured.

However, a serum measurement should be obtained if:
- The infant is <24 hours old
- transcutaneous bilirubinometer measurement >14.5 mg/dL (250 micromol/L)
- transcutaneous bilirubinometer (TcB) not available
- infant <34 weeks' gestational age.
- on treatment with phototherapy.

Further tests, other than total bilirubin, that may be required

- Direct bilirubin.
- Complete blood count, reticulocyte count, and smear for red cell morphology.
- Blood packed cell volume or hematocrit.
- Blood group (mother and baby).
- Direct antibody test (DAT or Coombs test).
  Consider:
- G6PD testing
- microbiological cultures of blood, urine and/or cerebrospinal fluid for infection
  However, in most infants no cause is identified.

Management

The need for treatment is ascertained by plotting the total bilirubin level on a graph of bilirubin against age in hours. This will determine if:
- no treatment is needed
- repeat bilirubin is required in 6–12 hours
- phototherapy or exchange transfusion is indicated.

Treatment will change according to the absolute level of bilirubin reached and the rate of rise on serial measurements (if bilirubin

rising > 0.5 mg/dL/hour, 8.5 micromol/L/hour). The evidence on which to base treatment thresholds is very limited; national guidelines have been published to assist uniformity of practice (American Academy of Pediatrics – Table 40.2, NICE guidelines in UK) Different cut-off criteria are used for preterm infants, for whom the treatment threshold is lower (NICE guidelines include graphs for different gestational ages).

If an exchange transfusion is being considered, a low serum albumin may be an additional risk factor for kernicterus.

Other treatment to be considered:
- Dehydration – associated with failure to establish breast-feeding or inadequate supply of breast milk; support for the mother to establish breast-feeding may be required.
- Sepsis – requires investigation and treatment.

Phototherapy

Blue-green light (wavelength 425–475 nm) converts unconjugated bilirubin to harmless isomers. The light is filtered to remove ultraviolet light.

Conventional phototherapy is with a phototherapy light source above the baby.

Continuous multiple phototherapy is used if the serum bilirubin is rising rapidly or is at a high level or does not fall within 6 hours of starting conventional phototherapy.

Phototherapy requires:
- effective light source
- high irradiance (usually $\geq 30\,\mu W/cm^2$ per nm)
- light as close to the infant as possible (if fluorescent tubes used, can be as close to about 10 cm from infant)
- widespread skin exposure.

Disadvantages of phototherapy
- Separates baby and parents.
- Eye coverage necessary, which may be disturbing to parents.
- Bronze-baby syndrome if phototherapy given with elevated conjugated bilirubin.
- Unstable body temperature possible while in open bassinet (cot) with majority of skin exposed.
- Increased insensible water loss, but less with use of LED light sources.
- Slightly loose, more frequent stools which may contribute to water loss.

Exchange transfusion

Baby's blood is removed in aliquots (usually twice blood volume, 'double volume exchange' = 2 × 80/kg) and replaced with transfused blood (see Chapter 77). Removes bilirubin and antibodies, and corrects anemia. Complications include thrombosis, embolus, volume overload or depletion, metabolic abnormalities, infection, coagulation abnormalities. Mortality is probably 0.1–.5% and procedure is time-consuming.

Intravenous immunoglobulin (IVIG)
Can be used in rhesus disease or ABO incompatibility when total bilirubin levels are rising despite continuous multiple phototherapy or level is near exchange transfusion level.

Table 40.2 Indications for phototherapy and exchange transfusion in infants ≥35 weeks' gestation (adapted from Management of hyperbilirubinemia in the newborn infant 35 or more weeks of gestation. *Pediatrics* 2004; **114**: 297–316).

Age	Phototherapy			Exchange transfusion		
	Higher risk	Medium risk	Lower risk	Higher risk	Medium risk	Lower risk
24 hours	>8 mg/dL (137 micromol/L)	>10 mg/dL (171 micromol/L)	>12 mg/dL (205 micromol/L)	>15 mg/dL (257 micromol/L)	>17 mg/dL (291 micromol/L)	>19 mg/dL (325 micromol/L)
48 hours	>11 mg/dL (188 micromol/L)	>13 mg/dL (222 micromol/L)	>15 mg/dL (257 micromol/L)	>17 mg/dL (291 micromol/L)	>19 mg/dL (325 micromol/L)	>22 mg/dL (376 micromol/L)
72 hours	>13 mg/dL (222 micromol/L)	>15 mg/dL (257 micromol/L)	>18 mg/dL (308 micromol/L)	>18 mg/dL (308 micromol/L)	>21 mg/dL (359 micromol/L)	>24 mg/dL (410 micromol/L)
96 hours	>14 mg/dL (239 micromol/L)	>17 mg/dL (291 micromol/L)	>20 mg/dL (342 micromol/L)	>19 mg/dL (325 micromol/L)	>22 mg/dL (376 micromol/L)	>25 mg/dL (428 micromol/L)

Lower risk –≥38 weeks and well. Medium risk –≥38 weeks and risk factors or 35–37 weeks and well. Higher risk – 35–37 weeks and risk factors. Risk factors – isoimmune hemolytic disease, G6PD deficiency, asphyxia, significant lethargy, temperature instability, sepsis, acidosis or albumin <3.0 g/dL (30 g/L) if measured.

Discharge and follow-up

In view of the re-emergence of kernicterus in otherwise healthy infants, particularly at 35–37 weeks' gestation, the American Academy of Pediatrics (2004) recommends predischarge measurement of bilirubin and/or assessment of clinical risk factors for the development of jaundice for all infants. The risk of developing significant hyperbilirubinemia in healthy term and near term newborns can be determined by plotting the bilirubin level on an hour-specific chart (Fig. 40.4). It also recommends a follow-up assessment for jaundice depending on their length of stay in the nursery:

- discharge at <24 hours, follow-up by 72 hours of life
- discharge at 24–48 hours, follow-up by 96 hours of life
- discharge at 48–72 hours, follow-up by 120 hours of life.

Earlier assessment may be needed if risk factors are present. Parents should also be given written and verbal information about jaundice.

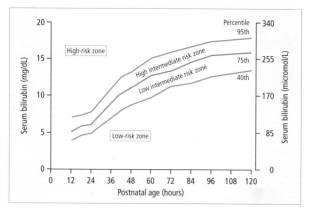

Fig. 40.4 Nomogram for determination of risk of development of severe hyperbilirubinemia for infants ≥35 weeks' gestation and ≥2.5 kg birthweight. (From Bhutani *et al.* Predictive ability of a predischarge hour-specific serum bilirubin for subsequent significant bilirubinemia in healthy term and near term newborns. *Pediatrics* 1999; **103**: 6–14.)

Question

What is the discharge follow-up policy in the UK?

Further assessment by 48 hours of age if risk factors present (gestational age <38 weeks, a previous sibling had neonatal jaundice requiring phototherapy, breastfed, visible jaundice in the first 24 hours of life), otherwise by 72 hours of age.

Key point

If the transcutaneous bilirubin (TcB) measurement is high (>14.5 mg/dL, 250 micromol/L), check with a total serum bilirubin (TSB) level.

Prolonged jaundice

Jaundice present at more than 2 weeks of age for term, 3 weeks for preterm infants can be considered as prolonged jaundice. It requires further assessment. First, it needs to be determined if the jaundice is unconjugated or conjugated.

Unconjugated jaundice causes are:
- breast milk jaundice – 15% of all breast-fed infants are still jaundiced at 2 weeks, gradually decreasing over several weeks
- hypothyroidism – should have been identified on routine biochemical screening on blood spots
- gastrointestinal obstruction, e.g. pyloric stenosis
- infection
- liver enzyme disorders.

Conjugated jaundice (>1.5 mg/dL, 25 micrograms/L) may be caused by:
- biliary atresia – uncommon, but important to identify as delay in surgery adversely affects outcome
- neonatal hepatitis syndrome.

The infant will pass pale stools (no stercobilinogen) and dark urine (from bilirubin).

Detailed investigation of infants with conjugated jaundice is required.

This is a common and serious problem in the neonatal period, affecting 1–5/1000 live births (Fig. 41.1). The highest incidence is in very low birthweight (VLBW) infants (see Chapter 33). Congenital infections are considered in Chapter 10.

Key point

Infection needs to be considered in all sick newborn infants. If suspected, a blood culture and other investigations should be performed and antibiotics and supportive therapy started immediately as it may progress and disseminate very rapidly.

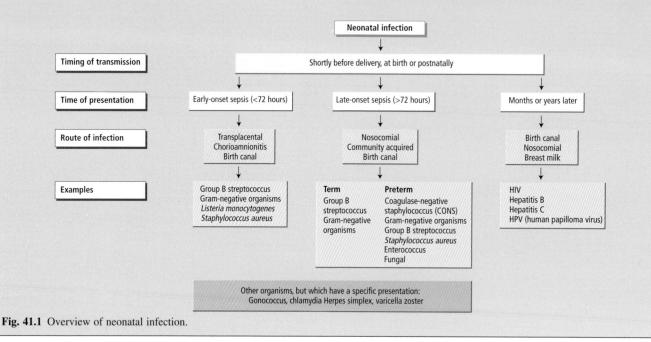

Fig. 41.1 Overview of neonatal infection.

Bacterial sepsis

Newborn infants are particularly susceptible to bacterial sepsis (systemic infection with positive blood or other central culture).

Early-onset sepsis (EOS): <72 hours of birth

Definitions range from 24 hours to 6 days, but most present within 72 hours of birth.

Results from vertical exposure to high bacterial load during birth and few protective antibodies.

Late-onset sepsis: >72 hours after birth

Within the hospital, mostly from organisms acquired by nosocomial transmission from person to person. May also be caused by community-acquired organisms.

Risk factors

Early-onset infection
• Preterm.
• Prolonged rupture of membranes (>18 hours).
• Maternal fever in labor (>38°C).

• Chorioamnionitis.
• Previous infected infant.

Late-onset nosocomial infection
• Preterm.
• Indwelling venous or arterial catheters or tracheal tube.
• Prolonged antibiotics.
• Damage to skin from tape, skin probes, etc.

Clinical presentation

• Usually non-specific deterioration.
• Apnea and bradycardia.
• Respiratory distress/increased ventilatory requirements.
• Slow feeding/vomiting/abdominal distension.
• Fever/hypothermia/temperature instability.
• Tachycardia/collapse/shock/purpura or bruising from disseminated intravascular coagulation (DIC).
• Irritability/lethargy/seizures.
• Jaundice.
• Rash.
• Reduced limb movement in bone or joint.

Neonatology at a Glance, 2nd edition. Edited by Tom Lissauer & Avroy A. Fanaroff. © 2011 Blackwell Publishing Ltd.

- In meningitis (late signs):
  - tense or bulging fontanelle
  - head retraction (opisthotonus).
- On monitoring:
  - hypo/hyperglycemia
  - neutropenia, neutrophilia, thrombocytopenia
  - acute phase reactants - raised C-reactive protein (CRP) or procalcitonin.

Investigations

Sepsis work-up:
- complete blood count (CBC), differential, platelets
- C-reactive protein/procalcitonin
- blood culture
- urine – microscopy and culture
- cerebrospinal fluid (CSF), if indicated
- chest X-ray, if indicated
- sites of infection – consider needle aspirate or biopsy for gram stain and direct microscopy
- tracheal aspirate if ventilated.
  Consider:
- maternal vaginal culture
- placental tissue culture and histopathology
- rapid antigen screen
- blood gases
- coagulation screen.

Question

When should a lumbar puncture (LP) be performed?
If blood culture is positive.
If there are clinical features of meningitis.
Consider whenever performing sepsis work-up, but delay if infant clinically unstable.
Skin over LP site needs to be sterile – otherwise may introduce infection.

Interpretation of laboratory investigations

Blood cultures:
- Gold standard but may be negative if insufficient volume of blood.
- If central line sepsis suspected, also take blood sample from it.

Blood count – infection is suggested by:
- neutropenia or neutrophilia
- increased ratio of immature (bands) : total neutrophils
- thrombocytopenia.

C-reactive protein/procalcitonin
- Raised in infection; also following meconium aspiration, asphyxia, post-surgery.
- Takes time to rise – may be normal initially.

CSF – in meningitis:
- More than 30 white blood cells (30×10^9/L); if more than 20/mm^3 white blood cells (20×10^9/L) and more than 5/mm^3 (5×10^9/L) neutrophils suspicious.
- Protein – term infants >200 mg/dL (>2 g/L).
- Glucose – less than 30% of blood glucose.
- May be able to observe group B streptococci on gram stain without any white cells present.

Treatment

- Supportive care – **A**irway, **B**reathing, **C**irculation. Check blood glucose.
- Treat with antibiotics immediately on suspicion of sepsis, immediately after taking cultures but whilst awaiting results.
- Antibiotic choice depends on local incidence and practice.

Early-onset sepsis
Cover gram-positive and gram-negative organisms.
For example:
- penicillin/amoxicillin + aminoglycoside (e.g. gentamicin/tobramycin).

Late-onset sepsis
Need to also cover coagulase-negative staphylococcus and enterococcus.
For example:
- methicillin/flucloxacillin + gentamicin or cephalosporin/gentamicin + vancomycin.

If central venous catheter in place, remove if unresponsive to antibiotics, persistent positive culture, gram-negative organisms or seriously ill.

Questions

How long should antibiotics be continued?
If blood cultures are negative and CRP/procalcitonin remains normal and clinical signs of sepsis have resolved – stop antibiotics at 48 hours.
If blood cultures negative but CRP/procalcitonin raised – treat as infected.
If blood cultures are positive – treat until clinical improvement and CRP has returned to normal (7–10 days, longer if gram-negative infection).
Meningitis – 14–21 days.
Septic arthritis/osteomyelitis – 3–6 weeks.

What supportive strategies are being evaluated?
Giving intravenous immunoglobulin if infected (giving it routinely as prophylaxis in VLBW infants – found to be ineffective). Targeted immunoglobulins are under development.
Giving granulocyte colony stimulating factor (GCSF) – raises white blood count, but efficacy unproven.
Exchange transfusion or extracorporeal membrane oxygenation (ECMO) – anecdotal evidence of benefit.

Group B streptococcal (GBS) infection

This is the leading cause of bacterial sepsis in term infants.
• Early-onset infection usually presents with respiratory distress and septicemia; more than 90% present in first 24 hours.
• Late-onset infection – higher proportion with meningitis; also causes focal infection in bones or joints.

It is a serious infection, with 4% mortality. Before active prevention, the incidence in the US of early-onset disease was approximately 1.5/1000 live births, late-onset disease 0.35/1000, causing 7600 cases of invasive disease per year, with 300 deaths. By 1999, the infection rate had declined to 0.3–0.6/1000 live births.

Up to 30% of pregnant women have rectal or vaginal carriage of group B streptococcus.

The 2002 CDC (Centers for Disease Control and Prevention) guideline recommends active prevention by culturing all mothers at 35–37 weeks and offering intrapartum prophylactic antibiotics to those who are positive for group B streptococcus (Fig. 42.1). However, the efficacy of this practice has not been demonstrated in a systematic review of well-designed clinical trials. Most infected infants are now preterm or have not been screened.

Listeria monocytogenes

• Rare. From maternal ingestion of unpasteurized milk, soft cheeses and undercooked poultry.

Question

What is the policy in the UK?

In the UK the incidence of early-onset GBS is about 0.5/1000 live births and routine culturing of mothers is not recommended (Royal College of Obstetricians and Gynaecologists, 2003). Their recommendation is that intrapartum antibiotics:
• should be offered – if previous baby with GBS infection
• should be considered – if preterm labor, prolonged rupture of membranes (PROM) >18 hours, or fever in labor >38°C.

• Mother develops flu-like symptoms. Fetal infection acquired transplacentally or from birth canal.
• Causes abortion, preterm delivery. Green staining of liquor even though preterm has been claimed to be characteristic.
• Early-onset infection – usually with pneumonia, septicemia and widespread rash. Mortality 30%.
• Late-onset infection – mostly with meningitis.

Gram-negative infection

• Less common than group B streptococcal infection.
• Presents as early- or late-onset infection.
• Significant morbidity and mortality.

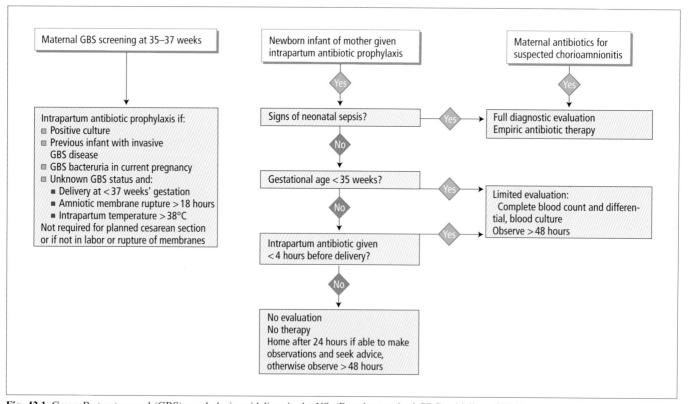

Fig. 42.1 Group B streptococcal (GBS) prophylaxis guidelines in the US. (Based on revised CDC guidelines, 2002.)

Neonatology at a Glance, 2nd edition. Edited by Tom Lissauer & Avroy A. Fanaroff. © 2011 Blackwell Publishing Ltd.

Some specific sites of bacterial infection (Fig. 42.2)

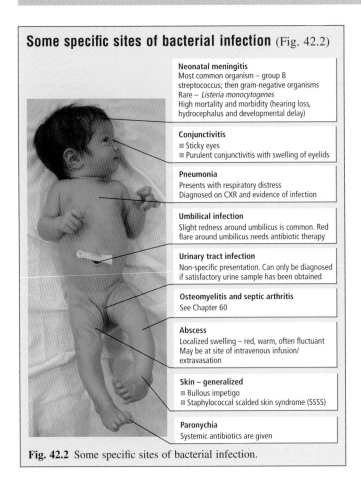

Neonatal meningitis
Most common organism – group B streptococcus; then gram-negative organisms
Rare – *Listeria monocytogenes*
High mortality and morbidity (hearing loss, hydrocephalus and developmental delay)

Conjunctivitis
▪ Sticky eyes
▪ Purulent conjunctivitis with swelling of eyelids

Pneumonia
Presents with respiratory distress
Diagnosed on CXR and evidence of infection

Umbilical infection
Slight redness around umbilicus is common. Red flare around umbilicus needs antibiotic therapy

Urinary tract infection
Non-specific presentation. Can only be diagnosed if satisfactory urine sample has been obtained

Osteomyelitis and septic arthritis
See Chapter 60

Abscess
Localized swelling – red, warm, often fluctuant
May be at site of intravenous infusion/extravasation

Skin – generalized
▪ Bullous impetigo
▪ Staphylococcal scalded skin syndrome (SSSS)

Paronychia
Systemic antibiotics are given

Fig. 42.2 Some specific sites of bacterial infection.

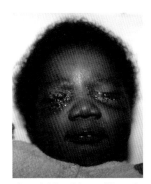

Fig. 42.3 Purulent conjunctivitis with swelling of eyelids at 6 days from *Chlamydia trachomatis*.

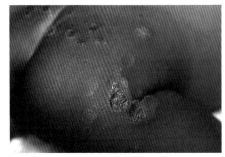

Fig. 42.4 Bullous impetigo. There are superficial blisters; some have been denuded.

Conjunctivitis

Sticky but white eyes

Common, 3rd–5th day of life. Clean with sterile water. If eye becomes red, may be staphylococcal or streptococcal and treat with a topical antibiotic ointment, e.g. neomycin. If persistent, usually due to failure of nasolacrimal duct to open, when the eye is sticky but conjunctiva is white and uninflamed.

Purulent conjunctivitis with swelling of eyelids (Fig. 42.3)

If onset within 48 hours of birth, likely to be gonococcal (ophthalmia neonatorum). The discharge should be gram-stained and cultured, and systemic treatment started immediately. Where penicillin resistance is troublesome, as in the US and UK, a third-generation cephalosporin is given. The eye is cleaned frequently.

In the US all infants are given eye prophylaxis with erythromycin or tetracycline eye ointment or silver nitrate eye drops. In the UK no prophylaxis is given, but the condition is rare.

Chlamydia trachomatis can cause a similar condition, usually at the end of the first week; may coexist with gonococcal infection. The diagnosis is made with a monoclonal antibody test or culture of the discharge. Treatment is with oral erythromycin. No topical treatment required. These conditions must be treated promptly to avoid damage to the eye. The mother and her partner also need treatment.

Herpes simplex must also be considered with this presentation.

Skin

Bullous impetigo

Superficial blisters, readily burst, to leave denuded skin (Fig. 42.4) with crust formation.

Staphylococcus aureus or streptococcal. Give systemic antibiotics to prevent spread. Remove crusts with warm water. Identify and treat source. Usually from nasal colonization.

Staphylococcal scalded skin syndrome (SSSS)

* Rare but serious infection. Toxin mediated.
* Fever.
* Bullae with shedding of skin leaving raw areas.
* Requires systemic antibiotics.
* Congenital candida may resemble SSSS.

43 Viral infections

Herpes simplex virus (HSV)

Infection in the newborn is rare; the incidence in the US is only 20–50/100000 live births; in the UK it is 2/100000 live births. Most (85%) are HSV type II in US, but in UK a higher proportion are HSV type I, associated with increased genital HSV type I infection.

Seroconversion rate in pregnancy is 4%.

At any time in pregnancy, 1% of HSV-2 seropositive women are excreting virus in genital tract.

Most infections (85%) are acquired by passage through infected birth canal, 10% are acquired postnatally from infected caregiver, and 5% are true intrauterine infections.

Risk of vertical transmission

- High (50%) with primary maternal infection, which may be symptomatic, with fever, systemic illness and painful genital lesions, though this is uncommon; usually asymptomatic. Risk of transmission is increased if membranes have ruptured for more than 6 hours or following birth canal interventions, e.g. scalp electrode. However, in 70% of infected neonates maternal infection is undiagnosed.
- Low (<4%) with recurrent maternal infection, which is often asymptomatic or genital lesions are localized.

Potential interventions to reduce transmission of symptomatic primary infection are:
- delivery by Cesarean section
- maternal aciclovir (acyclovir) therapy for primary infection.
- Reduced use of invasive obstetric procedures during delivery (mechanically assisted deliveries, fetal scalp electrodes).

Neonatal infection

There are three modes of presentation:
- **Disseminated infection** – presents in first week with pneumonia, hepatic failure, DIC (disseminated intravascular coagulation).
- **Encephalitis** – presents in second week. Lethargy is a prominent clinical feature, as well as seizures, lethargy and coma
- **Localized lesions** – skin, eye or mouth – presents with vesicles at 10–11 days. One-third progress to encephalitis.

Rarely there may be congenital infection - presents at birth with triad of eye, skin and neurologic signs.

Diagnosis

Difficult, as cause of maternal infection often undiagnosed and vesicles are present in only 60–80% of disseminated disease or encephalitis.

Rapid diagnosis now with PCR (polymerase chain reaction) of infant's blood, CSF (cerebrospinal fluid), nasaopharyngeal aspirates or local lesions.

Management of infected infant

- Intensive care support if required.
- High-dose aciclovir (acyclovir) therapy. Suppressive oral treatment is sometimes given during the first year of life to prevent CNS relapse, but evidence to support this is lacking.
- In spite of treatment, morbidity, mortality and risk of relapse remain high.

Hepatitis B (HBV)

- Highest incidence in the Far East and sub-Saharan Africa (Fig. 43.1). Increased risk with intravenous drug use.
- Screening of all mothers for HBsAg (hepatitis B surface antigen) is universal in the US and UK.
- HBV is transmitted from mother to infant during labor or at birth from ingestion of maternal blood and from breast milk. Also horizontal spread within families during childhood can occur.
- Infants are at high risk if their mother is hepatitis B e-antigen positive (HBeAg positive); the risk is markedly reduced if e-antibodies are present.
- Infants who become carriers are usually asymptomatic during childhood, but 30–50% develop chronic HBV liver disease, which in 10% progresses to cirrhosis. There is also a long-term risk of hepatocellular carcinoma.

Prevention

All infants born to HBsAg-positive mothers should be given HBV vaccination as soon as possible after birth with boosters during infancy. In the US this is part of the standard immunization program; in the UK it is restricted to these high-risk infants.

In the US, HBIG (hepatitis B immunoglobulin) for short-term protection from passive antibody is given within 12 hours of birth

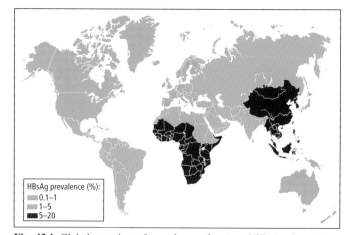

Fig. 43.1 Global overview of prevalence of maternal HbsAg (hepatitis B surface antigen).

Neonatology at a Glance, 2nd edition. Edited by Tom Lissauer & Avroy A. Fanaroff. © 2011 Blackwell Publishing Ltd.

to infants of HBsAg-positive mothers; in the UK it is confined to infants of mothers who are HBeAg-positive.

Immunization protects more than 90% of infants.

Hepatitis C

Vertical transmission is uncommon and almost exclusively in women with high Hep C viral load in late pregnancy (<5%) unless there is co-infection with HIV (when it is 10–20%). Although viral DNA is present in breast milk, transmission via breast milk has not been proven, so breast-feeding is not contraindicated. Carriers are at risk of chronic liver disease and hepatocellular carcinoma in later life.

HIV infection

The global scale of HIV infection is shown in Fig. 43.2 and how it is affecting children is shown in Fig. 43.3.

Main route of vertical transmission is at birth, but also transplacental and via breast-feeding.

Vertical transmission rate where mothers breast-feed and without any intervention is 25–40%.

Factors which increase transmission

- Advanced maternal disease.
- High plasma viral load.
- Primary infection during pregnancy or breast-feeding.
- Concomitant sexually transmitted infections.
- Rupture of the membranes longer than 4 hours.
- Chorioamnionitis.

- Vaginal delivery.
- Blood exposure/instrumental delivery.

Interventions that reduce transmission

- Antiretroviral therapy to mother antenatally and intrapartum and postnatally to the infant. For infants born to mothers with fully suppressed viral load at delivery post exposure prophylaxis with one drug (usually zidovudine), for 4 weeks is sufficient. For infants born to mothers with detectable viral load at delivery, triple therapy should be given (zidovudine for 4 weeks, lamivudine for 4 weeks and nevirapine for 2 weeks), or other antiretroviral therapy if there is a history of drug resistance in the mother.
- Treatment of other maternal sexually transmitted infections.
- Elective cesarean section with avoidance of labor and contact with the birth canal.
- Formula feeding instead of breast-feeding. Feeding strategies in resource-poor settings is described in Chapter 72.

These interventions can reduce transmission rate below 1%.

Diagnosis

Confirmation that the infant is uninfected relies on three negative tests for the viral antigen and/or genome (DNA PCR); antibody tests cannot be used as maternal antibody is detected until 18 months.

Management

Infants should receive cotrimoxazole as prophylaxis against *Pneumocystis carinii* pneumonia (PCP) from 4 weeks of age until negative HIV results are available.

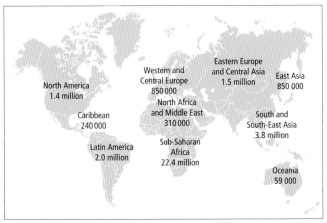

Total: 33.4 million adults and children
Children <15 years–2.1 million

Fig. 43.2 Global overview of number of adults and children with HIV infection. (UNAIDS, WHO, 2009.)

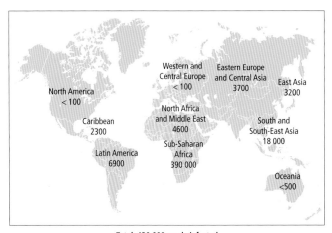

Total: 430 000 newly infected
AIDS Deaths in 2008 – 280 000

Fig. 43.3 Estimated number of newly HIV-infected children <15 years during 2008. Most are in sub-Saharan Africa. (UNAIDS, WHO, 2009.)

Hypoglycemia

Prolonged symptomatic hypoglycemia can cause neurologic damage. However, during the first few days of life, many breast-fed infants have low blood glucose levels but are asymptomatic; they are able to utilize ketones and other energy substrates. Therefore, the definition of hypoglycemia in the neonatal period has been the source of considerable controversy.

A serum glucose level of less than 45 mg/dL (<2.6 mmol/L) during the first days of life is currently accepted as a useful cut-off to establish the diagnosis of hypoglycemia and to initiate active evaluation and treatment. Normal newborn infants require 4–5 mg/kg/minute of glucose in order to maintain glucose homeostasis.

Risk factors

Antenatal

• Maternal diabetes mellitus – insulin-dependent or gestational (Fig. 44.1).
• Maternal obesity.
• Large or rapid infusions of glucose immediately before delivery.
• Maternal β-adrenergic agonist or antagonist therapy.

Neonatal

• IUGR (intrauterine growth restriction) (Fig. 44.2).
• Large for gestational age.
• Preterm.
• Ill infant – sepsis, etc.
• Iatrogenic – reduced feeds with inadequate intravenous glucose.
• Polycythemia.
• Hypoxic–ischemic encephalopathy (HIE).
• Hypothermia.
• Rhesus disease.

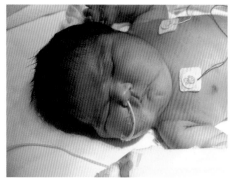

Fig. 44.1 Macrosomic infant of mother with diabetes mellitus. Maternal hyperglycemia causes β-cell hyperplasia of pancreas and hyperinsulinism in the fetus that lasts for up to 48 hours after birth.

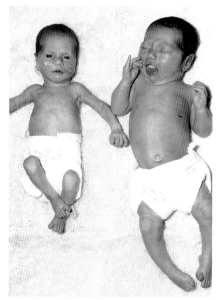

Fig. 44.2 Term twins, the one on the left with IUGR (intrauterine growth restriction). IUGR newborn infants are prone to hypoglycemia.

Causes

Risk factors for transient hypoglycemia are listed above. Persistent hypoglycemia is uncommon; its causes are shown in Fig. 44.3.

Clinical features

Most are asymptomatic. Clinical features include:
• jitteriness/irritability/high-pitched cry
• depressed consciousness/lethargy/hypotonia
• apnea
• seizures.

Some abnormal physical signs may assist in identifying the cause (Table 44.1).

Monitoring

Infants with risk factors are monitored before feeds until the blood glucose is above 45 mg/dL (>2.6 mmol/L) on two occasions. It is not necessary to monitor blood glucose levels in appropriately grown term infants establishing breast-feeding. All infants requiring intensive care should have their blood glucose monitored regularly.

Blood glucose determination should be performed at the bedside with a glucometer, which requires only a single drop of blood. If hypoglycemia is suspected, a laboratory sample must be checked as bedside monitors are not designed to measure low glucose levels accurately.

Neonatology at a Glance, 2nd edition. Edited by Tom Lissauer & Avroy A. Fanaroff. © 2011 Blackwell Publishing Ltd.

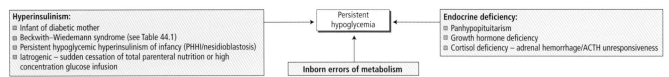

Fig. 44.3 Causes of persistent hypoglycemia.

Table 44.1 Clinical features associated with specific causes of hypoglycemia.

Clinical feature	Cause
Transient hypoglycemia	
Abnormal growth	Intrauterine growth restriction
	Macrosomia/large for gestational age
Plethora	Polycythemia
Persistent hypoglycemia	
Hepatomegaly with or without splenomegaly	Glycogen storage disease, infection
Hepatomegaly, large tongue, omphalocele, horizontal ear lobe crease	Beckwith–Wiedemann syndrome
Micropenis, hypoplastic optic disk	Panhypopituitarism
	Need to rule out midline brain defects, e.g. septo-optic dysplasia
Lethargy, coma, vomiting, unusual body odor	Hyperammonemia, lactic acidosis, urea cycle disorders or other inborn error of metabolism

Investigation

These are performed for persistent or symptomatic hypoglycemia.

Blood tests
- Plasma glucose concentration – true (laboratory) measurements must be taken.
- Serum insulin concentration.

If no features of hyperinsulinism (e.g. excessive glucose requirements to prevent hypoglycaemia), check:
- pituitary hormones
- for inborn error of metabolism (see Chapter 45)
- acylcarnitine (see Chapter 45).

Other investigations that may be indicated
- Ultrasound of brain and/or MRI – for structural anomaly.
- Ultrasound adrenals – for adrenal hemorrhage.
- Ophthalmologic examination – for septo-optic dysplasia.

Management

Prevention and treatment of hypoglycemia are shown in Fig. 44.4.

Hyperglycemia

No agreed definition, but >125–180 mg/dL (>7–10 mmol/L) on two occasions.

Frequent in extremely low birthweight infants:
- higher than needed rates of IV glucose infusion (>9 mg/kg/min)
- sepsis
- corticosteroid therapy (high doses)
- insufficient insulin secretion – neonatal diabetes
- absence of enteral feedings.

Management – treat cause or insulin therapy (but avoid hypoglycemia).

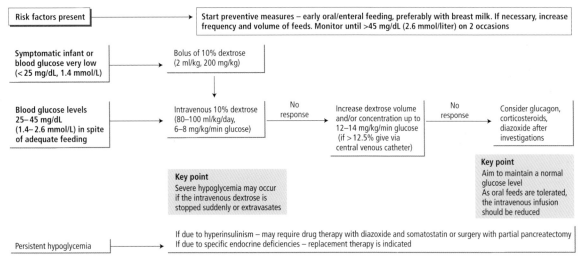

Fig. 44.4 An example of a guideline for the prevention and treatment of hypoglycemia.

45 Inborn errors of metabolism

There are almost a hundred inborn errors of metabolism that may present in the neonatal period (Table 45.1). They are rare (Table 45.2) but failure or delay in diagnosis can result in irreversible brain damage or death. In the US, tandem mass spectrometry on blood screening spots is used extensively to identify a wide range of metabolic disorders; in the UK screening for inborn errors of metabolism is mostly limited to phenylketonuria and medium-chain acyl CoA dehydrogenase deficiency (MCAD).

Age of presentation

As toxic metabolites are removed by the placenta, most cases present after feeding at several days of age, with acute deterioration of a previously well term infant. Occasionally presents as hydrops fetalis, or as sudden death in the first few days of life. Some present beyond the neonatal period.

Table 45.1 Examples of inborn errors of metabolism that may present in the neonatal period.

Amino acid disorders	Urea cycle – ornithine transcarbamylase
	Maple syrup urine disease (MSUD)
Carbohydrate disorders	Galactosemia
	Glycogen storage disease
Organic acidemias	Propionic acidemia (PA)
	Methyl malonic acidemia (MMA)
Fatty acid oxidation defects	LCAD (long-chain acyl CoA dehydrogenase deficiency)
	MCAD (medium-chain acyl CoA dehydrogenase deficiency)
Energy defects	Lactic acidosis (LA)

Table 45.2 Incidence of some inborn errors of metabolism.

Disorder	Frequency
Phenylketonuria	1 in 10 000
Homocystinuria	1 in 50 000
Galactosemia	1 in 100 000
Maple syrup urine disease	1 in 100 000
If screened with tandem mass spectrometry:	
Amino acid disorders	1 in 4800
Fatty acid oxidation defects	1 in 14 000
Organic acid disorders	1 in 20 000

When to suspect an inborn error of metabolism

Clinical features

These include:
- Neurologic:
  - poor feeding, vomiting, apnea, irritability, progressive lethargy, seizures, coma.
  - marked hypotonia.
- Acid–base abnormality:
  - persistent, unexplained metabolic acidosis, lactic acidosis or respiratory alkalosis
  - respiratory distress (from metabolic acidosis).
- Hypoglycemia:
  - severe and persistent.
- Acute liver disease:
  - jaundice (conjugated), hepatosplenomegaly.
- Cardiac disease:
  - heart failure, arrhythmias, cardiomyopathy, cardiac arrest.
- Dysmorphic infant.
- Failure to thrive.
- Abnormal body odor.

Suggestive clues

- Positive family history.
- Parental consanguinity.
- Sibling with unexplained severe illness or neonatal death.
- Maternal fatty liver of pregnancy (in fetal fatty acid oxidation defects).
- Sudden onset of symptoms in previously well term infant.
- Progressive deterioration or death despite supportive treatment.

Differential diagnosis

- Sepsis – ill with non-specific features.
- Congenital heart disease – heart failure.
- CNS catastrophe – seizures, encephalopathy, infection (herpes simplex virus).
- Gastrointestinal obstruction – vomiting.
- Metabolic derangement – non-specific features.
- Hypoxic–ischemic encephalopathy (HIE) – seizures and encephalopathy.

Neonatology at a Glance, 2nd edition. Edited by Tom Lissauer & Avroy A. Fanaroff. © 2011 Blackwell Publishing Ltd.

Investigations when inborn error of metabolism is suspected (Tables 45.3 and 45.4, Fig. 45.1)

Table 45.3 First-line investigations when inborn error of metabolism is suspected.

Investigation	Abnormality	Disorder
Blood gas	Metabolic acidosis	Organic acidemia (MSUD), disorders of carbohydrate metabolism
	Respiratory alkalosis	Urea cycle disorder
Glucose	Hypoglycemia with ketosis	Organic acidemias; glycogen storage
	Hypoglycemia without ketosis	Fatty acid oxidation
Ammonia	Hyperammonemia (Fig. 45.1)	Urea cycle defects, organic acidemia
Lactate	High	Respiratory chain defects, hypoxia
Urea nitrogen (blood urea)	Low	Urea cycle
Electrolytes	Raised anion gap	Lactic acidosis, organic acidemia
Liver transaminases	High	Tyrosinemia, galactosemia
Complete blood count	Neutropenia Thrombocytopenia	Organic acidemias
Coagulation	Prolonged	Liver disease
Urine	Abnormal odor	Organic acidemia
Urine reducing substances	Negative for glucose	Galactosemia
Urine ketones	Positive	Organic acidemias
	Low/negative	Fatty acid oxidation disorders

Table 45.4 Second-line investigations.

Urine organic acids
Urine amino acids
Plasma uric acid
Plasma amino acids
Plasma carnitine and acylcarnitine
Biotinidase
Galactosemia screening tests
CSF lactate and amino acids
More specialized tests, e.g. enzyme assay on skin fibroblasts or blood cells, DNA mutation analysis, special metabolite assays

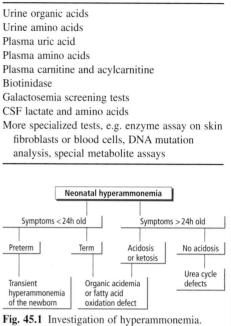

Fig. 45.1 Investigation of hyperammonemia.

Management

- Early intervention (Table 45.5) is imperative to prevent neurologic sequelae.
- Dialysis and medical management promote removal of toxic metabolites.
- Keep catabolism to a minimum.
- Empiric treatment may be indicated while awaiting results (Table 45.6). May include special diets, vitamins and carnitine; 5% respond to specific vitamins. Rapid diagnostic testing and clinical history now often allow specific rather than empiric management to be given.

Table 45.5 Immediate management.

Nutrition	Stop feeding, particularly protein and galactose Avoid catabolism – give intravenous glucose
Fluid and circulation	Fluid and circulatory support Correct metabolic acidosis with bicarbonate Correct hypoglycemia
Ventilatory support	Early mechanical ventilation if required
Toxin removal	Hemodialysis or hemodiafiltration
Hyperammonemia	Sodium benzoate, sodium phenylbutyrate and arginine
Insulin	Sometimes used to prevent catabolism
Empiric megavitamin therapy	(See Table 45.6)

Table 45.6 Empiric therapy.

Carnitine
Pyridoxine
Vitamin B_{12}
Biotin
Hydroxycobalamin
Riboflavin
Thiamin
Also coenzyme Q, sodium benzoate, biopterin

Key point

If an inborn error of metabolism is suspected, consult a specialized center for advice on management.

Question

What samples should be obtained if an inborn error of metabolism is suspected in an infant who is preterminal or has died?

Blood spot – on biochemical screening filter paper.
Plasma – heparinized, separated, deep-frozen.
Urine – deep-frozen.
Sample for DNA – blood in EDTA and deep-frozen.
Skin for fibroblast culture – sterile into medium, store at 4–8°C.
Liver for histochemistry or enzymes – snap-frozen.
Muscle and other tissues if indicated – snap-frozen.

Vomiting

This is the forceful return of gastric contents. It is in contrast to regurgitation or possetting, the effortless return of small quantities of milk, which is very common during the first few months of life.

The significance of the vomiting will depend on:
- infant's age
- frequency, amount and characteristics of vomiting, e.g. if projectile
- presence of bile (Fig. 46.1) or blood (Fig. 46.2)

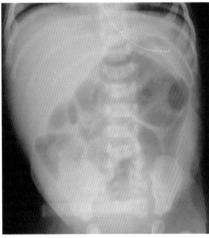

Fig. 46.1 Abdominal X-ray showing distended loops of bowel from meconium ileus. The infant presented with bile-stained vomiting at 30 hours of life.

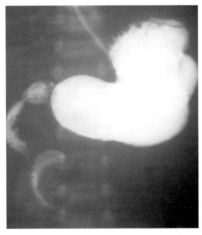

Fig. 46.2 Water-soluble contrast upper gastrointestinal study demonstrating coiled corkscrew appearance of second and third parts of duodenum due to midgut volvulus from malrotation. This infant presented with blood-stained vomiting at 12 hours of age. (Courtesy of Dr Annemarie Jeanes.)

- abdominal distension
- stool characteristics – delayed passage of meconium or absent transitional stools
- presence of dehydration, weight loss
- evidence of a systemic illness – poor feeding, fever, lethargy.

Causes

Physiologic:
- Gastroesophageal reflux.
- Ingestion of maternal blood.
- Overfeeding.
- Incorrectly positioned nasogastric tube.
  Infection:
- Systemic – septicemia, urinary tract infection, meningitis.
- Local – gastroenteritis.
  Mechanical/surgical:
- Intestinal obstruction – see Chapter 47.
- Paralytic ileus – sepsis, electrolyte disturbance.
- Necrotizing enterocolitis – see Chapter 35.
  CNS:
- Raised intracranial pressure – cerebral edema, intracranial or subdural bleed, hydrocephalus.
- Kernicterus.
  Drugs:
- Side-effects – caffeine, theophylline, antibiotics.
- Withdrawal (abstinence) – heroin, methadone.
  Cow's milk protein intolerance.
  Inborn errors of metabolism (rare).
  Endocrine:
- Congenital adrenal hyperplasia (rare).

Diagnostic clues

Bile-stained vomiting (yellow–green)
Causes:
- Intestinal obstruction – distal to ampulla of Vater.
- Necrotizing enterocolitis.
- Incorrectly positioned nasogastric tube.
- Feeding intolerance in very low birthweight infants establishing feeds (common and presence of bile not significant unless there is abdominal distension or features of necrotizing enterocolitis).

Key point

Bile-stained vomiting in term infants should always be regarded as intestinal obstruction until proven otherwise.

Neonatology at a Glance, 2nd edition. Edited by Tom Lissauer & Avroy A. Fanaroff. © 2011 Blackwell Publishing Ltd.

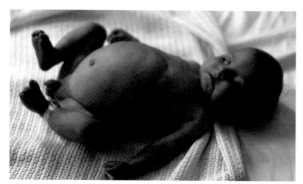

Fig. 46.3 Abdominal distension from Hirschsprung disease.

Vomiting with abdominal distension
Causes:
- Intestinal obstruction (Fig. 46.3).
- Paralytic ileus – sepsis, electrolyte disturbance.
- Necrotizing enterocolitis.

Blood-stained vomiting
Flecks of fresh blood or dark brown coffee grounds not uncommon in otherwise well infants and usually resolve spontaneously.
Causes:
- Swallowed maternal blood – from delivery or cracked nipple. Can be differentiated from fetal blood with the Apt test (see Table 46.1).
- Trauma – laryngoscopy at resuscitation, passing a nasogastric tube.
- Malrotation – uncommon but important to diagnose early (Fig. 46.2).
- Stress ulcer – hypoxic–ischemic encephalopathy.
- Abnormal coagulation – thrombocytopenia, hemorrhagic disease of the newborn, liver disease, DIC (disseminated intravascular coagulation), etc.
- Drug-induced – corticosteroids, indomethacin.

Investigations

Most infants will require no or limited investigations. Those to be considered are listed in Table 46.1.

Management

Depends upon severity and cause. Intravenous fluids may be required to correct electrolyte disturbances, acid–base imbalance and dehydration.

Gastroesophageal reflux in neonates

Incidence is increased in:
- preterm infants, particularly with bronchopulmonary dysplasia (chronic lung disease) or on caffeine
- following necrotizing enterocolitis and tracheoesophageal fistula repair
- infants with neurodevelopmental delay, e.g. following hypoxic–ischemic encephalopathy or hypotonia.

Associated features

- Failure to thrive.
- Irritability, arching of the back from esophagitis.
- Anemia (iron deficiency).
- Aspiration pneumonia.
- Apnea.
- Acute life-threatening events (ALTE).

Investigations

- Usually clinical diagnosis.
- Esophageal pH study, sometimes upper gastrointestinal contrast or endoscopy.

Management

Most do not need treatment. If required, use stepwise approach.
- Reduce interval between feeds, thicken feeds, alginate/antacid (Gaviscon), upright positioning.
- Prokinetic (domperidone).
- H_2 receptor antagonist, e.g. ranitidine; proton pump inhibitors, e.g. omeprazole – reduce gastric acidity.
- Surgery – fundoplication with or without gastrostomy.
  Evidence of efficacy of medication in neonates is limited.

Table 46.1 Vomiting-investigations to consider and their purpose.

Imaging	Blood tests	Urine and stool tests
Plain abdominal X-ray:	Electrolytes and acid–base – for imbalance	Urine – microscopy and culture
• intestinal obstruction – distended loops of bowel, bowel perforation	Sepsis work-up to exclude infection	Stool – for blood
• NEC (necrotizing enterocolitis)	Creatinine/blood urea nitrogen – for dehydration and renal function	Other:
Ultrasound scans:	Glucose – for hypoglycemia	Apt test of vomit/stool – to
• cranial for hemorrhage, ventricular dilatation	Calcium, magnesium, phosphorus, liver function tests	differentiate between
• abdominal for pyloric stenosis	Coagulation screen – if blood in vomit or sepsis	maternal and fetal blood.
Contrast X rays:	Consider:	Fetal hemoglobin is
• malrotation, strictures	• 17-hydroxyprogesterone – for congenital adrenal hyperplasia	alkali-resistant (remains pink
• site of intestinal obstruction	• blood ammonia – for urea cycle abnormalities	on addition of sodium
	• drug screen – for drug overdose or withdrawal	hydroxide)

Esophageal atresia

- More than 85% associated with tracheoesophageal fistula (Fig. 46.4).
- 1 in 3500 live births.
- Often associated with other abnormalities, e.g. VACTERL syndrome (**v**ertebral **a**nomalies, **a**nal atresia, **c**ardiac, **t**racheo-**e**sophageal, **r**enal, **l**imb).

Presentation

- Prenatal – polyhydramnios, absent stomach bubble, associated abnormalities.
- Birth onwards – frothing of oral secretions (Fig. 46.5) with choking and cyanosis.

Investigations

- Unable to pass wide-bore orogastric tube; confirmed on chest X-ray, shows tube in esophageal pouch. Air in the stomach indicates a fistula is present.

Management

- Pass large orogastric tube and aspirate pouch to avoid aspiration pneumonia.

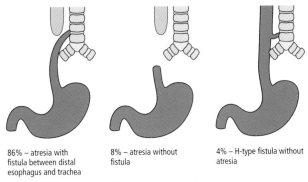

86% – atresia with fistula between distal esophagus and trachea

8% – atresia without fistula

4% – H-type fistula without atresia

Fig. 46.4 Different types of esophageal atresia.

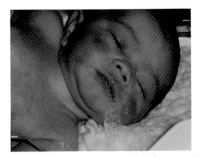

Fig. 46.5 Frothing of oral secretions after birth from esophageal atresia.

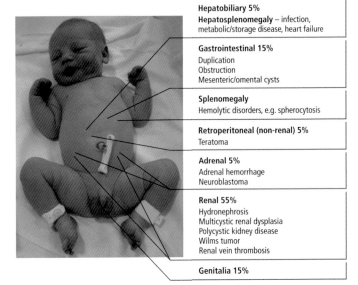

Hepatobiliary 5%
Hepatosplenomegaly – infection, metabolic/storage disease, heart failure

Gastrointestinal 15%
Duplication
Obstruction
Mesenteric/omental cysts

Splenomegaly
Hemolytic disorders, e.g. spherocytosis

Retroperitoneal (non-renal) 5%
Teratoma

Adrenal 5%
Adrenal hemorrhage
Neuroblastoma

Renal 55%
Hydronephrosis
Multicystic renal dysplasia
Polycystic kidney disease
Wilms tumor
Renal vein thrombosis

Genitalia 15%

Fig. 46.6 Abdominal masses and their causes.

- Intravenous fluids for resuscitation and maintenance. Early TPN (total parenteral nutrition).
- Surgical correction is required.

Abdominal masses

Often detected *in utero* on ultrasound screening. The causes are shown in Fig. 46.6.

Abdominal wall defects

Omphalocele

Defect in umbilicus with herniation of abdominal contents. The bowel is covered by peritoneum and amnion (Fig. 46.7). Vary in

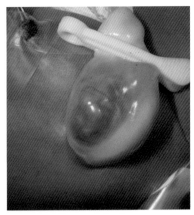

Fig. 46.7 Omphalocele.

size, from small defects where some bowel herniates into the umbilical cord to large defects where there is herniation of both bowel and liver. Occurs in 1 in 5000 fetuses. Most are diagnosed on prenatal ultrasound screening (see Fig. 3.4). In 40% it is associated with trisomy 13 or 18, Beckwith–Wiedemann (see Chapter 44) or other syndromes.

Management
- Pass a large-caliber nasogastric tube at delivery to limit passage of air into the bowel, and nothing by mouth.
- Place infant's lower body into a sterile plastic bag to limit heat and fluid loss and protect the bowel from damage and infection.
- Give intravenous fluids.
- Check for other anomalies, including echocardiography.
- Surgical repair is usually performed on the first day of life. If the defect is large, the viscera may be placed in a Silastic silo, and gradually placed in the abdomen over several days.

Gastroschisis

Defect in anterior abdominal wall, usually to right of umbilicus, with herniation of the bowel (Fig. 46.8). In contrast to omphalocele, there is no protective covering of the bowel and the incidence of associated anomalies is low, other than intestinal atresia. The condition is usually diagnosed on prenatal ultrasound scanning.

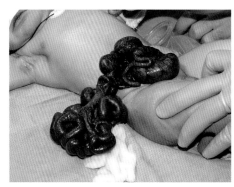

Fig. 46.8 Gastroschisis.

Management
- The infant's lower body is placed into a sterile plastic bag.
- Pass a large-caliber nasogastric tube at delivery to limit passage of air into the bowel.
- Give intravenous fluids; colloid may be required to replace fluid losses from the exposed bowel. Closely monitor electrolytes.
- Surgical repair can usually be performed directly.
- Prolonged parenteral nutrition is usually required to establish feeds. Prognosis is good.

Most of the conditions causing gastrointestinal obstructions are serious but their prognosis has improved with advances in medical, anesthetic and surgical care. They are relatively uncommon but are important to recognize because:
- failure or delay in diagnosis may result in electrolyte imbalance, dehydration and shock
- malrotation with midgut volvulus is a surgical emergency in order to avoid bowel necrosis.

Causes – see Fig. 47.1

Diagnostic clues

Prenatal:
- **Polyhydramnios** – from obstruction to the passage of amniotic fluid through the gastrointestinal tract.
- **Abnormal ultrasound** – dilated bowel, hyperechoic bowel, ascites, calcified lesions. May be difficult to diagnose.
- **Fetus with trisomy 21 (Down syndrome)** – 30% have associated duodenal atresia.
- **Family history of cystic fibrosis** – associated with meconium ileus.

Delivery room:
- **Bubbly oral secretions** – esophageal atresia.
- **Peri-umbilical abdominal wall discoloration** – *in utero* bowel perforation.

Clinical presentation

- Vomiting – usually bile (yellow–green stained). Bile is present if the obstruction is distal to ampulla of Vater. Presents within 24–48 hours of birth with high gastrointestinal lesions, may be delayed for several days for lower lesions.
- Feeding intolerance.
- Abdomen – distension with visible loops of bowel or peristalsis, erythema/edema of abdominal wall, abdominal mass, peritoitis and shock.
- Failure to pass meconium within 48 hours of birth.
- Blood in stool.

Diagnosis

Abdominal X-ray:
- Bowel obstruction – distended loops of bowel with air–fluid levels, with absence of gas distally (see Fig. 46.1).
- Bowel perforation – free air under diaphragm, intrahepatic or around falciform ligament.

Management

- Abdominal decompression with nasal or orogastric tube. In esophageal atresia, aspirate pouch to avoid aspiration pneumonia.
- Intravenous fluids for resuscitation and maintenance. Early TPN (total parenteral nutrition).
- Antibiotics preoperatively.
- Evaluate and correct bleeding diathesis.
- Surgical correction for most lesions.
- Evaluate for other anomalies. Karyotype may be necessary.

Some specific conditions

Esophageal atresia (Chapter 46)

Pyloric stenosis

Hypertrophy of circular smooth muscle of pylorus of stomach.
- **Presentation** – projectile vomiting in a hungry infant at 4–8 weeks of age. Occurs at same age in preterm infants.
- **Examination** – visible peristalsis. A firm, olive-like mass is palpable in right upper abdomen during feeds.
- **Investigation** – abdominal ultrasound – hypertrophy of pylorus.
- **Management** – correct electrolyte imbalance (hypochloremic hypokalemic alkalosis). Surgery muscle incision (pyloromyotomy).

Duodenal atresia

- **Lesion** – obstruction may be due to atresia, webs, stenosis or fibrous cord.
- **Incidence** – 1 in 7500 births. Check for trisomy 21 and other anomalies.
- **Antenatal** – polyhydramnios, distended fluid-filled stomach on ultrasound.
- **Presentation** – vomiting – bilious or non-bilious, upper abdominal distension and feeding intolerance.

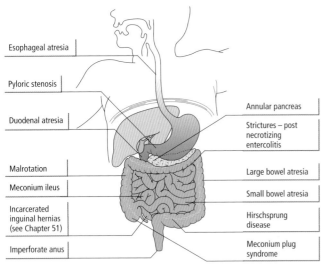

Esophageal atresia
Pyloric stenosis
Duodenal atresia
Malrotation
Meconium ileus
Incarcerated inguinal hernias (see Chapter 51)
Imperforate anus

Annular pancreas
Strictures – post necrotizing enterocolitis
Large bowel atresia
Small bowel atresia
Hirschsprung disease
Meconium plug syndrome

Fig. 47.1 Causes of intestinal obstruction.

Neonatology at a Glance, 2nd edition. Edited by Tom Lissauer & Avroy A. Fanaroff. © 2011 Blackwell Publishing Ltd.

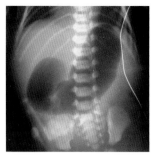

Fig. 47.2 Abdominal X-ray showing double bubble in duodenal atresia.

- **Diagnosis** – double bubble on X-ray (Fig. 47.2). May be accentuated by injecting 20 mL of air through gastric tube.

Malrotation

Failure of the developing bowel to undergo the normal counterclockwise rotation during the 4th to 10th weeks of embryogenesis. Peritoneal bands (which normally attach the bowel to the central body axis posteriorly and are also known as Ladd bands) compress the duodenum, partially obstructing it. Because the mesentery is not fixed, malrotation predisposes to midgut volvulus (twisting of a loop of bowel around its mesenteric attachment). In addition to intestinal obstruction, compression of the superior mesenteric artery leads to ischemia of the small bowel.

Presentation
Sudden bilious vomiting is malrotation until proven otherwise. Usually in first few weeks of life but can occur at any age. With acute volvulus also abdominal distension and tenderness followed by shock. Hematemesis (blood-stained vomit) may occur.

Investigation
Doppler ultrasound of mesenteric vessels may be helpful at the bedside. Upper gastrointestinal exam (contrast swallow) is diagnostic. The normal position of the duodenal–jejunal junction (Treitz angle) is to the left of the spine. Any other position indicates malrotation. Volvulus classically appears as a spiral corkscrew of the duodenum (see Chapter 46).

Management
Volvulus is a surgical emergency. Ischemia can lead to small bowel infarction requiring bowel resection. Extensive resection of the small bowel carries a poor prognosis.

To relieve the obstruction, the peritoneal bands around the duodenum are divided. Appendectomy is also performed to avoid future confusion if the child has abdominal pain.

Meconium ileus

- Small bowel obstruction from inspissated, putty-like, sticky meconium.
- Affects 10–15% of patients with cystic fibrosis, whereas 95% of infants with meconium ileus have cystic fibrosis.

Presentation
Bilious vomiting, failure to pass meconium, abdominal distension, abdominal mass. Edema of abdominal wall suggests peritonitis. Complications include volvulus and perforation.

Investigation and management
- Abdominal X-ray – dilated loops of bowel, air fluid levels and ground glass soap-bubble appearance of meconium (see Fig. 46.1).
- Intra-abdominal calcification indicates intrauterine perforation and peritonitis.
- Gastrograffin (water-soluble contrast) enema may wash out the meconium, otherwise surgery is required.
- Check for cystic fibrosis.

Meconium plug syndrome

Presentation – low bowel obstruction, as in Hirschsprung disease.

Hirschsprung disease

- Congenital absence of ganglionic cells in the myenteric plexus secondary to defective migration of ganglion cell precursors from neural crest to hind gut. Proximal bowel is normal.
- Incidence – 1 in 5000 births, male : female ratio 5 : 1.
- May be associated with trisomy 21 (Down syndrome).
- Accounts for 20–25% of cases of neonatal intestinal obstruction.

Presentation
- Delayed passage of stools – more than 50% do not stool for 48 hours.
- About 50% of affected children present with abdominal distension (see Fig. 46.3) and vomiting in neonatal period, others when older with constipation.
- May present with enterocolitis – explosive liquid stools, fever and shock.

Investigation
Abdominal X-ray shows distal bowel obstruction – multiple distended loops of bowel with lack of air in the rectum.

Diagnosis
- Rectal suction biopsy for histology.
- Barium enema – excludes other causes of intestinal obstruction and may show transition zone between normal and aganglionic bowel.

Treatment
Surgical repair.

Imperforate anus

- Incidence 1 in 5000 births. Associated anomalies of genitourinary and gastrointestinal tract common, and in VACTERL association.
- In boys most often with fistula to urethra, in girls to vestibule adjacent to vagina. Some lesions are complex.
- Surgery is with anoplasty or colostomy followed by repair.

Congenital heart disease:
- is the most common group of structural malformations
- affects 6–8 per 1000 live births
- accounts for 30% of all congenital abnormalities.

Risk factors

- Chromosomal disorders and syndromes, e.g. trisomy 21 (Down syndrome), microdeletion chromosome 22 abnormalities (for aortic arch abnormalities and Di George sequence), Turner, Noonan, Williams, syndromes and many others.
- Maternal – diabetes mellitus, teratogenic drugs, e.g. anticonvulsants, fetal alcohol syndrome.
- Congenital infection, e.g. rubella.
- Siblings of affected child – only slight increase in risk.

Presentation

- Antenatal detection on ultrasound screening.
- Detection of a heart murmur.
- Heart failure – respiratory distress/shock.
- Cyanosis.

Antenatal diagnosis

Many lesions are diagnosed antenatally, especially the severe abnormalities detectable on the four-chamber view used for antenatal ultrasound screening (Fig. 48.1), e.g. hypoplastic left heart. Lesions such as transposition of the great arteries and coarctation of the aorta are difficult to identify.

If risk is increased or an abnormality detected, referral to a perinatal cardiac specialist is indicated. Antenatal detection allows parents to be counseled and postnatal management planned.

Key point

About a quarter of infants with congenital heart disease present in the neonatal period and usually have severe lesions.

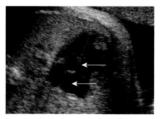

Fig. 48.1 Fetal ultrasound showing atrioventricular septal defect (AVSD).

Classification (Table 48.1)

Table 48.1 Classification of cardiac disorders.

Acyanotic	Cyanotic
Shunts ('holes')	**Transposition of the great**
VSD (ventricular septal defect) 32%	**arteries** 5%
PDA (patent ductus arteriosus) 12%	**Reduced pulmonary blood**
ASD (atrial septal defect) 6%	**flow**
Obstruction ('narrowing')	Tetralogy of Fallot 6%
Pulmonary stenosis 8%	Pulmonary atresia
Aortic stenosis 5%	Tricuspid atresia
Coarctation of the aorta 6%	**Total anomalous**
Hypoplastic left heart	**pulmonary venous**
Pump failure	**connection (TAPVC)**
Supraventricular tachycardia (SVT)	
Cardiomyopathy	

In infants with congenital heart disease:
- 10–15% have complex heart disease with multiple lesions
- 10–15% of children with congenital heart disease have abnormalities of other systems.

Heart murmur

Detected in 1–2% of normal infants on routine examination.

The cause may be:
- **A transient flow murmur** related to circulatory changes following birth. The murmur is soft, systolic, at the left sternal edge or pulmonary area in a well infant whose examination, including four limb blood pressure measurements, is otherwise normal.
- **Pulmonary artery branch stenosis.** The murmur is best heard in the pulmonary area and radiates to the axilla and back. Resolves in a few weeks.
- **Congenital heart disease.** Though uncommon, the most worrying of these are duct-dependent lesions, which may result in circulatory failure or cyanosis when the ductus arteriosus closes. The femoral pulses may be palpable even in coarctation of the aorta shortly after birth as the ductus arteriosus is still patent.

The definitive diagnosis is by echocardiography. A chest X-ray and ECG are of limited value in establishing a specific diagnosis, but abnormalities may lead one to suspect congenital heart disease. Pulse oximetry will establish if the arterial oxygen saturation is normal (>95%). If there are features of an innocent flow murmur, reassess infant within days to check that the murmur has disappeared. The parents need to be informed that they should seek medical assistance should the infant develop symptoms suggestive of heart failure, i.e. slow feeding, breathlessness and sweating. If the murmur persists or has pathologic features or if abnormal clinical

Key point

The absence of a murmur does not exclude congenital heart disease.

Neonatology at a Glance, 2nd edition. Edited by Tom Lissauer & Avroy A. Fanaroff. © 2011 Blackwell Publishing Ltd.

Heart failure

Causes of heart failure and clinical features are shown in Table 48.2 and Fig. 48.2.

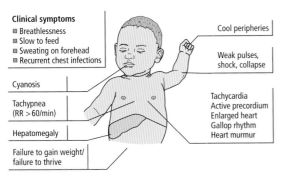

Fig. 48.2 Clinical features of heart failure.

Clinical symptoms
- Breathlessness
- Slow to feed
- Sweating on forehead
- Recurrent chest infections

Cyanosis

Tachypnea (RR > 60/min)

Hepatomegaly

Failure to gain weight/ failure to thrive

Cool peripheries

Weak pulses, shock, collapse

Tachycardia
Active precordium
Enlarged heart
Gallop rhythm
Heart murmur

Table 48.2 Causes of heart failure in the neonatal period.

Left-to-right shunting (high-output failure)
Patent ductus arteriosus
Atrioventricular septal defect (AVSD)/large ventricular septal defect (VSD)
Left ventricular outflow obstruction (duct-dependent systemic circulation)
Severe coarctation of the aorta
Critical aortic valve stenosis
Hypoplastic left heart syndrome
Myocarditis/cardiomyopathy
Arrhythmias
Supraventricular tachycardia (SVT)
Non-cardiac
Severe anemia, polycythemia, arteriovenous malformation, e.g. vein of Galen malformation

features develop, referral to a pediatric cardiologist and echocardiography are indicated.

Selected causes of heart failure

Left-to-right shunting (high-output failure)

Patent ductus arteriosus in preterm infants
See Chapter 32.

Atrioventricular septal defect (AV canal defect)
- Common (40%) in trisomy 21 (Down syndrome).
- Surgery at 2–4 months.

Large ventricular septal defect
- Only presents at about 1–3 months, when pulmonary vascular resistance is low and left-to-right shunt maximal.
- Surgery if medical therapy fails.

Left ventricular outflow obstruction (low-output heart failure/shock when duct closes)

Severe coarctation of the aorta/interruption of the aortic arch
Key clinical sign is weak or absent femoral pulses. Blood pressure in the arms is markedly higher than in the legs (>20 mmHg). Surgery is required.

Less severe lesions may present as hypertension in adults.

Hypoplastic left heart (Fig. 48.3)
Presents with signs of low cardiac output when ductus arteriosus closes. Pulses are weak at presentation, and there is severe metabolic acidosis. Fatal without treatment – requires a series of palliative operations (Norwood procedure) or heart transplantation.

Supraventricular tachycardia
- Heart rate 220–300 beats/min (Fig. 48.4).

Hypoplastic left heart

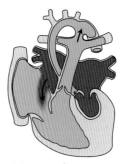

Fig. 48.3 Hypoplastic left heart syndrome.

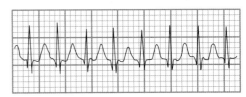

Fig. 48.4 ECG showing supraventricular tachycardia.

- Heart is usually structurally normal, but accessory pathway (Wolff–Parkinson–White syndrome) is present in 40%.
- If no response to placing ice pack on face, give the drug adenosine, or DC cardioversion.

Cyanosis

Central cyanosis

Central cyanosis:
- is clinically detectable if there is over 5 g/dL of reduced hemoglobin
- is best detected in tongue/mucous membranes

- in the absence of respiratory distress is usually due to cyanotic congenital heart disease (Table 48.1).

If there is respiratory distress, the cause may be:
- congenital heart disease
- pulmonary disease
- PPHN (persistent pulmonary hypertension of the newborn)
- polycythemia.

Peripheral cyanosis (acrocyanosis)

Hands and feet are blue. Common in infants in the first couple of days of life and in children of any age when cold. The tongue and mucous membranes are pink. It is of no clinical significance in the absence of hypovolemia or shock.

'Traumatic' cyanosis

Cyanosis of the head, often with petechiae from venous congestion, e.g. caused by umbilical cord around baby's neck or face presentation. Tongue is pink. Resolves spontaneously.

Selected causes of cyanotic congenital heart disease

Transposition of the great arteries

In transposition of the great arteries there are two parallel circulations – the aorta arises from the right ventricle and the pulmonary artery from the left ventricle (Fig. 48.5). For survival, mixing of blood between the two circulations must occur, e.g. via the foramen ovale or ductus arteriosus. The less mixing between the circulations, the more severe the cyanosis and the earlier the presentation.

Presentation
Profound cyanosis occurs in the first day or two of life when the duct closes, but may be delayed if there is appreciable mixing of blood from an associated anomaly, e.g. atrial septal defect.

Management
This is to promote mixing of the two circulations:

Complete transposition of the great arteries

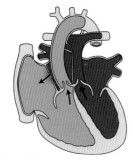

Fig. 48.5 Transposition of the great arteries.

Balloon septostomy

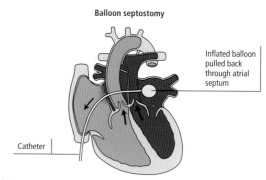

Inflated balloon pulled back through atrial septum

Catheter

Fig. 48.6 Balloon atrial septostomy to enlarge the foramen ovale.

- by maintaining ductal patency with a prostaglandin infusion
- by performing a balloon atrial septostomy to enlarge the foramen ovale (Fig. 48.6).

An operation will subsequently be required. This is usually the switch operation, in which the pulmonary artery and aorta are switched over. The coronary arteries also have to be transferred to the new aorta, which is technically demanding.

Total anomalous pulmonary venous connection (TAPVC)

The pulmonary veins, instead of connecting into the left atrium, connect into the right side of the circulation, sometimes below the diaphragm.

If the connection is narrow (obstructed) they present with cyanosis, respiratory distress and poor cardiac output. This may be difficult to distinguish from surfactant deficiency. Treatment is surgical, sometimes in an emergency.

Investigations

The immediate problem is to distinguish between a respiratory disorder, congenital heart disease (CHD) and persistent pulmonary hypertension of the newborn (PPHN).

Chest X-ray

Helpful to confirm if lung disease is the cause of respiratory distress, but rarely diagnostic of congenital heart disease as heart size and shape and pulmonary vasculature are difficult to determine in neonatal period. An enlarged heart border may be due to normal thymus.

However, a chest radiograph may show:
- heart enlarged (>60% diameter of thorax), e.g. outflow obstruction from coarctation of the aorta or volume overload
- abnormal shape (e.g. boot shape with tetralogy of Fallot, 'egg on side' with TGA) but often recognized only after the diagnosis has been made
- prominent pulmonary vascular markings (plethoric) from excess blood flow to the lungs, e.g. left-to-right shunt from patent ductus

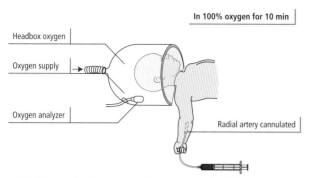

In 100% oxygen for 10 min

Headbox oxygen

Oxygen supply

Oxygen analyzer

Radial artery cannulated

Fig. 48.7 Hyperoxia (nitrogen washout) test to identify cyanotic congenital heart disease.

arteriosus, but this only occurs later when the pulmonary vascular resistance falls
• reduced pulmonary vascular markings (oligemic) from reduced blood flow to the lungs, e.g. tetralogy of Fallot.

ECG

• Seldom diagnostic; interpretation requires considerable skill.
• Can be useful if there is a superior axis (e.g. AVSD, tricuspid atresia)
• Helpful for arrhythmias and as baseline.

Hyperoxia test

May be helpful to distinguish respiratory from cardiac causes (Fig. 48.7).
Interpretation of right radial artery oxygen tension is:
• If PaO_2 >110 mmHg (15 kPa):
  – unlikely to be cyanotic heart disease
  – usually lung disease or PPHN (persistent pulmonary hypertension of the newborn).
• If PaO_2 <110 mmHg (15 kPa):
  – likely to be cyanotic heart disease, but can be severe lung disease or PPHN.

Echocardiography and Doppler

Allow definitive anatomic diagnosis and identification of shunts in most instances. Need good equipment and experienced operator.

Cardiac catheterization

Sometimes required for hemodynamic measurements and increasingly used for interventional procedures, e.g. valvuloplasty.

Management

• Maintain **A**irway, **B**reathing, **C**irculation. Provide ventilatory support if necessary.

• Correct metabolic acidosis, hypoglycemia and hypocalcemia.
• In the first few days of life, give prostaglandin intravenously to keep the ductus arteriosus patent.
• If duct-dependent defect – do not give additional oxygen unless SaO_2 falls below 75%.
• If in heart failure:
  – high-output failure (after first week of life) – fluid restriction (acute only), diuretics, ACE inhibitors, e.g. captopril
  – low-output failure/shock – inotropes, volume support; arrhythmias require specific treatment.
• Refer to pediatric cardiac center.

Question

Why may giving prostaglandin be life-saving?
By keeping the ductus arteriosus patent when the circulation is duct-dependent. This occurs:
• with obstruction to outflow of the left ventricle, when the systemic circulation is maintained by blood flowing right to left across the patent ductus, e.g. severe coarctation of the aorta (Fig. 48.8)
• with reduced pulmonary blood flow, when the pulmonary circulation is maintained by blood flowing from left to right through the duct, e.g. pulmonary atresia (Fig. 48.9).

Duct-dependent coarctation

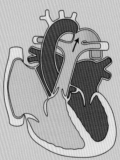

Fig. 48.8 Severe coarctation of the aorta, an example of duct-dependent systemic circulation.

Pulmonary atresia with intact septum

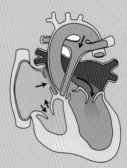

Fig. 48.9 Pulmonary atresia, an example of duct-dependent pulmonary circulation.

Most significant structural abnormalities of the kidneys and urinary tract are now identified prenatally on ultrasound screening. They account for 20–30% of all prenatally detected abnormalities. Early recognition and treatment may prevent or ameliorate complications such as urinary tract infection, failure to thrive and renal failure. When indicated, it may allow prenatal referral to a tertiary center. The disadvantage is that many minor or transient genitourinary anomalies are identified, resulting in unnecessary concern for the parents and additional investigations for the child.

Embryology

The kidneys and genitourinary tract are embryologically interdependent. If one system is abnormal, look for abnormalities of the other.

Structural abnormalities of the kidneys

Outflow obstruction

In the fetus with outflow obstruction (Fig. 49.1) there may be:
• hydronephrosis – unilateral or bilateral, with renal parenchyma that may be normal or malformed or dysplastic
• dilatation of the ureters and/or bladder
• reduced or absent amniotic fluid volume.

Unilateral hydronephrosis
• Hydronephrosis is dilatation of the proximal collecting system (Fig. 49.2).
• It is the commonest abnormality diagnosed antenatally, and accounts for 50% of all prenatally detected urologic anomalies. It occurs in 1 in 500–700 infants. Most common cause is physiologic hydronephrosis, but others are obstruction at the ureteropelvic or vesicoureteric junction or urinary reflux.
• Management is shown in Fig. 49.3.
• Most but not all resolve spontaneously. Prognosis is dependent on degree of kidney damage resulting from obstruction.

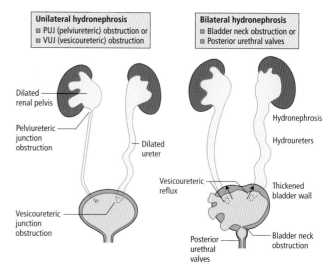

Fig. 49.1 Features of unilateral and bilateral outflow obstruction.

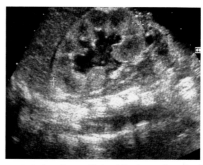

Fig. 49.2 Ultrasound showing unilateral hydronephrosis. As a measure of its severity, the anteroposterior renal pelvis diameter is measured. (Courtesy of Dr Annemarie Jeanes.)

• If the anteroposterior diameter does not exceed 15 mm either antenatally or postnatally, intervention is rarely needed.

Bilateral hydronephrosis
Less common than unilateral hydronephrosis but more likely to be serious.

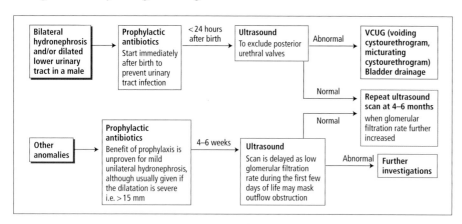

Fig. 49.3 Example of a guideline of the initial management of renal and urinary tract abnormalities detected on antenatal ultrasound.

Neonatology at a Glance, 2nd edition. Edited by Tom Lissauer & Avroy A. Fanaroff. © 2011 Blackwell Publishing Ltd.

Posterior urethral valves

• Mucosal folds or a membrane obstruct urine flow causing bilateral hydronephrosis, hydroureter and thickened bladder. One third develop end-stage renal failure.

• Incidence is 1 in 5000–8000 live male births.

• Most are diagnosed on prenatal ultrasound, when antenatal intervention may be considered. Options include percutaneous vesicoamniotic shunt placement, bladder aspiration, and drainage of a severely distended kidney. However, outcome after intervention has been disappointing. As amniotic fluid is mainly derived from fetal urine, there may severe oligohydramnios resulting in Potter syndrome (Fig. 49.4); the dominant features are from compression of the fetus and pulmonary hypoplasia resulting in stillbirth or early neonatal death.

• Presentation in the infant not diagnosed antenatally includes a palpable, distended bladder, poor urinary flow, renal and pulmonary failure.

• Management postnatally is shown in Fig. 49.3. It is with prophylactic antibiotics, renal and urinary tract ultrasound within 24 hours of birth and VCUG (voiding cystourethrogram, micturating cystourethrogram).

• Treatment – drainage of the urinary tract, initially by urinary catheter, later by ablation of the valves.

> **Key point**
>
> Bilateral hydronephrosis with bladder distension in a boy should be assumed to be posterior urethral valves until proven otherwise.

Polycystic kidney disease

Autosomal dominant polycystic kidney disease (ADPKD)
(Fig. 49.5a)

• Common: 1 in 500–1000.

• Wide spectrum of severity; usually asymptomatic in childhood, causes renal failure in late adulthood.

• Extrarenal features: cysts in liver and pancreas, cerebral aneurysms and mitral valve prolapse.

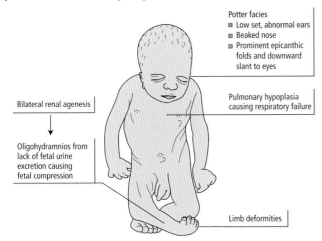

Fig. 49.4 Potter syndrome.

Bilateral renal agenesis ↓ Oligohydramnios from lack of fetal urine excretion causing fetal compression

Potter facies
▪ Low set, abnormal ears
▪ Beaked nose
▪ Prominent epicanthic folds and downward slant to eyes

Pulmonary hypoplasia causing respiratory failure

Limb deformities

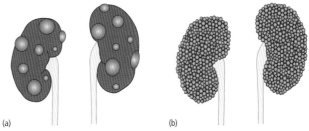

Fig. 49.5 (a) Autosomal dominant polycystic kidney disease (ADPKD). There are separate cysts of varying size between normal renal parenchyma. (b) Autosomal recessive polycystic kidney disease (ARPKD). There is diffuse bilateral enlargement of the kidneys.

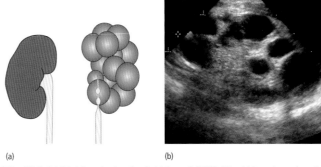

Fig. 49.6 (a) Multicystic dysplastic kidney (MDK). The kidney is replaced by cysts of variable size, with atresia of the ureter. (b) Renal ultrasound shows discrete cysts of variable size in multicystic dysplastic kidney (MDK).

Autosomal recessive polycystic kidney disease (ARPKD)
(Fig. 49.5b)

• Rare: 1 in 10 000–40 000.

• Cysts form in the collecting duct.

• Presents with abdominal masses, hypertension and renal failure.

• Associated with congenital hepatic fibrosis.

• May cause renal failure requiring renal transplant.

Multicystic renal dysplasia (MCD)

• Uncommon: 1 in 4000 live births.

• Renal parenchyma replaced by cysts of various sizes (Fig. 49.6a and b).

• Kidney is functionless, accompanied by atresia of the ureter.

• If bilateral, it causes Potter syndrome.

• Kidney may be large and palpable, but more often is small. Contralateral kidney is usually normal, should have undergone compensatory hypertrophy, but at increased risk of vesicoureteric reflux.

• Half will have involuted by 2 years. Nephrectomy is only indicated if cysts increase in size or hypertension develops, both of which are rare.

Renal agenesis

• Unilateral agenesis/dysplasia (present in 1 in 1000) is only important if the contralateral kidney is abnormal.

• Bilateral agenesis is fatal from pulmonary hypoplasia from severe oligohydramnios.

Renal function in the newborn

Almost all infants void by 24 hours of life. If it is suspected that urine has not been passed within the first day, it is usually that voiding has not been recorded, especially immediately after birth.

Consider obstruction or intrinsic renal problem, but they are usually detected on antenatal ultrasound screening.

Some key points regarding renal function are listed in Fig. 50.1.

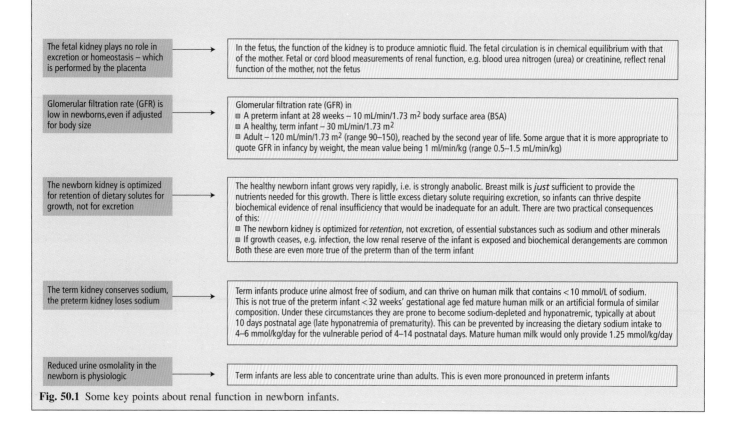

Fig. 50.1 Some key points about renal function in newborn infants.

Electrolyte problems

Sodium

Normal range 135–145 mmol/L.

Hyponatremia – Na < 130 mmol/L.

Results from excess water over sodium or insufficient sodium over water.

Key is to assess fluid status overall. If detailed assessment required, measure paired urinary and serum sodium, osmolality and creatinine to establish fractional excretion of sodium. (Fractional excretion of sodium, $FENa = UNa/PNa \times PCr/UCr \times 100$, where UNa is urinary sodim, PNa plasma sodium, PCr is plasma creatinine, UCr urinary creatinine).

Term infants, hyponatremia – usually from giving excessive volume of IV water. Especially in first 48 hours of life and when there is intravascular volume depletion with water reabsorption. Also excess IV fluids to mother during labor; oliguric renal failure (renal impairment with little urine output and fluid overload).

Preterm – marked Na loss in urine, poor at conserving sodium as tubular reabsorptive capacity not fully developed. This results in hyponatremia of prematurity (see Fig. 50.1).

Other causes include:
• insufficient Na supplementation (low FENa)
• gastrointestinal losses – diarrhea, vomiting (low FENa)

Neonatology at a Glance, 2nd edition. Edited by Tom Lissauer & Avroy A. Fanaroff. © 2011 Blackwell Publishing Ltd.

- renal losses – diuretics (high FENa), renal dysplasia, congenital adrenal hyperplasia, renal tubulopathies
- SIADH, syndrome of inappropriate antidiuretic hormone (high FENa, low POsm and high UOsm) – probably rare in newborn infants.

Hypernatremia – >150 mmol/L

Result of excessive water loss over sodium or excess sodium intake over water.

If detailed assessment required, assess fluid status and measure FENa.

Hypernatraemic dehydration may be from:
- insufficient input of fluids e.g. insufficient breast milk
- excessive water losses, e.g. evaporative through skin as extremely preterm, phototherapy, radiant heater or gastrointestinal
- excess sodium intake, e.g. sodium containing flushes of lines, sodium bicarbonate, sodium phosphate, etc (high UOsm and high FENa)

Rare causes – diabetes insipidus (central, e.g. septo-optic dysplasia or nephrogenic, no ADH or ADH effect) (low UOsm, low FENa).

Potassium (normal range 3.5–5.5 mmol/L)

Hyperkalemia – K > 6.0 mmol/L

Serious condition as can result in arrhythmias and death. But most common reason is hemolyzed blood sample.

Other causes – renal impairment (transient is relatively common in extremely preterm infants), excess K supplementation, congenital adrenal hyperplasia.

Neonates tolerate hyperkalemia better than older children, so only treat if K > 6.5. Seldom required.

Treatment involves giving calcium gluconate to stabilize myocardium, salbutamol IV or nebulized, correcting acidosis, stopping all K, changing to low K feed, calcium resonium orally or rectally but can cause gastrointestinal obstruction.

Hypokalaemia – K < 3.0 mmol/L

Causes include insufficient supplementations, diuretics, diarrhea, vomiting, renal tubular losses (e.g. Bartter syndrome), drugs, e.g. amphotericin.

Calcium and phosphate

Hypocalcemia

Relatively common problem and can lead to seizures.

Causes: birth trauma/asphyxia, infants of diabetic mothers, exchange transfusion with blood reconstituted in citrate, maternal hyperparathyroidism, Di George syndrome, associated with hypomagnesemia.

Hypophosphatemia

Usually results from insufficient supplementation in feeds or total parenteral nutrition.

Urinary tract infection (UTI)

- Commoner in boys than in girls – the reverse of older children.
- Should be suspected in any infant who is non-specifically unwell.

Presentation

- Fever or sometimes low temperature or temperature instability.
- Poor feeding.
- Vomiting.
- Prolonged jaundice.
- Diarrhea.
- Failure to thrive.

Investigations

Urine – collecting urine samples:
- adhesive bags – high false positive rate, helpful if negative
- clean catch specimen
- urethral catheterization
- suprapubic aspiration (see Chapter 75).

Blood culture and sepsis work-up (with or without lumbar puncture) should be performed as urinary tract infection is often accompanied by septicemia in neonates.

Diagnosis

Is made by culture of a single strain of any organism on a catheter sample or suprapubic aspirate. However, may get false positive suprapubic aspirate result from skin commensal or bowel perforation.

White cells may or may not be present on microscopy or urinalysis.

E. coli is the commonest organism (>75%); remainder caused by *Klebsiella*, *Proteus*, *Enterobacter*.

Management

Intravenous antibiotics – started immediately whilst awaiting the result of the urine culture. Subsequent choice of antibiotics will depend on the sensitivities of the cultured organism. Should be continued at full dosage until the infant has been well for 2–3 days and a negative follow-up urine culture obtained. Prophylactic antibiotics, e.g. trimethoprim or cefalexin, should be given until the results of imaging of the kidneys and urinary tract are known.

Imaging – if culture is positive, ultrasound of the kidneys and urinary tract is performed to detect renal tract abnormalities. A VCUG (voiding cystourethrogram, micturating cystourethrogram) is performed to identify bladder outflow obstruction, e.g. from posterior urethral valves or vesicoureteral reflux (Fig. 50.2). A radionuclide scan (DMSA, dimercaptosuccinic acid) is performed 3 months later to identify renal scarring (Fig. 50.3).

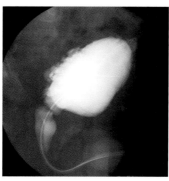

Fig. 50.2 VCUG (voiding cystourethrogram, micturating cystourethrogram) showing trabeculation of the bladder wall, hypertrophy of the bladder and dilated posterior urethra from posterior urethral valves.

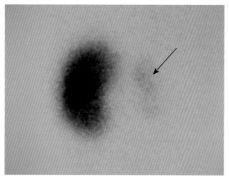

Fig. 50.3 Renal scarring of right kidney (arrow) on DMSA scan on investigation following a urinary tract infection.

Acute renal failure

In acute renal failure there is sudden impairment in renal function leading to inability of the kidney to excrete nitrogenous wastes. It is defined as a rise in the plasma creatinine concentration to twice the upper limit of normal, i.e. 1.5 mg/dL (130 mmol/L) accompanied by a reduction in urine flow rate to <1 mL/kg/hour. However, renal failure can occur without oliguria. It results from a significant fall in glomerular filtration rate with failure of tubular reabsorption of salt and water.

Causes

Different in neonates to children and adults as usually prerenal (Table 50.1). Mild renal impairment is not uncommon in the first few days of life, particularly in preterm infants, and is usually transient.

Clinical features

- Usually identified by rise in plasma creatinine.
- Urinary features – oliguria, hematuria, proteinuria.
- Clinical features – hypertension, edema, dehydration, vomiting, lethargy and seizures.
- Other biochemical features – hyperkalemia, acidosis, hyperphosphatemia and hypocalcemia.

Ultrasound of kidneys and urinary tract

Identifies abnormal kidneys, outflow obstruction, abnormal blood flow in renal arteries and veins.

Table 50.1 Causes of acute renal failure in neonates.

Prerenal	Renal	Post-renal
Hypovolemia	Acute tubular necrosis secondary to an uncorrected prerenal cause	Congenital obstructive uropathy – posterior urethral valves, etc.
Dehydration, sepsis, necrotizing enterocolitis	Congenital renal abnormality, e.g. polycystic kidney disease, renal agenesis, renal hypodysplasia	
Blood loss: antepartum, neonatal		Neurogenic bladder
Heart failure	Vascular insult – renal vein thrombosis, renal artery thrombosis (associated with use of umbilical arterial lines)	
Hypoxia including birth asphyxia	Nephrotoxins	
	Infection – pyelonephritis	

Management

Prevention

• Monitor the creatinine, blood urea nitrogen (urea) and electrolytes of newborn infants who have been exposed to risk factors for acute renal failure, such as birth asphyxia or sepsis.
• Early treatment of hypovolemia.
• Relief of obstruction.
• Avoid nephrotoxic agents if possible, discontinue if renal failure.

Electrolyte and fluid management

• Restrict sodium, potassium and phosphate. Use calcium carbonate as phosphate binder. Correct metabolic acidosis.

• High dose furosemide 2–5 mg/kg to convert oliguric into non-oliguric renal failure.
• Nutritional support.
• Dialysis – rarely needed, only if fluid and metabolic abnormalities cannot be corrected. Peritoneal dialysis is preferable but may not be possible (e.g. abdominal wall defects or necrotizing enterocolitis). Hemodialysis is difficult due to vascular access and risks associated with anticoagulation.

51 Genital disorders

Features of the normal male genitalia are listed in Table 51.1. Most abnormalities of the male genitalia arise from abnormal embryology (Fig. 51.1).

Inguinal hernia

This results from the processus vaginalis remaining patent. Much more common in males than females and usually on the right side.

Common in preterm infants, particularly those with bronchopulmonary dysplasia (chronic lung disease) as they have weak muscles and raised intra-abdominal pressure.

Presents as a swelling in the groin or scrotum on crying (Fig. 51.2). It should be repaired promptly to avoid the risk of strangulation in both term and preterm infants, unless the anesthetic risk necessitates delaying the operation.

If the hernia becomes irreducible, the lump is firm and tender. The infant vomits and becomes unwell. It can usually be reduced after sustained gentle compression with opioid analgesia. If possible, surgery is delayed for 24–48 hours to allow the edema to resolve. If reduction is unsuccessful, emergency surgery is required to avoid bowel strangulation and damage to the testis.

Table 51.1 Features of normal male genitalia.

Length and diameter – normal size
Meatus – at tip
Testes – palpable in scrotum
Scrotum – rugae

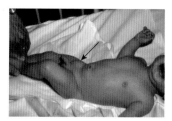

Fig. 51.2 Inguinal hernia in a newborn infant (arrow). (Courtesy of Dr Mike Coren.)

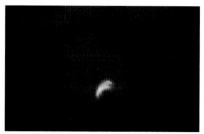

Fig. 51.3 Hydrocele on transillumination. (Courtesy of Dr Mike Coren.)

Hydrocele

This is fluid around the testis from a processus vaginalis that is wide enough to allow peritoneal fluid to flow down it but too narrow to form an inguinal hernia.

Tense, transilluminates (Fig. 51.3). Often bilateral. Most resolve spontaneously.

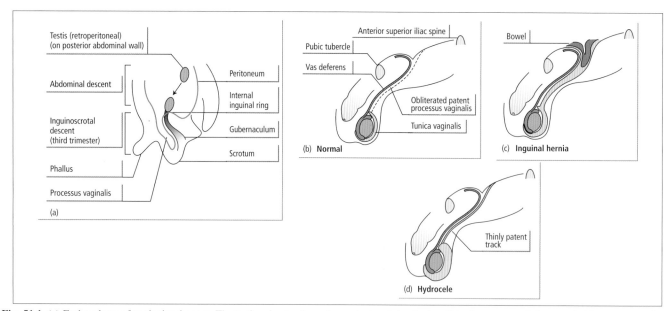

Fig. 51.1 (a) Embryology of testicular descent. The testis migrates from the posterior abdominal wall to the scrotum. It is preceded by a tongue of peritoneum, the processus vaginalis. This is obliterated in the normal infant (b). It remains widely patent in an inguinal hernia (c). With a hydrocele, it is patent but narrow (d).

Neonatology at a Glance, 2nd edition. Edited by Tom Lissauer & Avroy A. Fanaroff. © 2011 Blackwell Publishing Ltd.

Undescended testis

Failure of the testis to descend into the scrotum. Present in 5% of term male infants. Incidence is higher in preterm infants as testicular descent through the inguinal canal only occurs in the third trimester of pregnancy. Testicular descent may continue after birth; by 3 months of age only 1.5% are affected, but few descend thereafter.

Examination

With warm hands the contents of the inguinal canal are gently massaged towards the scrotum. If undescended, no testis is palpable in the scrotum, and the overlying scrotum is often poorly formed. The undescended testis may be palpable in the groin, but may sometimes be in the abdomen or outside the normal line of descent. A descended testis sometimes subsequently retracts upwards into the inguinal region (retractile testis).

Investigations

For bilateral undescended testes, pelvic ultrasound and karyotype may be needed to establish the infant's gender, i.e. male and not a virilized female. The presence of testicular tissue can be confirmed by detecting testosterone production after hormonal stimulation. Sometimes laparoscopy is required to locate the testis.

Management

Surgery to place the testis in the scrotum (orchidopexy) is usually performed during the second year of life because:
• fertility is optimized – the testis needs to be in the scrotum to be below body temperature
• malignancy – there is increased risk, which for a unilateral undescended testis is probably reduced to nearly the same as for a normal testis
• it is cosmetic and avoids psychologic upset.

Torsion of the testis

There is interruption of the blood supply to the testis and epididymis. Occasionally occurs in newborn infants. The testis and surrounding area may be inflamed and the scrotum is black. Must be differentiated from a strangulated hernia and scrotal hematoma. The torsion must be relieved expediently for the testis to remain viable. Doppler ultrasound of testicular blood supply is helpful to determine testicular viability. The testis is seldom viable if torsion is present at birth.

Hypospadias

Common, affecting 1 in 300 boys. In the fetus, the urethra is created by flat tissue folding over from the perineum towards the tip. If this is not completed, the meatal opening may not reach the normal site at the tip of the penis (Fig. 51.4).

In hypospadias there is:
• a ventral urethral meatus – usually on the glans of the penis, but can be on the shaft or perineum (Fig. 51.5)

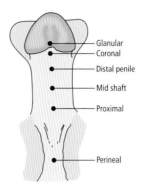

Glanular
Coronal
Distal penile
Mid shaft
Proximal
Perineal

Fig. 51.4 Classification of hypospadias.

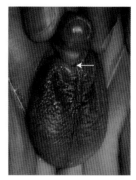

Fig. 51.5 Hypospadias. The urethral meatus is shown by the arrow.

• a hooded foreskin – from failure to fuse
• chordee – tethering resulting in ventral curvature of the penis, most obvious on erection. This is associated with the more severe forms.

Surgical correction is performed by 2 years of age so that the urethral meatus is at the tip of the penis, erection is straight and the penis looks normal. In most cases of hypospadias affecting only the glans, surgery is not required, except sometimes for cosmetic reasons.

Circumcision

At birth, the foreskin adheres to the surface of the glans penis. These adhesions subsequently separate, allowing the foreskin to become retractile. The foreskin cannot be retracted in 50% of boys at 1 year of age and in 10% at 4 years, but in only 1% by 16 years.

In the US, circumcision is widely performed. In the UK, the main indication is religious, among Jews and Muslims. Its advantages and disadvantages are controversial and emotive.

Advantages are:
• hygiene – easier to keep clean
• prevents the possibility of developing pathologic phimosis (scarring) or recurrent balanitis (infection) of the foreskin requiring circumcision at a later age
• slightly reduced incidence of urinary tract infection and sexually acquired HIV infection.

However, it is not a trivial operation, as healing can take up to 10 days. Complications include:
• pain during and after the operation – adequate analgesia should be provided
• bleeding
• infection
• damage to the glans penis, although this is rare.

Key point

Infants with hypospadias must not be circumcised as the foreskin may be needed at surgery.

In newborn infants, disorders of sexual differentiation present with ambiguous genitalia. There may be:
- virilized female – clitoromegaly, labial fusion
- undervirilized male – micropenis, bilateral undescended testes, poorly developed or bifid scrotum
- true hermaphrodite, now called ovotesticular DSD (disorders of sex development) – complex external phenotype with both testicular and ovarian tissue present.

They are rare but require prompt evaluation and skilled management to avoid emotional turmoil for parents. Family support and counseling are of utmost importance.

Sexual differentiation

The fetal gonad is initially bipotential (Fig. 52.1).

The testis-determining gene on the Y chromosome (*SRY*) causes differentiation of gonads into testes. Production of testosterone and its metabolite dihydrotestosterone results in the development of male genitalia.

Undervirilization in the male may result from:
- inadequate androgen action from:
  - abnormal testes
  - inability to convert testosterone to dihydrotestosterone (5α-reductase deficiency)
  - abnormalities of the androgen receptor (androgen insensitivity syndrome)
- gonadotropin insufficiency from:
  - congenital hypopituitarism
  - several syndromes, e.g. Prader–Willi syndrome.

In the absence of the *SRY* gene the gonads become ovaries and the genitalia female.

Virilization is from excessive androgens; the most common cause of this is congenital adrenal hyperplasia.

Hermaphroditism is from chromosomal rearrangement and is rare.

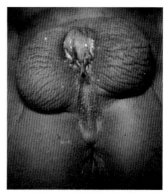

Fig. 52.2 Ambiguous genitalia at birth. Do not guess the gender. (Courtesy of Dr David Clark.)

Birth

When a baby is born, the parents immediately want to know if they have a girl or boy.

If the genitalia are ambiguous (Fig. 52.2), it is imperative not to guess but to inform the parents that further evaluation is needed. Birth registration must be delayed until this has been completed.

Investigations

Detailed assessment may include:
- karyotype
- sex and adrenal hormones:
  - blood glucose and electrolytes
  - 17α-hydroxyprogesterone
  - testosterone, dihydrotestosterone and androstenedione
  - hormone (GnRH or HCG) stimulation tests
- ultrasound of internal genitalia and gonads.

Laparoscopic examination and biopsy of internal structures are sometimes required.

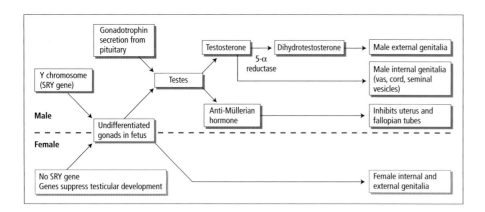

Fig. 52.1 Sexual differentiation in the fetus.

Neonatology at a Glance, 2ⁿᵈ edition. Edited by Tom Lissauer & Avroy A. Fanaroff. © 2011 Blackwell Publishing Ltd.

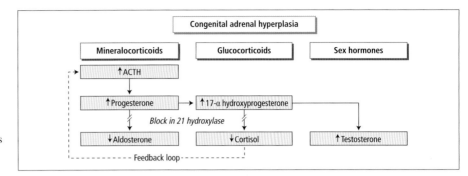

Fig. 52.3 Abnormal adrenal steroid biosynthesis in the commonest form of congenital adrenal hyperplasia (21-hydroxylase deficiency).

Management

Ensure good communication between all health-care professionals so that they do not ascribe a gender to the infant inadvertently.

Most are reared as females, as it is easier to create female external genitalia than a functioning penis, but it is increasingly recognized that this may not necessarily be in the long-term best interest of the child. There is increasing evidence of problems with gender identity as teenagers and adults of males reared as females, and evidence of good sexual functioning and satisfaction in males who had a poorly formed penis in the neonatal period. Early referral, expert multidisciplinary assessment and long-term management are required.

Congenital adrenal hyperplasia

- Autosomal recessive condition.
- About 1 in 5000 live births.
- Most common cause is a deficiency of an enzyme, 21-hydroxylase, required for cortisol biosynthesis (Fig. 52.3). There is a deficiency

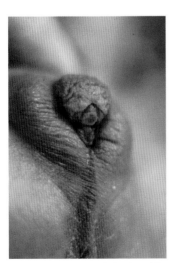

Fig. 52.4 Virilized female from congenital adrenal hyperplasia. There is clitoral hypertrophy and fusion of the labia. (Courtesy of Dr David Clark.)

in the production of cortisol, aldosterone (salt loss) and an excess of adrenal steroids (virilization).

Presentation

May be with:
- virilization of female external genitalia (Fig. 52.4)
- enlarged penis and pigmented scrotum in male, but rarely recognized
- salt-losing adrenal crisis at 1–3 weeks of age; there is vomiting, weight loss, circulatory collapse which may be fatal; may be accompanied by hypoglycemia
- tall stature, precocious puberty in males.

Diagnosis

Raised blood level of 17α-hydroxyprogesterone.

Management

Short term:
- Salt-losing crisis – requires intravenous saline, dextrose, hydrocortisone.
- Corrective surgery of external genitalia in females.
  Long term:
- Glucocorticoids throughout life.
- Mineralocorticoids if salt loss; infants may need extra oral sodium chloride.
- Monitoring of growth and pubertal development.
- Additional hormone replacement (stress doses) if ill or prior to surgical procedures.
- Further corrective surgery in adolescence to external genitalia in females.
- Psychologic support.

Prenatal testing and screening

Prenatal testing and treatment of affected fetuses are available.

Screening (17α-hydroxyprogesterone concentration) is now performed in most routine biochemical screening programs of newborns in the US but not in the UK.

Anemia

Physiology

In the fetus, the oxygen tension is low. To compensate for this, the oxygen affinity of fetal red cells containing hemoglobin F (HbF) is increased compared to adult red cells (Fig. 53.1) and this favors uptake of more oxygen. The hemoglobin concentration (Hb) is also much higher than in adults.

After birth, the concentration of Hb is greatly affected by the time of cord clamping and the position of the infant relative to the placenta. If the cord is clamped immediately the Hb may be up to 6 g/dL lower than if the infant receives a placental 'transfusion' by delaying cord clamping and placing the baby lower than the placenta.

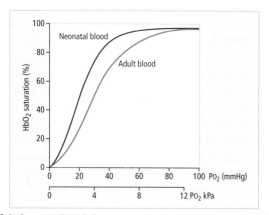

Fig. 53.1 Oxygen dissociation curve showing the higher oxygen affinity of neonatal than adult hemoglobin.

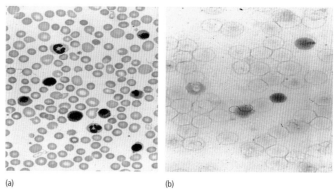

Fig. 53.3 Fetomaternal hemorrhage. (a) Anemia (number of red cells are reduced), nucleated red cells (erythroblasts) and reticulocytes on a blood smear (film) from a term neonate with severe anemia at birth (4.5 g/dL) due to fetomaternal hemorrhage. (b) Kleihauer test on maternal blood from of the same baby showing several intensely pink-stained cells containing HbF, which is resistant to acid lysis.

Clinical features (Table 53.1) and management

Blood transfusion

Kept to a minimum because of potential hazards but often required for VLBW (very low birthweight) infants. Erythropoietin is used only occasionally in preterm infants to reduce the need for blood transfusions as its efficacy is modest and it acts slowly.

Oral folic acid

Given as prophylaxis if chronic hemolysis (e.g. hereditary spherocytosis). Some neonatal units prescribe it for VLBW infants for the first few months as their folate stores are low, the folate content of breast milk is low and there is increased demand from rapid growth.

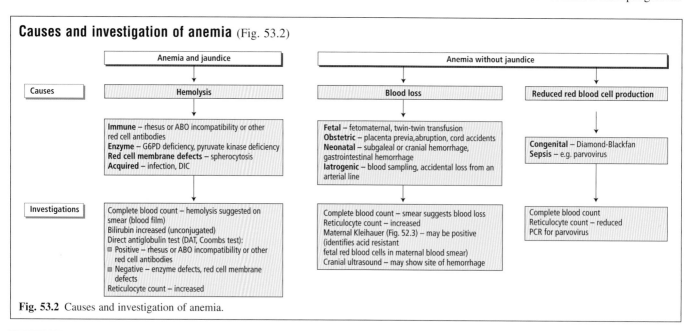

Causes and investigation of anemia (Fig. 53.2)

Anemia and jaundice		Anemia without jaundice	
Causes **Hemolysis**		**Blood loss**	**Reduced red blood cell production**
Immune – rhesus or ABO incompatibility or other red cell antibodies **Enzyme** – G6PD deficiency, pyruvate kinase deficiency **Red cell membrane defects** – spherocytosis **Acquired** – infection, DIC		**Fetal** – fetomaternal, twin-twin transfusion **Obstetric** – placenta previa, abruption, cord accidents **Neonatal** – subgaleal or cranial hemorrhage, gastrointestinal hemorrhage **Iatrogenic** – blood sampling, accidental loss from an arterial line	**Congenital** – Diamond-Blackfan **Sepsis** – e.g. parvovirus
Investigations Complete blood count – hemolysis suggested on smear (blood film) Bilirubin increased (unconjugated) Direct antiglobulin test (DAT, Coombs test): ▫ Positive – rhesus or ABO incompatibility or other red cell antibodies ▫ Negative – enzyme defects, red cell membrane defects Reticulocyte count – increased		Complete blood count – smear suggests blood loss Reticulocyte count – increased Maternal Kleihauer (Fig. 52.3) – may be positive (identifies acid resistant fetal red blood cells in maternal blood smear) Cranial ultrasound – may show site of hemorrhage	Complete blood count Reticulocyte count – reduced PCR for parvovirus

Fig. 53.2 Causes and investigation of anemia.

Neonatology at a Glance, 2nd edition. Edited by Tom Lissauer & Avroy A. Fanaroff. © 2011 Blackwell Publishing Ltd.

Table 53.1 Clinical features of anemia.

History	Examination
History – blood loss	Pallor
Family history – anemia, jaundice, splenomegaly from hemolytic disease	Jaundice from hemolysis
	Apnea and bradycardia
Obstetric history – antepartum hemorrhage	Tachycardia
Maternal blood type – rhesus or other red cell antibodies, potential for ABO incompatibility (mother O, infant A or B)	Heart murmur – systolic flow murmur
	Respiratory distress, heart failure
Ethnic origin – hemoglobinopathies and G6PD deficiency more common in certain ethnic groups	Hepatomegaly and/or splenomegaly, hydrops
	Inadequate weight gain from poor feeding

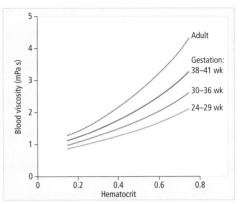

Fig. 53.4 Hematocrit is the main determinant of blood viscosity. Blood viscosity rises exponentially when hematocrit is >0.65.

Oral iron therapy

In preterm infants given after the age of 4–6 weeks to prevent anemia of prematurity. Not given if the infant has recently had a blood transfusion or is on iron-supplemented formula feeding.

Polycythemia

Usually defined as a venous hematocrit (Hct) above 0.65. The hematocrit depends on the site of sampling: capillary hematocrit > peripheral venous > central venous > arterial.

Potential danger of high hematocrit is hyperviscosity, which causes sludging of red blood cells and formation of microthrombi, leading to vascular occlusion (Fig. 53.4).

Causes

Increased erythropoietin production
- Intrauterine hypoxia – IUGR (intrauterine growth restriction).
- Maternal diabetes.
- Trisomy 21 (Down syndrome).
- High altitude.

Increased blood volume
- Excessive placental transfusion from delayed cord clamping.
- Twin–twin transfusion.

Clinical features

These are:
- plethora (Fig. 53.5)
- hypoglycemia/hypocalcemia
- irritability, lethargy, seizures
- poor feeding
- hyperbilirubinemia
- respiratory distress
- heart failure
- priapism
- intestinal – necrotizing enterocolitis
- renal – renal vein thrombosis, hematuria, oliguria
- thrombocytopenia.

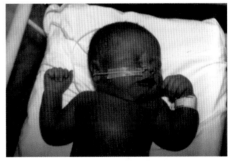

Fig. 53.5 Plethoric term infant. Nasogastric tube is because of poor feeding.

Treatment and management

There is an increased risk of long-term neurologic impairment in polycythemic infants. However, it is not established that treatment is of benefit. Treatment is to reduce the hematocrit by replacing a proportion of the infant's blood with 0.9% saline (plasma is no longer used for this purpose to minimize blood product usage). This is done by partial exchange transfusion (see Chapter 77).

If the venous hematocrit is greater than 0.65 and the infant is symptomatic or the hematocrit is above 0.70 even if asymptomatic – generally agreed that a partial dilutional exchange transfusion should be performed.

If venous hematocrit 0.65–0.70 and asymptomatic – observe and treat only if the infant becomes symptomatic.

Question

Should one screen for polycythemia?
At-risk infants (intrauterine growth restriction, macrosomia, twins) should have their hematocrit checked. Routine screening of all infants is not recommended because of lack of evidence of benefit of treatment (American Academy of Pediatrics).

Anemia and polycythemia 133

Neutrophil disorders

There is a physiologic rise in neutrophils between 12 and 24 hours of life and thereafter the number falls (Fig. 54.1).

Neutrophilia
The most common causes are:
- acute bacterial infection
- maternal chorioamnionitis (usually without active infection in the baby).

Much less common causes are fungal infection and postnatal corticosteroid therapy. When neutrophilia is accompanied by a left shift, i.e. increase in immature neutrophils, such as band forms (Fig. 54.2), it is used as a marker for bacterial infection. The combination of an abnormal absolute neutrophil count and immature:total neutrophil ratio increases the likelihood of infection to about 65%. Neutrophilia from bacterial infections often develops 12–24 hours after the onset of infection. Serial measurements are more informative than isolated values. However, interpretation of the blood smear requires technical expertise. In the UK band counts have largely been replaced by measuring acute phase reactants (C-reactive protein or procalcitonin). In many units in the US both band counts and acute phase reactants are measured.

Neutropenia
This is a neutrophil count of less than 1500 cells/mm³ (1.5 × 10^9/L). Neutropenia is usually caused by sepsis, necrotizing enterocolitis, cytomegalovirus (CMV) and other congenital infections, intrauterine growth restriction (IUGR), maternal pre-eclampsia and the chromosome trisomies (13, 18 and 21). Alloimmune neutropenia and inherited causes are uncommon. Most types of neonatal neutropenia are self-limiting and treatment is primarily of the underlying cause. Intravenous immunoglobulin is non-specific and has not been shown to be beneficial. Recombinant hemopoietic growth factors, in particular recombinant G-CSF (granulocyte colony stimulating factor) and GM-CSF (granulocyte macrophage colony stimulating factor) will increase the neutrophil count, but have not been shown to improve outcome. White cell transfusions are rarely effective.

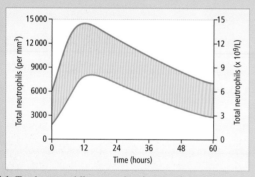

Fig. 54.1 Total neutrophil count, showing the rise with age and the normal range. (From Manroe *et al. J Pediatr* 1979; **95**: 89.)

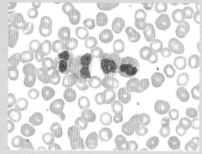

Fig. 54.2 Blood smear showing four neutrophil 'band' cells in a neonate with bacterial sepsis. The 'band' cells also show toxic granulation in the cytoplasm, another useful sign of acute bacterial infection.

Thrombotic disorders (thrombophilia)

These are a group of disorders characterized by an increased tendency for abnormal clot formation. Thrombosis occurs in approximately 5 per 100 000 births; 50% of episodes are arterial and 50% are venous.

Predisposing factors

These are:
- indwelling catheters (80–90% of episodes)
- acute bacterial and viral infection
- asphyxia (ischemia), shock
- cardiac abnormality
- diabetes mellitus
- polycythemia
- prematurity
- twin–twin transfusion
- genetic.

Maternal and familial conditions associated with thrombophilia

These include:
- multiple fetal losses
- anticardiolipin antibodies

Neonatology at a Glance, 2nd edition. Edited by Tom Lissauer & Avroy A. Fanaroff. © 2011 Blackwell Publishing Ltd.

- SLE (systemic lupus erythematosus)
- maternal diabetes
- placental abruption
- myocardial infarction
- deep venous thrombosis
- pulmonary embolism.

Inherited causes of thrombosis

Gene mutations have been identified for some of the most common thrombotic disorders:
- protein C deficiency (Fig. 54.3)
- protein S deficiency
- antithrombin deficiency
- factor V Leiden mutation (APC resistance)
- prothrombin gene mutation.

Diagnosis

Most thrombi are asymptomatic

Clinical signs of thrombosis depend on location of the clot, which may embolize:
- Arterial – limb may become mottled in color, cool and discolored. Pulses reduced. In time may be gangrenous with zone of

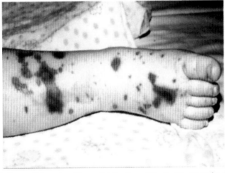

Fig. 54.3 Infant with microthrombi in the skin from protein C deficiency.

demarcation (see Fig. 65.5). Thrombus in aorta may lead to heart failure or stroke.
- Venous – portal vein, renal vein thrombosis causing abdominal mass, hematuria, oliguria and hypertension. Thrombus in right atrium may lead to stroke.

Imaging
Depends on site:
- Ultrasound, echocardiography, MRI for diagnosis and follow-up.
- Angiography is the gold standard but may be difficult or impossible to perform or not justified, e.g. for stroke. MR angiography is now available.

Management

Options include:
- If catheter-related, may be due to arterial spasm or too large a catheter or hypovolemia. If does not respond promptly to partial withdrawal of the catheter or correction of hypovolemia, the catheter should be removed.
- Observe and follow up for increase in clot size and functional compromise.
- Anticoagulation with unfractionated or low molecular weight heparin (e.g. enoxaparin).
- Clot lysis with fibrinolytic agents (tissue plasminogen activator).
- Surgical thrombectomy – rarely required or possible.
- Factor concentrate if thrombosis and inherited deficiency (e.g. protein C, antithrombin).

Question

Which neonates should be screened for inherited thrombophilia?

Any neonate with clinically significant thrombosis, e.g. severe purpura, renal vein thrombosis, extensive thrombosis or a family history of severe neonatal purpura.

55 Coagulation disorders

In the newborn, abnormal bleeding may be due to:
- a platelet abnormality (number or function)
- abnormal coagulation system
- vascular endothelial damage.

Thrombocytopenia

This is the most common platelet disorder. It is defined as a platelet count of less than $150\,000/mm^3$ ($150 \times 10^9/L$). It is usually identified on the complete blood count (CBC), but, if severe, may cause petechiae (Fig. 55.1) or bleeding.

A convenient classification is according to the time of onset (Table 55.1). The most common causes are maternal pre-eclampsia and diabetes mellitus, intrauterine growth restriction and neonatal infection.

Treatment is directed to the underlying cause.

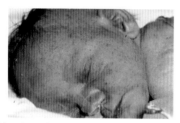

Fig. 55.1 Petechiae from thrombocytopenia in an infant.

Table 55.1 Classification of fetal and neonatal thrombocytopenia (most common causes in bold type).

Time of presentation	Condition
Fetus	**Neonatal alloimmune thrombocytopenia (NAITP)**
	Maternal autoimmune thrombocytopenia (ITP, SLE)
	Congenital infection (CMV, rubella, herpes, syphilis)
	Severe rhesus disease
	Chromosome abnormalities (trisomy 21, 18, 13)
	Inherited (very rare)
Neonatal (<72 h)	**Placental insufficiency (PIH, IUGR, diabetes)**
	Neonatal infection
	Birth asphyxia
	Neonatal alloimmune thrombocytopenia (NAITP)
	Maternal autoimmune thrombocytopenia (ITP, SLE)
	Thrombosis (renal vein, aortic)
	Congenital infection (CMV, rubella, herpes, syphilis)
	Inherited (very rare)
Neonatal (>72 h)	**Late-onset bacterial infection, necrotizing enterocolitis**
	Disseminated intravascular coagulation (DIC)
	Giant hemangioma (Kasabach–Merritt syndrome)

ITP, idiopathic thrombocytopenic purpura; SLE, systemic lupus erythematosus; CMV, cytomegalovirus; PIH, pregnancy-induced hypertension; IUGR, intrauterine growth restriction.
Adapted from Murray N, *Semin Neonatol* 1999; **4**: 27–40.

For infants who are sick or septic, where production may be compromised, platelet transfusion is given if:
- platelets $<30\,000/mm^3$ ($30 \times 10^9/L$) in term infants
- platelets $<50\,000/mm^3$ ($50 \times 10^9/L$) in preterm infants
- if actively bleeding or before surgery, platelets $<100\,000/mm^3$ ($100 \times 10^9/L$).

These values are a guide.

Abnormal coagulation

Coagulation factors are a group of proteins that upon activation will lead to the formation a fibrin-rich clot or hemostatic plug (Fig. 55.2). These proteins are formed early in gestation in the fetus and do not cross the placenta.

The most common acquired cause of coagulopathy is a combination of coagulation activation and poor liver reserve in a sick or septic infant.

Deficiency of some of the coagulation factors will lead to bleeding disorders (Table 55.2).

Indications for performing clotting studies

These are:
- family history of bleeding disorder
- clinical signs of abnormal bleeding:
  - oozing from venepuncture sites
  - bleeding umbilical cord stump
  - extensive bruising or large cephalhematoma or subgaleal (subaponeurotic) bleed
  - excessive bleeding after circumcision
  - gastrointestinal bleeding
- septic infant
- necrotizing enterocolitis

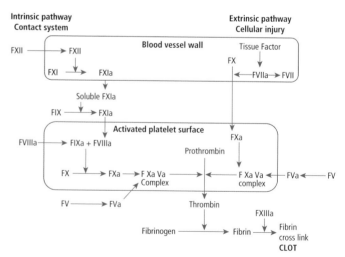

Fig. 55.2 The coagulation pathway.

Neonatology at a Glance, 2nd edition. Edited by Tom Lissauer & Avroy A. Fanaroff. © 2011 Blackwell Publishing Ltd.

Table 55.2 Bleeding disorders.

Deficiency	Disorder	Comments
Vitamin K	Hemorrhagic disease of newborn	From deficiency of the vitamin K-dependent factors (factors II, VII, IX and X) Associated with breast-feeding or severe liver disease in the infant or maternal use of anticonvulsants
Factor VIII	Classic hemophilia A	X-linked inheritance – positive family history in 80%. Mild and moderate forms usually asymptomatic during the newborn period, but 20% of cases present in the newborn, usually after circumcision or other surgery. Severe form may result in life-threatening hemorrhage
Factor IX	Christmas disease – hemophilia B	X-linked inheritance. Similar presentation to hemophilia A
Von Willebrand factor	Von Willebrand disease	Most common inherited bleeding disorder Autosomal dominant inheritance Only rare subtypes present in the newborn period

- rapidly falling platelet counts in a sick infant
- severe hypoxic ischemic encephalopathy.

Investigations

Coagulation screen consists of:
- PT (prothrombin time) or INR (international normalized ratio of PT)
- APTT (activated partial thromboplastin time)
- TT (thrombin time).
  May include:
- fibrinogen
- D-dimers – a measure of fibrin breakdown, may be useful for diagnosis of disseminated intravascular coagulation (DIC).

Interpretation of abnormal clotting studies (Table 55.3)

The normal values for preterm and term infants are derived locally, as different hospitals use different assays.

The coagulation values in preterm and term neonates differ significantly from older children and adults:
- Prothrombin time tends to be a few seconds longer at birth but will be normal within a week.
- Activated partial thromboplastin time may not reach adult normal ranges for several months because of low levels of the 'liver' factors (e.g. IX, XI, XII).

Table 55.3 Interpretation of abnormal clotting studies.

Test	Vitamin K deficiency	DIC	Liver impairment	Hemophilias
Platelets	Normal	Reduced	Normal	Normal
PT	Prolonged	Prolonged	Prolonged	Normal
PTT	Prolonged	Prolonged	Prolonged	Prolonged
TT	Normal	Prolonged	Prolonged	Normal
Fibrinogen	Normal	Reduced	Reduced	Normal

The prothrombin time (PT) may be reported in the form of an INR (international normalized ratio). A normal INR is ≤1.0; an INR >1.1 is equivalent to a prolonged PT. PTT, partial thromboplastin time; TT, thrombin time.

- Thrombin time may be slightly prolonged in early life due to the presence of a fetal form of fibrinogen. This is of no clinical significance.

Management of abnormal clotting

If there is active bleeding a correct diagnosis must be established. Vitamin K should be given while results are awaited, and fresh-frozen plasma (FFP) may be given if there is severe bleeding. Intramuscular injections must **not** be given to any neonate with a known or suspected major coagulation disorder (e.g. hemophilia), and care must also be taken after venepuncture and/or heelprick testing in such babies – pressure for >5 minutes is recommended.

If there is disseminated intravascular coagulation (DIC), treat the underlying cause. In the interim, platelets, FFP and cryoprecipitate (only if the fibrinogen level is low) may be indicated. Their need is determined by the coagulation tests, which should be repeated regularly as this is an evolving disorder.

FFP contains all coagulation factors and is suitable for emergencies, but does not contain sufficient of any single factor for severe single factor deficiencies. Replacement by a suitable concentrate is optimal, once a firm diagnosis has been established.

Severe congenital coagulation factor deficiencies – consult pediatric hematologist.

Question

What is special about taking blood samples for coagulation studies?

Blood sample must be free-flowing. Poor samples cause tissue activation and can give abnormal results, including a normal result in a baby with severe hemophilia.

If the sample is taken from a heparinized line, it may not be possible to interpret the thrombin time. Instead, fibrinogen levels and reptilase time must be used as they are unaffected by heparin.

If an inherited coagulation disorder is suspected, it is advisable to test the parents as well as the baby since neonatal coagulation tests are often difficult to interpret.

Functions of the skin include:
- mechanical protection
- barrier against microorganisms and toxins
- thermoregulation and fluid balance
- sensory input and tactile communication with the environment.

There are marked differences in the structure and function of the skin of preterm infants, term infants and adults (Table 56.1).

Goals of neonatal skin care

- Avoid traumatic injury during routine care.
- Prevent skin dryness leading to cracking and fissures.
- Minimize exposure to topical agents that are potentially toxic when absorbed (Table 56.2).

Diaper (napkin) dermatitis

Much less of a problem since disposable diapers (nappies).
- Keep skin dry with superabsorbent diapers and frequent changes.
- Treat underlying cause of excessive stooling, such as infectious diarrhea, malabsorption, opiate withdrawal.
- Apply petrolatum to reddened, intact skin to promote healing.
- Apply zinc oxide and pectin paste barriers liberally to excoriated skin to prevent reinjury from fecal enzymes and allow skin to heal.
- Identify candida dermatitis with distinctive pattern of redness on perineum, groin and thighs, and red pustular satellite lesions; apply antifungal ointment or cream. Also, consider oral antifungal treatment. Add 1% hydrocortisone if unresponsive.

Table 56.2 Toxicity reported from topical antiseptic use in preterm infants.

Antiseptic	Toxicity
Hexachlorophene	Spongiform encephalopathy
Povidone-iodine	Hypothyroidism, goiter
Chlorhexidine in alcohol	Scalds (avoid alcohol containing solution in preterm)

Question

Does the application of an occlusive barrier to the skin of preterm infants reduce transepidermal water loss and desquamation?

This has been demonstrated in a randomized controlled trial using Aquaphor (petrolatum/lanolin). However, it was associated with an increased risk of coagulase-negative staphylococcal infection and is no longer used for this purpose.

Infection

- **Bacterial** – bullous impetigo, staphylococcal scalded skin syndrome (SSSS) (see Chapter 42).
- **Viral** – herpes simplex virus infection (see Chapter 43), CMV and rubella (see Chapter 10).
- **Fungal** – (see Chapter 33).

Table 56.1 Developmental differences between the skin of infants and adults.

Developmental differences	Significance
Stratum corneum	
Term infants and adults: 10–20 layers	*Preterm infants, susceptible to:*
<30 weeks of gestation: 2–4 layers	• evaporative and transepidermal water loss
24 weeks of gestation: virtually no stratum corneum. Also, diminished cohesion between epidermis and dermis as fewer fibrils	• transcutaneously transmitted infection and toxicity from topical agents
	• epidermal stripping with adhesives
Dermis	
Term – only 60% the depth of adults	*Preterm* – excess fluid (edema) accumulates in the dermis, which is prone to injury
Preterm – even thinner dermis, less collagen and fewer fibrils	
Sweating	
Term – limited ability during first few days	Thermal sweating in adults is important to avoid overheating, but newborn infants cannot do this
Preterm – unable to sweat before 31 weeks' gestational age in response to heat, although sweat glands are present	
Emotional sweating of hands and feet – present at term, poorly developed in preterm infants	Emotional sweating to measure response to pain – can be used in term infants, but not in preterm

Neonatology at a Glance, 2nd edition. Edited by Tom Lissauer & Avroy A. Fanaroff. © 2011 Blackwell Publishing Ltd.

Vascular skin lesions

Port wine stain (nevus flammeus)

Present at birth in 0.3% of newborns. Most often on the face. Permanent malformation of the capillaries in the dermis. Laser therapy may improve the appearance of disfiguring lesions.

Rare associations:
• trigeminal nerve distribution (Sturge–Weber syndrome) as shown in Fig. 56.1a, intracranial vascular anomaly in 10% (Fig. 56.1b)
• severe limb lesions – bone hypertrophy (Klippel–Trenaunay syndrome).

Strawberry nevus (hemangioma)

Not usually present at birth. Appears in first month of life (Fig. 56.2). Preterm infants at increased risk. Increases in size until 8–18 months of age then gradually regresses. May ulcerate. No treatment indicated unless it interferes with vision or the airway, when laser therapy or steroids systemically or intralesional may be indicated.

Congenital melanocytic nevus (CMN) (pigmented nevus)

Small lesions (<1.5 cm) – observe, may remove when older for cosmetic reasons. Small but possible increased risk of malignant melanoma; this contrasts with the much higher risk of giant lesions

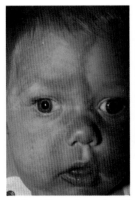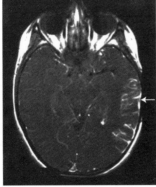

Fig. 56.1 (a) Port wine stain with trigeminal distribution (Sturge–Weber syndrome). (b) MRI scan showing intracranial vascular anomaly (arrow).

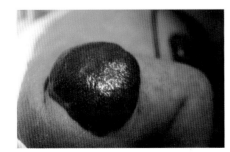

Fig. 56.2 Strawberry nevus. (Courtesy of Dr David Clark.)

(>20 cm) (Fig. 56.3), which are usually treated aggressively by surgical removal.

Genetic syndromes

There are a large number of rare conditions (Table 56.3).

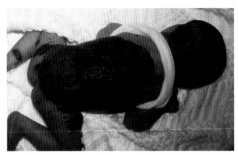

Fig. 56.3 Giant congenital melanocytic nevus (GCMN). Rare but serious condition because of 5–15% risk of malignant melanoma in first decade of life. The lesion may be hairy and satellite lesions are often present.

Table 56.3 Some skin lesions associated with genetic syndromes.

Skin lesion	Diagnostic group
Unformed skin	Aplasia cutis (absent patch of skin ± bony defect); may be associated with trisomy 13
Thin skin	Dermal hypoplasia, collagen disorders
Blisters/erosions	Bullous disorders, e.g. epidermolysis bullosa (Fig. 56.4)
Thick/scaly skin	Ichthyoses, e.g. collodion infant, or more severe, harlequin fetus
White skin/hair	Pigment deficient disorders, e.g. oculocutaneous albinism, piebaldism, tuberous sclerosis
Palpable brown patches	Syndromes with melanocytic nevi
Flat brown patches	Syndromes with café-au-lait macules, e.g. neurofibromatosis
Deficient hair, nails, sweat	Ectodermal dysplasias. Syndromes with abnormal hair

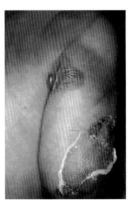

Fig. 56.4 Epidermolysis bullosa. Rare group of disorders. Bullae, or blisters, are caused by trauma or friction to the skin. There are scarring and non-scarring subgroups. (Courtesy of Prof. Julian Verbov.)

Seizures (Table 57.1)

Table 57.1 Recognition, causes, investigation and management of seizures.

Recognition	Seizures may present with clonic or tonic involuntary movements of one or more limbs. Often difficult to recognize with certainty, as manifestations are often subtle: • apnea or transient cyanosis, or episodes of oxygen desaturation • lip smacking • transient eye rolling, altered consciousness, floppiness.

Causes

Cerebral	Metabolic	Sepsis	Drugs	Others
Hypoxic–ischemic: encephalopathy, birth trauma, vascular anomaly Subarachnoid or subdural hemorrhage Parenchymal hemorrhage in preterm infants Congenital malformations of the brain	Hypoglycemia Hypocalcemia Hypomagnesemia Hyponatremia Hypernatremia Hyperammonemia	Septicemia Meningitis or encephalitis	Drug withdrawal: • maternal abuse • following neonatal narcotic therapy Side-effect of drugs	Kernicterus Pyridoxine deficiency Benign

Investigation

Always performed	EEG	To be considered
Blood glucose (immediate at bedside) Urea and electrolytes Calcium and magnesium Complete blood count Blood cultures Lumbar puncture – protein, glucose, gram stain and culture Blood gases Cranial ultrasound to identify hemorrhage or parietal infarcts or cerebral malformation or abnormalities (may miss subarachnoid hemorrhage)	EEG (Fig. 57.1) or aEEG (amplitude integrated EEG, cerebral function monitoring), which should ideally be combined with video observation – useful to identify seizures (See Chapter 13 for seizures on aEEG) 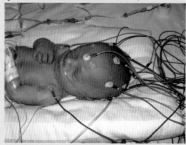 **Fig. 57.1** EEG being performed.	CT/MRI scan of brain to identify malformations, ischemic injury Metabolic screen – plasma for ammonia, amino acids, lactate; urine for amino acids and organic acids Screen for congenital infection Urine for drug toxicology

Management

Airway, Breathing, Circulation.
Check for hypoglycemia.
Anticonvulsants:
• Administer if seizure is prolonged (more than about 5 minutes) or recurs.
• No drug shown to be superior to others. Those used include phenobarbital, clonazepam, phenytoin, midazolam, paraldehyde, lidocaine (lignocaine; with ECG monitoring).
• Acute seizures often respond poorly.
• Use as few anticonvulsants as possible.
• Treat the underlying cause, if possible, e.g. sepsis.
• If resistant to treatment, consider therapeutic trial of pyridoxine.
If caused by acute brain insult, most seizures resolve and anticonvulsant therapy can usually be slowly withdrawn. If maintenance anticonvulsant therapy required – is usually with phenobarbital, clonazepam or sodium valproate.

Neonatology at a Glance, 2nd edition. Edited by Tom Lissauer & Avroy A. Fanaroff. © 2011 Blackwell Publishing Ltd.

Strokes

Probably occur in as many as 0.2–1 per 1000 live births.

Etiology

May be prenatal, but in most symptomatic infants is perinatal, characteristically in primigravid mother with long or difficult labor and slightly lower Apgar scores and umbilical artery pH compared to normal.

Types

- Arterial ischemic stroke (AIS).
- Parasagittal or border zone.
- Cerebral sinovenous thrombosis (CSVT).
  Maternal or fetal risk factors – none in 40–50%.

Clinical presentation

Poor feeding initially, focal signs or seizures on days 1–3, but many are asymptomatic.

Diagnosis

- Cranial ultrasound abnormal in 80–90% infants after day 3 but not always diagnostic.
- MRI for accurate diagnosis and prognosis (Fig. 57.2).

Prognosis

25% of infants with strokes identified in the neonatal period develop a neurologic disability, e.g. hemiplegia later in infancy or childhood from a unilateral lesion, visual impairment from occipital lesions, generalized learning difficulties and seizures with large strokes.

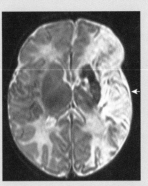

Fig. 57.2 MRI scan showing left cerebral infarct. (Courtesy of Dr Frances Cowan.)

Neural tube defects

In the embryo, the flat neural plate folds to become the brain and spinal cord. Neural tube defects arise from a deficiency in this process:
- anencephaly – from failure of cranial development of most of the cranium and brain
- spina bifida – from failure of caudal development of the vertebral bodies and spinal cord
- midline defects – from failure of fusion, e.g. of the skull as an encephalocele.

Most are now diagnosed antenatally, by ultrasound or α-fetoprotein measurement in maternal serum.

Prevalence

There is a combination of environmental and genetic factors. The risk of having a second affected infant is 3–5% and of a third 5–10%. The risk is reduced by maternal folic acid supplementation periconceptually and during early pregnancy.

In the US folic acid has been added to bread and other grain products since 1998 and the birth prevalence has dropped from 38 to 30 per 100000 live births, a 19% reduction. Other reasons for this are a natural decline and antenatal diagnosis and termination of pregnancy.

In the UK, food is not fortified with folic acid, so folic acid supplementation in low dose is recommended for all women planning a pregnancy, but compliance is poor. High-dose folic acid is given after a previously affected infant. The birth prevalence in the UK is 14 per 100000 live births.

Anencephaly

The condition is lethal; most are stillborn. There has been considerable debate about the ethics of the use of their organs for donor transplantation. However, the situation rarely arises because few

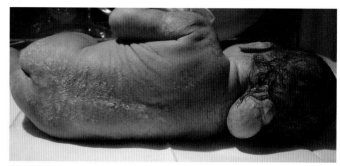

Fig. 58.1 Occipital encephalocele.

anencephalic infants are now born as most are diagnosed antenatally and parents opt for termination of pregnancy.

Encephalocele

Herniation of sac, which may contain brain, through a midline skull defect. Most are occipital (Fig. 58.1). Developmental impairment is likely if brain tissue is in the sac or there are other cerebral malformations.

Spina bifida

There are several types, of increasing severity:
- spina bifida occulta (Fig. 58.2a)
- meningocele (Fig. 58.2b)
- myelomeningocele (Figs 58.2c and d).

Spina bifida occulta

If skin lesion is over lower spine there is no neurologic deficit at birth but tethering of the spinal cord may occur during childhood.

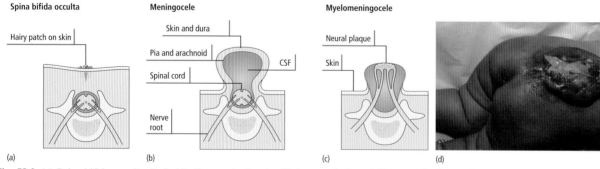

Fig. 58.2 (a) Spina bifida occulta. Defect in the vertebral arch with intact spinal cord. Frequent finding on X-rays – asymptomatic. More extensive lesions indicated by overlying patch of hair or nevus or other skin abnormality. (b) Meningocele. Bony defect with herniation of meninges but not the spinal cord. The lesion is covered with skin. (c) Myelomeningocele. Defect in the lumbar or thoracic spine with herniation of the meningeal sac and spinal cord tissue with leakage of CSF. (d) Photograph of myelomeningocele (myelo = cord; meninges = covering, cele = sac) showing exposed neural tissue and patulous, neuropathic anus.

Neonatology at a Glance, 2nd edition. Edited by Tom Lissauer & Avroy A. Fanaroff. © 2011 Blackwell Publishing Ltd.

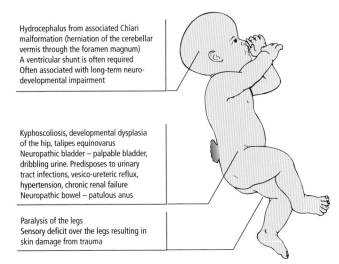

Hydrocephalus from associated Chiari malformation (herniation of the cerebellar vermis through the foramen magnum) A ventricular shunt is often required Often associated with long-term neuro-developmental impairment

Kyphoscoliosis, developmental dysplasia of the hip, talipes equinovarus Neuropathic bladder – palpable bladder, dribbling urine. Predisposes to urinary tract infections, vesico-ureteric reflux, hypertension, chronic renal failure Neuropathic bowel – patulous anus

Paralysis of the legs Sensory deficit over the legs resulting in skin damage from trauma

Fig. 58.3 Complications associated with severe myelomeningocele. These depend on the extent and level of the lesion.

An ultrasound or MRI scan of the spine is indicated and a neurosurgical opinion should be sought.

Meningocele

Prognosis following surgery is usually good.

Myelomeningocele

Wide range of complications (Fig. 58.3). Most lesions are detected antenatally and a management plan made before the baby is born.

Management requires an extensive multidisciplinary team (pediatrics, orthopedics, neurosurgery, urology, child development) and the parents and family.

The back lesion is usually closed immediately after birth to minimize the risk of infection and monitoring performed for hydrocephalus.

Hydrocephalus

This is from an excessive volume of cerebrospinal fluid (CSF). It is usually from blockage of CSF flow or a defect in CSF reabsorption.

Causes

Congenital
- Aqueduct stenosis.
- Chiari malformation.
- Atresia of outflow foramina of fourth ventricle (Dandy–Walker syndrome).
- Congenital infection.

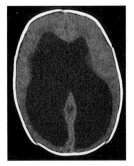

Fig. 58.4 CT scan showing ventricular dilatation in a term infant. (Courtesy of Dr Richard Nicholl.)

Acquired
- Post-intrventricular hemorrhage in preterm infants.
- Post-intracranial infection.
- Post-subdural/subarachnoid hemorrhage.

Clinical features

- Ventricular dilatation on imaging precedes symptoms or signs (Fig. 58.4).
- Increasing head circumference.
- Separation of sutures.
- Vomiting.
- Apnea, abnormal muscle tone, seizures, depressed consciousness.
- Dilatation of head veins.
- Setting-sun sign (eyes deviate downwards).
- Full then bulging fontanelle.

Monitoring and treatment

In neonates, hydrocephalus is monitored by serial cranial ultrasound measurements of ventricular size and head circumference.

If severe and progressive or the infant becomes symptomatic, a ventricular shunt is inserted surgically.

Hydrocephalus in preterm infants

This is usually secondary to intraventricular hemorrhage, which may cause obstruction but mainly interferes with CSF reabsorption. The ventricular dilatation may regress, but if it progresses a ventricular shunt will be required. Ventricular shunt insertion in small infants may have to be delayed because of the risk of skin breakdown, or shunt blockage if the CSF protein is high. If the infant becomes symptomatic but a shunt cannot be inserted, CSF may need to be removed by lumbar or ventricular puncture. A large randomized trial showed no difference in long-term outcome between repeated lumbar/ventricular taps compared with removal of CSF only when symptomatic. Drug treatment with acetazolamide, which reduces CSF production, is not used as it has been shown to be ineffective and carries a risk of electrolyte imbalance. Therapy with fibrinolytic agents is under investigation.

The 'hypotonic infant' describes marked hypotonia or floppiness, i.e. less resistance to passive movement than normal, and is usually accompanied by muscle weakness (Fig. 59.1a, b and c). The cause of the hypotonia is either:

• **central** – central nervous system, or
• **peripheral** – lower motor neuron, neuromuscular junction or muscle disorders.

The level of dysfunction needs to be established.

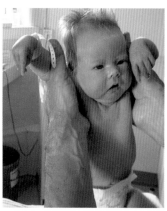

(a)

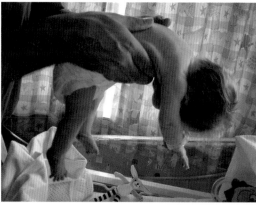

(b)

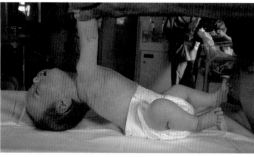

(c)

Fig. 59.1 (a) When held upright, the hypotonic infant slides through one's hands. (b) When held prone, the infant flops like a rag doll. (c) On traction of the arms, there is marked head lag.

Transient hypotonia resulting from systemic infection, electrolyte disorders, hypermagnesemia, seizures or drugs administered to the infant or mother and the reduced tone and power of preterm infants are not included in the definition of the hypotonic infant.

Clues from the history

• Family history – may be consanguinity, unexplained deaths.
• May be increasing severity with succeeding generations, e.g. muscular dystrophy.
• Clinical features in mother – ptosis in myasthenia gravis, absence of facial expression and weak grip in myotonic dystrophy and family history of cataracts.
• Pregnancy – polyhydramnios and reduced fetal movements.

Causes and clinical features (Table 59.1)

Table 59.1 Causes and clinical features of central and peripheral hypotonia.

	Central hypotonia	**Peripheral hypotonia**
Causes	Cerebral malformation Encephalopathy: • Hypoxic–ischemic encephalitis • Meningitis/encephalitis • Hypoglycemia. Chromosomal/syndromes: • Trisomy 21 (Down syndrome) • Prader–Willi syndrome Metabolic: • Hypothyroidism • Inborn errors of metabolism, e.g. hyperammonemia, amino acidopathy	Anterior horn cell: • Spinal muscular atrophy (Werdnig–Hoffmann syndrome) Neuromuscular junction: • Neonatal myasthenia gravis Muscles: • Congenital myopathies • Myotonic dystrophy
Clinical features	Antigravity movements present Normal or brisk tendon reflexes Features of brain dysfunction may be present	Weak or absent antigravity movements from severe muscle weakness Reduced or normal tendon reflexes Other features – see Fig. 59.2

Investigations

May include:
• karyotype/DNA analysis
• imaging of brain – MRI, CT or ultrasound
• blood glucose, calcium, magnesium and lactate

Neonatology at a Glance, 2nd edition. Edited by Tom Lissauer & Avroy A. Fanaroff. © 2011 Blackwell Publishing Ltd.

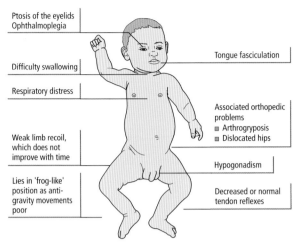

Fig. 59.2 Clinical features that may be present with a peripheral neuromuscular disorder.

Ptosis of the eyelids
Ophthalmoplegia

Difficulty swallowing

Respiratory distress

Weak limb recoil, which does not improve with time

Lies in 'frog-like' position as anti-gravity movements poor

Tongue fasciculation

Associated orthopedic problems
■ Arthrogryposis
■ Dislocated hips

Hypogonadism

Decreased or normal tendon reflexes

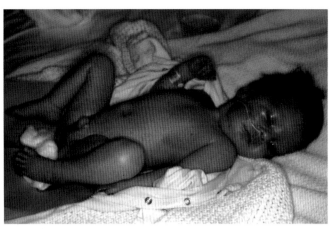

Fig. 59.3 Prader–Willi syndrome. Characteristic facies and hypogonadism. The nasogastric tube is required because of poor feeding. (Courtesy of Dr Mike Coren.)

- acid–base status, urine and plasma amino acids, urine organic acids, plasma ammonia, lactate
- CPK (creatine phosphokinase) – raised in muscular dystrophy
- thyroid function tests
- congenital infection screening tests
- EMG (electromyogram)
- muscle biopsy.

Some specific conditions

Central

Hypoxic–ischemic encephalopathy
Hypotonia may be replaced by spasticity when older.

Prader–Willi syndrome
- 70% have partial chromosomal deletion (imprinting from a paternal deletion or uniparental disomy of two maternal chromosomes).
- Characteristic facies (Fig. 59.3).
- Hypotonia.
- Hypogonadism/cryptorchidism.
- Obesity beyond neonatal period.
- Developmental delay.

Peripheral (rare)

Spinal muscular atrophy type 1 (Werdnig–Hoffmann syndrome)
- Autosomal recessive – anterior horn cell degeneration.
- Pregnancy – decrease or loss of fetal movements.

- At birth – arthrogryposis (contractures) may be present.
- Characteristic feature – fasciculation of tongue.
- Severe, progressive disorder, death from respiratory failure during first year of life.
- DNA test available.

Neonatal myasthenia gravis
- Affects 10–20% of infants of mothers with myasthenia gravis.
- Transient condition, from maternal anti-acetylcholine antibodies.
- Neonate – generalized weakness, facial diplegia, rarely ptosis, weak suck and cry, tendon reflexes normal.
- Use neostigmine, not tensilon, to confirm diagnosis.

Myotonic dystrophy
- Autosomal dominant – inherited from the mother (trinucleotide repeat expansion mutations). Earlier and more severe presentation in successive generations.
- Pregnancy – polyhydramnios and decreased fetal movement.
- Neonate – weakness, edema and petechiae at birth with or without arthrogryposis.
- Facial diplegia, ptosis, tent-shaped mouth, club foot.
- Brain abnormalities present in some forms of muscular dystrophies.
- CPK may be elevated, EMG and biopsy are diagnostic.

Congenital myopathies
- Most are recessively inherited.
- Neonate – weak, hypotonic, areflexic.
- Abnormal swallowing, normal extra-ocular movements.
- Muscle weakness usually slowly progressive.

60 Bone and joint disorders

Congenital abnormalities of the hip and feet

Developmental dysplasia of the hip, DDH (congenital dislocation of the hip, CDH)

Hip is dislocatable, dislocated and/or has shallow acetabulum.

Incidence
- 6 per 1000 live births have abnormal clinical examination on screening.
- 1.5 per 1000 live births are treated.

Risk factors, clinical examination and initial management
These are described in Chapter 16.

Treatment
- Double diapering (double nappies) – efficacy is questionable.
- Pavlik harness for 1–3 months (Fig. 60.1):
  - maintains flexion and abduction
  - redirects femoral head towards acetabulum.
- Traction, splinting or open reduction and derotation femoral osteotomy may be required.

Outcome
- 80–95% identified on screening do not need surgery.
- 5% of treated cases develop avascular necrosis (ischemic damage) of the femoral head.
- The impact of routine neonatal screening on the need for surgery is uncertain.

Talipes equinovarus

Anatomy
Foot held in rigid equinovarus position (Fig. 60.2a and b). Needs to be distinguished from positional talipes (see Chapter 20).

Incidence
1 in 1000 live births.

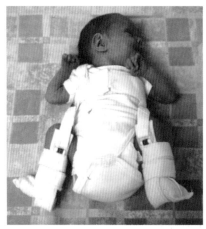

Fig. 60.1 Pavlik harness for treatment of developmental dysplasia of the hip.

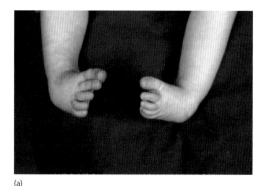

(a)

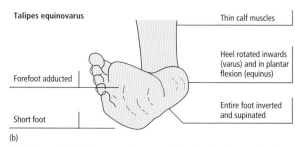

Talipes equinovarus

Forefoot adducted

Short foot

Thin calf muscles

Heel rotated inwards (varus) and in plantar flexion (equinus)

Entire foot inverted and supinated

(b)

Fig. 60.2 (a and b) Talipes equinovarus. The foot is inverted and supinated and the forefoot is adducted. The affected foot is shorter and the calf muscles thinner than normal. The position of the foot is fixed and cannot be corrected by passive manipulation.

Risk factors
- Multifactorial inheritance.
- 20–30% risk if affected parent.
- 3% risk for subsequent siblings.
- May be congenital or secondary (teratologic) to:
  - oligohydramnios
  - neuromuscular disorder, e.g. spina bifida
  - malformation syndrome.
- May be associated with developmental dysplasia of the hip.

Management
- Refer to orthopedic surgeon.
- Neonatal treatment – stretching, strapping or serial plaster casts started in first few days (Fig. 60.3).

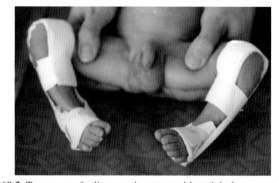

Fig. 60.3 Treatment of talipes equinovarus with serial plaster casts.

Neonatology at a Glance, 2nd edition. Edited by Tom Lissauer & Avroy A. Fanaroff. © 2011 Blackwell Publishing Ltd.

- Maximal correction is by 3 months of age.
- Corrective surgery may be required at 6–12 months.

Infection

Septic arthritis

- Rare in newborn.
- Usually from extension from underlying bone infection, rather than primary infection of the joint or from hematogenous spread.

Signs
- Decreased joint movement.
- Joint is swollen, warm, red (Fig. 60.4).
- Effusion may be present.

Diagnosis
Joint aspiration for cell count, >50 000 white blood cells/mm³ (>50 white blood cells × 10⁹/L), gram stain, culture, protein, glucose (<30% of serum level).

Imaging
- Ultrasound – fluid in joint space.
- Radionuclide bone scan, if indicated – hot spot.
- MRI scan of bone if necessary.
  Plain X-ray is of limited value – may show widened joint space.

Treatment
- Single or repeated needle aspiration.
- Surgical drainage of hip joint if no improvement.
- Antibiotics – prolonged course for 3–6 weeks.

Long-term complications
- Erosion of articular surface.
- Joint ankylosis.

Osteomyelitis

- Rare in newborn.
- Most are hematogenous in origin, in metaphysis.
- Usually presents within first 2 weeks of life.

Pathogens
Commonest are *Staphylococcus aureus* and streptococci.

Signs
- No movement (pseudoparalysis) of limb.
- Red, warm, swollen, painful limb.

Diagnosis
- Blood culture positive.
- Bone aspiration for cultures if indicated.

Imaging
- Ultrasound – periosteal elevation and soft tissue swelling.
- Radionuclide bone scan, if indicated – hot spot (needle aspiration does not produce positive bone scan).
- Plain X-ray – limited use at this stage, as only shows periosteal elevation and soft tissue swelling.
- MRI scan of bone if necessary.

Treatment
Antibiotics – prolonged course for 3–6 weeks. Continue for 2–3 weeks after symptoms resolve and ESR (erythrocyte sedimentation rate) or CRP (C-reactive protein) normalizes.

Skeletal dysplasias

There are several hundred, with shortening of the limbs and spine resulting in short stature.

Achondroplasia

- Short bowed limbs, normal trunk, large head.
- Midface hypoplasia, frontal bossing.
- Trident hand (short and broad), protuberant abdomen.

Osteogenesis imperfecta

- Inherited disorder of type 1 collagen formation.
- Rare – 1 in 20 000 live births.

Clinical features
- Increased bone fragility, susceptibility to fracture (Fig. 60.5).
- Blue sclerae, defective tooth formation in some patients.
- Hearing loss.
- Scoliosis, kyphosis.

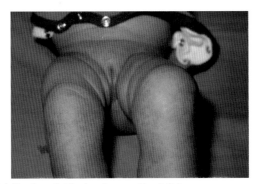

Fig. 60.4 Septic arthritis showing swollen left knee.

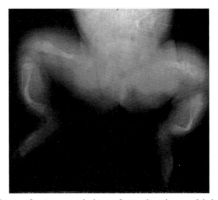

Fig. 60.5 X-ray of osteogenesis imperfecta showing multiple fractures.

Hearing

Congenital hearing loss affects 1–2/1000 live births. If the infant receives neonatal intensive care, risk is increased 10-fold.

Hearing loss is:
- **conductive** – involves conduction of sound in the middle or outer ear, often occurs in childhood from secretory otitis media;
- **sensorineural** – involves the hair cells of the cochlea in the inner ear, or the cochlear branch of cranial nerve VIII, as in congenital or neonatal hearing loss.

The speech and language of children with severe hearing impairment is delayed or does not develop. The earlier in life hearing can be restored or specialist assistance provided, the better the outcome. Screening infants with risk factors (Table 61.1) identifies only 40–60% of significant bilateral hearing loss. Universal screening in the first few days of life, and certainly by the age of 3 months is therefore recommended (Table 61.2).

Table 61.1 Risk factors for hearing loss.

Family history
Syndromes with hearing loss
Malformations of the ears, including pits and tags
Perinatal
Very low birthweight
Congenital infection – e.g. CMV (cytomegalovirus), rubella
Severe hyperbilirubinemia
Ototoxic medications, e.g. furosemide
Mechanical ventilation or extracorporeal membrane oxygenation
Hypoxic–ischemic encephalopathy
Bacterial meningitis

Table 61.2 Rationale for universal hearing screening.

Is hearing impairment common?
Yes – more common than hypothyroidism, phenylketonuria or hemoglobinopathy
Is the condition serious?
Yes. Results in marked speech and language delay
Is treatment available?
Yes. Sound amplification including cochlea implantation, finger-spelling, lip-reading, use of gestures and sign language to maximize early development of language skills
Are reliable screening tests available?
Yes. Acceptable sensitivity and specificity
Are other methods of detection available?
Other methods, e.g. parental concern, are unreliable
Does it improve outcome?
Yes. The earlier amplification and specialist intervention for infant and family, the better the outcome
Also offers possibility of preventing progression in certain cases and anticipating other difficulties, e.g. visual deterioration in Usher syndrome
Can it be done at reasonable cost?
Yes, but requires skilled facilities for diagnostic confirmation and habilitation

Neonatal hearing screening

Can be performed using the automated auditory brainstem response (AABR) (Fig. 61.1) or evoked otoacoustic emissions (EOAE) (Fig. 61.2).

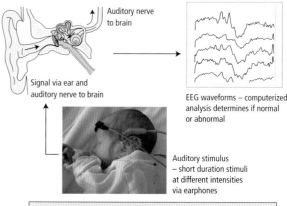

Automated auditory brainstem response audiometry (AABR)

Auditory nerve to brain

Signal via ear and auditory nerve to brain

EEG waveforms – computerized analysis determines if normal or abnormal

Auditory stimulus – short duration stimuli at different intensities via earphones

Advantages
- Screens hearing pathway from ear to brainstem
- Good for testing speech wavelengths
- Detects moderate hearing loss
- Few false negatives, false positive rate <3%, the lowest referral rate of the screening tests available

Disadvantages
- Affected by movement, so infants need to be asleep or very quiet, so time consuming
- Complex computerized equipment, but is mobile
- Requires electrodes applied to infant's head, which parents may dislike

Fig. 61.1 Automated auditory brainstem response (AABR).

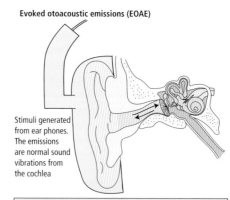

Evoked otoacoustic emissions (EOAE)

Stimuli generated from ear phones. The emissions are normal sound vibrations from the cochlea

Advantages
- Simple and quick to perform, though is affected by ambient noise

Disadvantages
- Misses auditory neuropathy
- False positive rate of up to 30% in first 24 hours after birth as vernix or amniotic fluid are still in ear canal
  Referral rate of 6–8%, with risk of loss to follow-up
  Can reduce referral rate to 1% by doing AABR if fail EOAE testing but adds complexity to screening program

Fig. 61.2 Evoked otoacoustic emissions (EOAE).

Neonatology at a Glance, 2nd edition. Edited by Tom Lissauer & Avroy A. Fanaroff. © 2011 Blackwell Publishing Ltd.

Vision

The normal term infant will fix and follow horizontally a moving face, a brightly colored object (e.g. a red ball) or a picture of a target of black and white concentric circles by about 6 weeks. They prefer to look at high contrast patterned objects rather than plain ones.

Visual acuity is initially poor – only about 6/200. It improves over the first few months, to 6/60 at 3 months, but adult visual acuity is not reached until about 3 years. At birth, many have mild hypermetropia (far-sightedness), which persists through early childhood; clarity of vision is achieved by accommodation. This contrasts with preterm infants, who often become myopic (nearsighted).

The eyes of newborn infants are often not aligned, and an intermittent squint (strabismus) is common during the first weeks of life. A constant squint or one persisting beyond 12 weeks post term should be referred to an ophthalmologist.

Lesions needing urgent ophthalmologic referral

During early childhood, failure of focused visual images to reach the retina, e.g. from a cataract or glaucoma, results in permanent loss of vision (amblyopia). Optimal vision is achieved if surgery and optical correction are performed soon after birth. Affected infants must therefore be referred urgently to an ophthalmologist for surgery.

Cataracts (Fig. 61.3)
Cataracts may be detected by parents or on checking the red reflex with an ophthalmoscope during the routine examination of the newborn, but may otherwise present with blindness at several months of age. Many are genetic, but congenital infection and other causes must be excluded. They are infrequent.

Congenital glaucoma (Fig. 61.4)
Intraocular pressure is raised. There is watering of the eyes, photophobia and irritability. The eye becomes enlarged and the cornea hazy. Most are bilateral.

Other congenital abnormalities

There are numerous, rare, congenital abnormalities of the eye, including:
- anophthalmos/microphthalmos (absent or extremely small eye)
- coloboma (Fig. 61.5) may affect iris, ciliary body, choroid and optic nerve. Vision may be normal in mild cases, but poor if optic nerve involved
- aniridia (absence of iris)
- albinism (lack of melanin pigment in iris and retina) – may be ocular or generalized, often resulting in macular hypoplasia, nystagmus and poor vision
- white pupil (leukocoria) or white reflex on ophthalmoscopy – causes include retinoblastoma, cataract, retinopathy of prematurity.

Affected infants should be referred to an ophthalmologist.

The causes of severe visual impairment and blindness in children are listed in Table 61.3. Most visually disabled children also have other disabilities.

Other eye conditions

- Retinopathy of prematurity – see Chapter 34.
- Conjunctivitis – see Chapter 42.
- Chorioretinitis in congenital infection – see Chapter 10.

Table 61.3 Causes of severe visual impairment and blindness in children (<16 years).

Whole globe and anterior segment	7%
Glaucoma, cornea, lens (cataract)	10%
Congenital infection	2%
Retina	29%
Retinopathy of prematurity	3%
Oculocutaneous albinism	4%
Optic nerve, cerebral/visual pathways	76%

In some children there was more than one cause.
From Rahi *et al.* Severe visual impairment and blindness in children in the UK. *Lancet* 2003; **362**: 1359–1365.

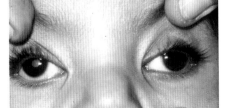

Cataract

Fig. 61.3 Cataract in right eye of a newborn infant. (Courtesy of Prof. Alistair Fielder.)

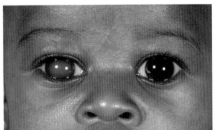

Glaucoma

Fig. 61.4 Congenital glaucoma of right eye. (Courtesy of Prof. Alistair Fielder.)

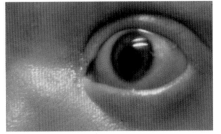

Coloboma

Fig. 61.5 Iris coloboma. Keyhole-shaped pupil due to defect of the iris inferiorly.

Pain is a subjective cortical experience. Although neonates cannot describe a painful experience to us, there is good evidence from physiologic and behavioral responses that they respond to pain and it causes distress (Table 62.1). Pain is one of the main parental concerns for infants in intensive care or undergoing procedures. Parents often also worry about long-term consequences. There is evidence that children who undergo repeated painful experiences as neonates show increased sensitivity to pain in childhood, e.g. to an immunization, and are more fearful of pain than their peers.

Development of pain pathways in the fetus and preterm infant

Although it was thought for many years that preterm and newborn infants were unable to feel pain as their nerves were unmyelinated, it has now been shown that at:
• 20 weeks' gestation – sensory receptors and cortical neurons have developed
• 24 weeks – cortical synapses are present
• 30 weeks – myelination of pain pathways and development of spinal cord synapses with sensory fibers.

Implications

• Even preterm infants have anatomic, neurophysiologic and hormonal components to perceive pain.
• Central descending inhibitory control is less well developed – so response to painful stimuli is actually greater than in older children and adults.

Factors that modify pain responses

Infants requiring intensive care are subjected to an average of two to ten painful procedures per day. They are also repeatedly disturbed, e.g. for examination, nursing care, etc.

The pain they experience will be affected by:
• procedure being performed (Fig. 62.1), the skill of the operator and their concern about minimizing pain and discomfort
• gestational age and postnatal age

Table 62.1 Some milestones in neonatal pain.

1987	Thoracotomy for surgical ligation of patent ductus arteriosus – greater physiologic and hormonal responses if performed without analgesia
2000	American Academy of Pediatrics Policy Statement on Prevention and Management of Pain and Stress in the Neonate. Updated 2006
2001	International Consensus Statement for the Prevention and Management of Pain in the Newborn

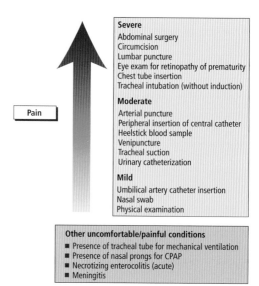

Fig. 62.1 Postulated hierarchy of pain from procedures. (Adapted from Porter F *et al.* Procedural pain in newborn infants: the influence of intensity and development. *Pediatrics* 1999; **104**: 1–10.)

• behavioral state
• number of previous painful experiences
• time since last painful experience
• severity of their illness.

Assessment of pain

Pain can be assessed clinically according to:
• Physiologic responses:
  – heart rate, respiratory rate, oxygen requirement, blood pressure, palmar sweating.
• Behavioral responses:
  – facial expression, body movements, crying.
• Metabolic responses:
  – stress hormones, e.g. cortisol
  – blood glucose, lactate.

These may be used as proxy measures of pain. Obtaining reliable results is problematic and their interpretation is difficult.

Pain assessment scales

A variety of neonatal pain assessment scales have been developed (Table 62.2), mainly for clinical research or postoperative pain assessment (CRIES score). The simpler scales can also be used for regular, systematic pain assessment for infants undergoing intensive care, or as guidance for staff on pain assessment.

Neonatology at a Glance, 2nd edition. Edited by Tom Lissauer & Avroy A. Fanaroff. © 2011 Blackwell Publishing Ltd.

Table 62.2 Some validated pain assessment scales in newborn and preterm infants.

Neonatal Pain, Agitation and Sedation Scale (NPASS)	Premature Infant Pain Profile (PIPP)	Neonatal Facial Coding Scale (NFCS)	CRIES score
Behavioral cues: • Sleep in preceding hour • Facial expression of pain • Motor activity, tone • Consolability, cry Physiologic cues: • Heart rate • Systolic blood pressure • Respiratory frequency and pattern • Oxygen saturation	Gestational age Behavioral state Brow bulge Eye squeeze Nasolabial furrow Heart rate Oxygen saturation	Brow bulge Eye squeeze Nasolabial furrow Open lips Stretch mouth Lip purse Taut tongue Chin quiver Tongue protrusion	**C**rying **R**equires increased oxygen **I**ncreased vital signs **E**xpression **S**leeplessness

Minimizing pain

There are both non-pharmacologic and pharmacologic approaches. Always consider:
• is any procedure really necessary?
• timing the procedure for when the infant is awake, if possible
• grouping procedures together, **but** limit the number of procedures occurring within a short time of each other (as with physical training, we all need recovery time!)
• using equipment or methods designed to minimize discomfort (e.g. appropriate heel lancets, non-invasive monitoring, venous or arterial catheters to avoid repeated skin punctures, avoiding intramuscular injections unless essential, etc.).

Non-pharmacologic

These include:
• environmental modification:
  – quiet, shade for baby's eyes, talking to baby, slow stroking, rocking, skin-to-skin contact
• non-nutritive sucking on a pacifier (dummy) or sucking on breast
• sucrose – high-concentration sucrose shown to reduce pain response; breast milk may also be helpful
• positioning on side, wrapping (not tight), comfort holding with still hands (Fig. 62.2)
• opportunities for the baby to grasp and to brace feet.

Pharmacologic approaches

Infants on mechanical ventilation
In neonates, use of analgesic/anesthetic agents differ between units. The most widely used are:
• morphine – side effects include drop in blood pressure, respiratory depression and abstinence (withdrawal) syndrome if too rapid dose reduction after prolonged use
• fentanyl – side effects include respiratory depression, tolerance, glottic and chest wall rigidity.

Procedures
Optimal analgesia aims to prevent rather than treat pain. In the past, fear of side effects limited the use of opioids and anesthetic

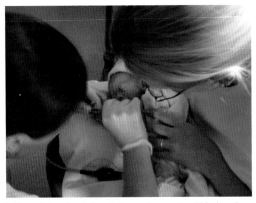

Fig. 62.2 Containing the infant helps reduce pain. This involves secure, supported, non-restrictive positioning, not tight swaddling to prevent moving. Here, during the insertion of a nasogastric tube, the mother is containing her baby and the infant is grasping the nurse's finger.

agents, but it should now be possible to provide adequate pain relief, especially postoperatively. Options include:
• opioids – additional boluses may be required if on continuous opioid infusion
• general anesthesia – all major or surgical procedures
• regional anesthesia – e.g. peripheral nerve blocks, spinal or epidural, local infiltration – increasingly used in neonates for some surgical procedures and postoperative analgesia
• non-opioids – e.g. acetaminophen (paracetamol); sometimes used for a minor procedure or postoperatively.

Question

How can the pain of heelsticks be minimized?
Pain is mainly from squeezing the foot, so keep to minimum.
Autostylets are less painful than lancets. Venepuncture is less painful than heelsticks and adequate samples are obtained twice as often, but not suitable for repeated sampling.
Topical analgesia – not effective for heelsticks and not licensed in US in newborns. Theoretical concern about methemoglobinemia, but not a problem in practice.
Analgesia – sucrose or breast milk or nurse at breast.

Pharmacology includes the study of:
- the effects of drugs on the body (pharmacodynamics)
- the effect of the body on drugs (pharmacokinetics – *a*bsorption, *d*istribution, *m*etabolism, *e*limination)
- the use of drugs.

The pharmacology, and in particular the pharmacokinetics of drugs in neonates differs significantly from that in children and adults. Primarily this is the result of their different physiology (Fig. 63.1).

Drug prescription and administration

The wide variation in absorption, metabolism, excretion and body composition is mainly related to the neonate's gestational age and postnatal age together with their variation in size, from less than 500 grams in the extreme preterm to 5000 grams in the large term infant. As a result, drug regimens are complex and vary according to age and are usually calculated as a dose per kilogram.

Drug monitoring

Monitoring plasma levels of drugs is useful if there is a known concentration range within which the drug works and has no toxicity. This applies to only a few drugs, but some of them are in routine use in neonatology (e.g. gentamicin, vancomycin). Monitoring may involve the measurement of peak and trough plasma concentrations, or trough levels only. Measurements are made once the drug has reached steady-state (Fig. 63.2).

Drugs in breast milk

Neonates may be exposed to maternal drugs through their consumption of breast milk. Breast milk has a lower pH than blood (pH 7.0 versus pH 7.4) and a high fat content and will therefore concentrate basic and fat soluble drugs. Highly protein-bound drugs do not tend to transfer into milk as easily. The concentration of a drug in breast milk will vary with its concentration in maternal

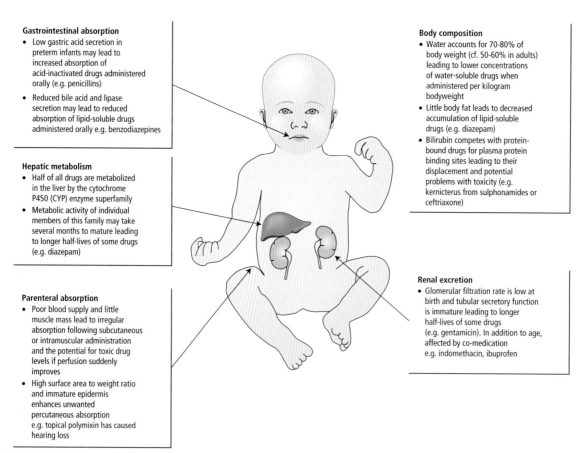

Gastrointestinal absorption
- Low gastric acid secretion in preterm infants may lead to increased absorption of acid-inactivated drugs administered orally (e.g. penicillins)
- Reduced bile acid and lipase secretion may lead to reduced absorption of lipid-soluble drugs administered orally e.g. benzodiazepines

Hepatic metabolism
- Half of all drugs are metabolized in the liver by the cytochrome P450 (CYP) enzyme superfamily
- Metabolic activity of individual members of this family may take several months to mature leading to longer half-lives of some drugs (e.g. diazepam)

Parenteral absorption
- Poor blood supply and little muscle mass lead to irregular absorption following subcutaneous or intramuscular administration and the potential for toxic drug levels if perfusion suddenly improves
- High surface area to weight ratio and immature epidermis enhances unwanted percutaneous absorption e.g. topical polymixin has caused hearing loss

Body composition
- Water accounts for 70-80% of body weight (cf. 50-60% in adults) leading to lower concentrations of water-soluble drugs when administered per kilogram bodyweight
- Little body fat leads to decreased accumulation of lipid-soluble drugs (e.g. diazepam)
- Bilirubin competes with protein-bound drugs for plasma protein binding sites leading to their displacement and potential problems with toxicity (e.g. kernicterus from sulphonamides or ceftriaxone)

Renal excretion
- Glomerular filtration rate is low at birth and tubular secretory function is immature leading to longer half-lives of some drugs (e.g. gentamicin). In addition to age, affected by co-medication e.g. indomethacin, ibuprofen

Fig. 63.1 Key physiologic factors affecting neonatal pharmacology.

Neonatology at a Glance, 2nd edition. Edited by Tom Lissauer & Avroy A. Fanaroff. © 2011 Blackwell Publishing Ltd.

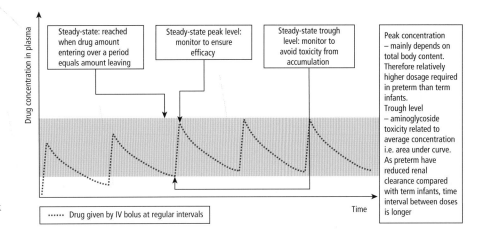

Fig. 63.2 Drug monitoring – steady-state, peak and trough levels.

Steady-state: reached when drug amount entering over a period equals amount leaving

Steady-state peak level: monitor to ensure efficacy

Steady-state trough level: monitor to avoid toxicity from accumulation

Peak concentration – mainly depends on total body content. Therefore relatively higher dosage required in preterm than term infants. Trough level – aminoglycoside toxicity related to average concentration i.e. area under curve. As preterm have reduced renal clearance compared with term infants, time interval between doses is longer

Drug concentration in plasma

Drug given by IV bolus at regular intervals

Time

plasma; drugs with a short half-life that may be given after feeding are to be preferred. The majority of drugs are transferred into breast milk in concentrations too low to affect neonatal health; certain drugs must be avoided and general advice should be to avoid the use of any medications wherever possible (Table 63.1).

Drug licensing and neonatalogy

Up to 80% of drugs administered in neonatal intensive care are not licensed by a national licensing body (FDA, Food and Drug Administration, in the US; EMEA, European Medicines Agency in Europe) for use in this population (*unlicensed*), or are used outside their license, e.g. other dosing regimens, other formulation

(*off-label*). Doctors can prescribe and nurses can administer unlicensed and off-label medicines, but, it imposes additional responsibility on prescribers to ensure that the use of a particular drug is supported by the best available evidence. Considerable effort and finance is now being devoted to the development, research and licensing of medicines for children.

Question

What lessons in neonatal pharmacology have been learnt from the past?

1886: Aniline dyes used to stamp names on diapers absorbed percutaneously and cause methemoglobinemia.

1956: Sulfonamides displace bilirubin from plasma protein binding sites and cause kernicterus.

1959: Chloramphenicol causes the 'gray baby' syndrome of circulatory collapse due to immature glucuronidation.

1982: Benzyl alcohol, added to intravenous flush solutions as a bacteriostatic agent, accumulates in newborns causing death, intraventricular hemorrhage and the 'gasping baby' syndrome.

1985: Polysorbate 80, a carrier in a parenteral vitamin E preparation, associated with liver failure.

1989: Topical iodine-containing antiseptics noted to be absorbed and may cause hypothyroidism – now used sparingly and excess removed.

Table 63.1 Examples of drugs used in breast-feeding mothers that may affect nursing infant. A formulary should always be consulted.

Maternal drug	Effect on infant
Examples of drugs to avoid	
Radioactive iodine	May cause thyroid suppression
Cytotoxic agents	Risk of cytotoxic effect
Diazepam	May cause sedation and may accumulate
Tetracycline	Possibility of permanent staining of teeth
Lithium	Risk of neurological effects, cardiac malformations

Quality assurance

Quality assurance (clinical governance) is a framework for accounting for the quality of clinical services and for their improvement (Fig. 64.1). It is a key issue for all who provide care for newborn infants.

Clinical audit

Aims to improve patient care and outcomes through systematic review against explicit criteria followed by change. The audit cycle is shown in Fig. 64.2, and questions about audit are addressed in Table 64.1. The PDSA cycle (Plan, Do, Study, Act), shown in Fig. 64.3, is used to implement improvements rapidly.

Critical incident reporting (Table 64.2)

Reporting critical incidents, not only those that have caused harm but also those that could have caused harm are a key component of quality assurance. The most common and serious critical incidents in neonatal practice and ways to minimize the risk of them occurring are considered in Chapter 65.

Simulation

Simulation has become an important component of quality assurance in neonatal care. It is widely used for multidisciplinary life support courses, e.g. for neonatal resuscitation and emergencies. It is also increasingly used to simulate emergencies or other situations in the workplace, whether in the neonatal unit, delivery room or lying-in (postnatal) wards. It can be used to improve not only medical management, but also leadership skills, multidisciplinary teamwork and communication skills. It also allows training in some practical procedures before performing them on patients.

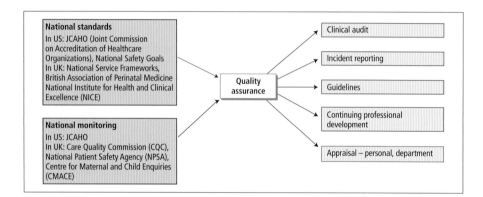

Fig. 64.1 Framework for quality assurance.

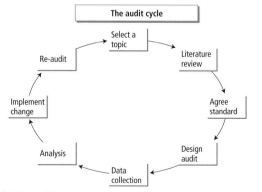

Fig. 64.2 The audit cycle.

Table 64.1 Questions about audit.

Who?	All health professionals
How are topics selected?	Observing current practice Clinical incidents, complaints and claims, etc.
Design?	Agree standards Multidisciplinary Identify data sample Only collect relevant data
Analysis and recommendations	Were standards met? Feedback results Identify improvements Develop an action plan Re-audit to check improvement

Neonatology at a Glance, 2nd edition. Edited by Tom Lissauer & Avroy A. Fanaroff. © 2011 Blackwell Publishing Ltd.

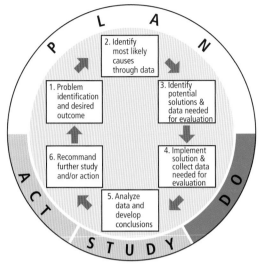

Fig. 64.3 The PDSA cycle to rapidly initiate change in practice and evaluate it.

Table 64.2 Questions and answers about critical incidents.

What are they?	Unexpected events that cause or could cause harm to the patient. Include near-misses
Who should report them?	Everyone
What should be reported?	The facts
Why report?	To identify causes To develop a strategy to prevent recurrence To act as warning for complaints/litigation To provide information for external monitoring
Who is to blame?	A no-blame culture should be developed – disciplinary action will not follow *except* where acts or omissions are malicious, criminal, or constitute professional misconduct
What level of investigation is required?	Depends on extent of harm to the patient and assessment of likelihood of recurrence by taking the whole circumstance of the event into account, not just the incident itself If risk of harm or recurrence is high, perform root cause analysis
What is root cause analysis?	Asks why it occurred rather than focusing on the problem
What if major harm has occurred or major damage to the organization?	Because of potential litigation, the hospital risk management group and senior managers should be informed. A more detailed, formal causal analysis (FMEA, failure mode and effect analysis) should be undertaken

Question

Are there any quality improvement initiatives specifically for neonatal care?

Many local and national initiatives, but the most comprehensive dedicated to neonatal care is the Vermont–Oxford Neonatal Intensive Care Quality Network.

It aims to improve the quality and safety of medical care for newborn infants and their families by:
• providing an information resource which also uses material from other disciplines in health-care and other professions, e.g. aviation industry
• providing expert faculty
• promoting four key habits to improve outcome (Fig. 64.4)
• organizing collaborative safety improvement projects, e.g. reducing nosocomial infection, by visits between units or via the internet
• voluntary, anonymous collection of errors on internet.

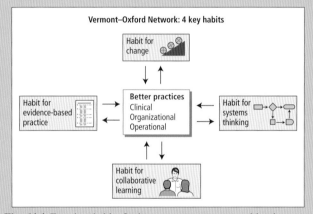

Fig. 64.4 Four key habits for better outcomes promoted by the Vermont–Oxford Network. (Reproduced with permission of J. Horbar, Vermont–Oxford Network.)

A survey in the US showed that medical errors were responsible for 98 000 deaths per year, i.e. more people die in a year in the US from medical errors than from motor vehicle accidents or breast cancer.

In a prospective study of pediatric admissions to hospital, potential adverse events were highest in the NICU (neonatal intensive care unit):

- 91% of admissions had a medication error
- 46% of admissions had a potential adverse event
- 74% of errors involved physician ordering.

Neonatal critical incidents which may relate to fetal or obstetric care will need to be considered in conjunction with maternal–fetal medicine, e.g. hypoxic–ischemic encephalopathy or seizures within 48 hours of birth. Other critical incidents involving neonatal care are considered in Chapter 64 on neonatal quality assurance.

The most common critical incidents are medication errors and extravasation injuries, but a selection of frequent or important examples follows. Some approaches to their prevention are given, but each critical incident will need to be considered by the multidisciplinary risk management team.

Prevention of critical incidents requires a culture of safety throughout the unit (Fig. 65.1).

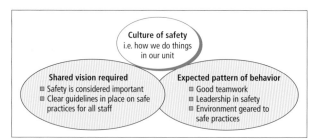

Fig. 65.1 Requirements of a culture of safety in the neonatal unit. (Adapted from J. Horbar, Vermont–Oxford Network.)

Extravasation of intravenous infusions (Figs 65.2 and 65.3)

Cause

- Fragile tissues.
- Small catheter, difficult to fix securely.
- Movement by infant.
- Irritant infusion – e.g. calcium, high concentration of dextrose, total parenteral nutrition.

Prevention

- Expert fixation of catheters.
- Leave potential extravasation area uncovered to be visible.
- Avoid occluding limb with tape.

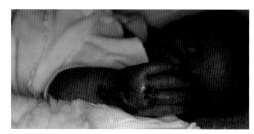

Fig. 65.2 Extravasation injury.

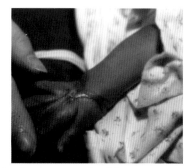

Fig. 65.3 Scarring from extravasation injury.

Medication errors

Why?

- Prescription errors occur as there is a wide range of dosage – varies 10-fold if baby weighs 0.5 kg or 5 kg (unlike adults, where there is usually a standard dose).
- Dilutions often needed – common source of error.
- Use of potentially dangerous drugs – insulin, inotropes, aminophylline, digoxin, narcotics, heparin.

Prevention

- Staff training, with input and checking by pediatric pharmacist.
- Clear formulary.
- Minimize range of drugs used.
- Computer-assisted guidance on dosage and dilutions.
- Avoid abbreviations, e.g. micrograms, not μg.
- Use limited number of standard dilutions, drawn up in pharmacy where possible.
- Clear differentiation between vials, e.g. by color.
- Checking by two trained professionals (but do not rely on this).
- Remove undiluted dangerous drugs, e.g. strong KCl.
- Pay special attention to dangerous drugs.

Neonatology at a Glance, 2nd edition. Edited by Tom Lissauer & Avroy A. Fanaroff. © 2011 Blackwell Publishing Ltd.

- Regular checks, pressure-sensitive alarms.
- Give irritant infusions via central lines if possible.

What to do if extensive

- Flush affected area with saline via several skin punctures. Elevate affected limb.
- Consult plastic surgeons if concern about long-term scarring.

Excessive fluid volume infused

Cause

- Incorrect settings on pump.
- Malfunction of pump.

Prevention

- Check and monitor infusion.

Giving wrong breast milk to wrong patient

Cause

- Similar names.
- Poor labeling.

Prevention

- Clear labeling.
- Double-checking.
- Warning mechanism (name alert tags) for staff if similar names.

Complications of umbilical arterial catheters (UAC)

Incorrect vessel

- Inserted into umbilical vein instead of artery.

Prevention
- Check for presence of arterial pulsation to confirm in artery.
- Check position on abdominal X-ray (Fig. 65.4).

    This is important – if in umbilical vein by mistake, excessively high oxygen will be given, which could damage eyes (retinopathy of prematurity, ROP) if preterm.

Thrombosis/emboli/vasoconstriction

Consequences
- Occlusion of the artery causes mottling of skin and cyanosis in one or both legs. May result in gangrene/amputation of limb.
- Emboli may affect distant organs.

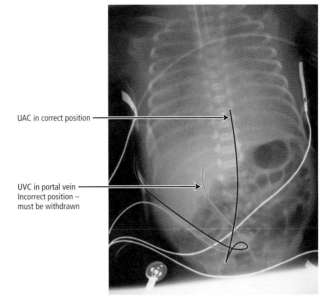

UAC in correct position

UVC in portal vein
Incorrect position –
must be withdrawn

Fig. 65.4 X-ray showing umbilical arterial and venous catheters. Catheter in umbilical artery (red line) – initial course caudally towards groin, then cranially up middle of spine. Catheter in umbilical vein (blue line) – cranial course to right of spine. This catheter is in the portal vein, a potentially dangerous position, and must be withdrawn. In addition, overlapping catheters, as shown here, can easily lead to misinterpretation.

Prevention
- Regular observation. If skin becomes discolored, reposition or remove catheter.
- Position catheter either high at T6–10 or low at L3–4 to avoid catheter tip near renal vessels to reduce risk of renal artery thrombosis (hematuria, renal failure, hypertension).
- Flush catheter gently, heparinize line.
- Ensure infant's intravascular volume is adequate.

Blood loss from arterial catheters

Cause

- Disconnection of catheter.

Prevention

- Clear labeling that catheter is arterial.
- Connections screwed together.
- Pressure-sensitive alarm.

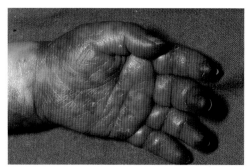

Fig. 65.5 Ischemic damage from radial artery catheter.

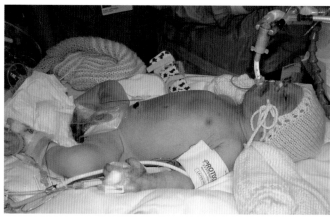

Fig. 65.6 Scalding of skin from excessive heat from radiant warmer on dislodging of skin temperature probe. It resolved within a few hours.

Ischemic damage from peripheral artery catheters

Cause

• Small size of vessel.

Prevention

• Choose suitable artery:
  – use radial artery only if ulnar artery shown to be patent (Fig. 65.5) (see Chapter 75 for Allen test)
  – avoid superficial temporal artery as can cause ischemia of parietal lobe
  – avoid brachial artery as end artery and occlusion may result in loss of distal limb, and median nerve may be damaged.
• Only use for sampling, not injecting.
• Remove if blanching, other than transient.

Portal vein thrombosis from umbilical venous catheters

Cause

• Catheter in portal vein causing portal vein thrombosis.

Prevention

• Check on X-ray that catheter is in the inferior vena cava and not the portal vein (Fig. 65.4).

Extravasation of total parenteral nutrition (TPN) from central venous lines

Cause

• Catheters may migrate and TPN may be infused into:
  – the tissues, causing swelling and inflammation
  – the lungs, causing pleural effusion
  – the pericardium, causing pericardial effusion and tamponade.

Prevention

• Check catheter tip is in the inferior or superior vena cava, not the right atrium.

Burns and scalds

Cause

• Overheating of humidifier in CPAP/ventilator circuit.
• Disconnection of temperature probe or malfunctioning of radiant warmer (Fig. 65.6).
• Failure to regularly move transcutaneous O_2/CO_2 probes.

Prevention

• Temperature alarms.

Scarring of skin

Cause

• Poorly keratinized skin prone to long-term scarring, especially if black ethnicity (keloid formation).

Prevention

• Minimize skin damage:
  – care with adhesive tape, probes and pressure from attachments for tracheal tubes, nasal CPAP, etc.
  – if transcutaneous O_2/CO_2 electrodes used, rotate to different skin sites regularly
  – procedures, e.g. chest tube for pneumothorax, incise skin along line of skinfold (Fig. 65.7).

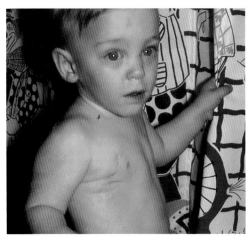

Fig. 65.7 Scarring from chest tubes.

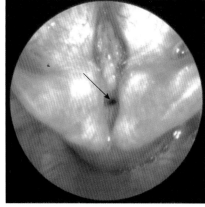

Fig. 65.8 Tracheal stenosis following prolonged mechanical ventilation. The narrowed trachea is shown with an arrow.

Nasal damage from tracheal tube

Cause

- Dilatation of nostril or damage to the nasal septum by tube.

Prevention

- Avoid excessively large tracheal tubes.
- Avoid leaving in situ for long periods.
- Fix tube securely to prevent leverage.

Nasal damage from nasal CPAP

Cause

- Pressure on nostrils or nasal septum.

Prevention

- Correct positioning and fixing of nasal prongs, avoiding excessive pressure on the nostrils or nose.

Tracheal stenosis

Cause

- Damage to subglottic area from tracheal tube (Fig. 65.8).

Prevention

- Avoid excessively large tubes.
- Minimize time left in place.
- Secure to prevent tube movement and irritation.

Infection

Cause

- Nosocomial infection – inadequate hand-washing.
- Catheter related – at insertion or subsequently, e.g. breaking of long line.
- Procedures – infection where skin denuded from monitor probes or tape.

Prevention

- **Meticulous hand-washing**.
- Sterile insertion.
- Minimize interference of lines.
- Remove lines as soon as possible.

Aspiration pneumonia from misplaced gavage (nasogastric) feeding tubes

Cause

- Tube inserted into trachea instead of stomach.

Prevention

- Check correct position with pH indicator paper.

What is evidence-based medicine (EBM)?

It is the conscientious, explicit and judicious use of current best evidence in making decisions about the care of individual patients.

Steps in the practice of evidence-based medicine

See Fig. 66.1.

Examples of evidence-based medicine in neonatology

The following are some examples from neonatal medicine of therapy proven to be beneficial or harmful. However, for most decisions in clinical practice, guidance from evidence-based medicine is not available, is inconclusive or may be conflicting. Clinicians have to base their decisions on the best available information, clinical experience and the evaluation of potential benefits and risks for the individual patient.

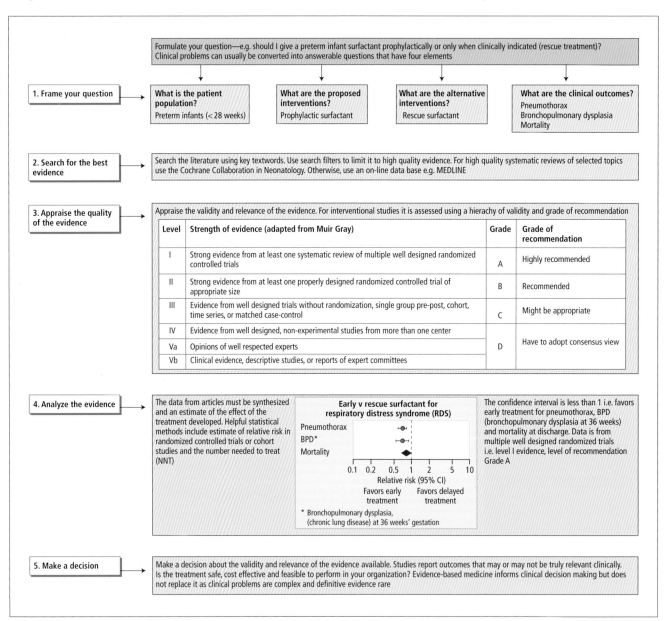

Fig. 66.1 Steps in the practice of EBM (evidence-based medicine). (Data on surfactant from Yost CC, Soll RF. Early versus delayed selective surfactant treatment for neonatal respiratory distress syndrome (Cochrane Review). In: *The Cochrane Library,* Issue 1, 2004. Chichester, UK: John Wiley & Sons, Ltd.)

Neonatology at a Glance, 2nd edition. Edited by Tom Lissauer & Avroy A. Fanaroff. © 2011 Blackwell Publishing Ltd.

Beneficial therapies

Examples of therapies shown to be beneficial are:
- Maternal prophylactic corticosteroids for preterm birth.
- Maternal anti-D (Rho) immunoglobulin – to rhesus negative mothers to prevent rhesus disease of the newborn.
- Surfactant therapy in preterm infants.
- Natural versus synthetic surfactant – natural produces greater reduction in ventilator support, fewer pneumothoraces and fewer deaths, but a possible increase in intraventricular hemorrhage (but not for severe hemorrhages).
- Moderate hypothermia for moderate or severe HIE (hypoxic-ischemic encephalopathy).

Harmful therapies

Examples of therapies shown to be harmful are:
- Uncontrolled oxygen therapy and blindness in preterm infants. This demonstrates the dangers of the introduction of a new therapy, oxygen, followed by changes in its use, without evidence from randomized controlled trials for either change in clinical practice (Fig. 66.4).
- Antibiotic side effects:
  - chloramphenicol (unmonitored) – gray baby syndrome (circulatory collapse)
  - sulfonamides – displacement of bilirubin, resulting in kernicterus
  - tetracycline – yellow staining of teeth and bones.
- Aquaphor, to cover the skin of preterm infants to reduce evaporative heat and water loss – increased risk of sepsis.
- Early prophylactic corticosteroids in preterm infants to reduce severity of respiratory distress syndrome and BPD (bronchopulmonary dysplasia) – gastrointestinal perforation, growth failure, hypertension and possible neurodevelopmental deficit.

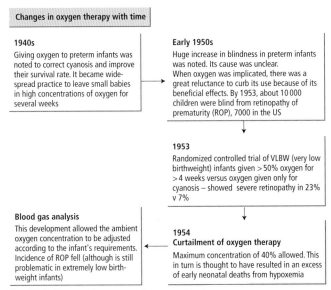

Fig. 66.4 Changes in oxygen therapy with time.

Question

What is the effect of antenatal corticosteroids on early neonatal morbidity and mortality in preterm infants?

The meta-analysis (Fig. 66.2) shows that corticosteroids given before preterm birth reduce the incidence of respiratory distress syndrome, intraventricular hemorrhage and neonatal mortality.

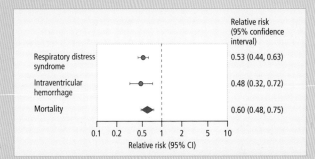

Fig. 66.2 Prophylactic corticosteroids for preterm birth. (Data from Crowley P. Prophylactic corticosteroids for preterm birth (Cochrane Review). In: *The Cochrane Library*, Issue 1, 2004. Chichester, UK: John Wiley & Sons.)

Question

What is the effect of moderate hypothermia for moderate or severe HIE (hypoxic-ischemic encephalopathy) on outcome?

Meta-analysis (Fig. 66.3) on outcome at 18 months of age, mainly of three large multicenter international trials of cooling from before 6 hours of age for 72 hours, showed a reduction of death and severe disability (risk ratio 0.81, number needed to treat 9) and improved survival with normal neurological function (risk ratio 1.53, number needed to treat 8).

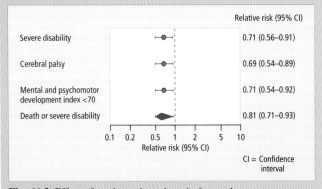

Fig. 66.3 Effect of moderate hypothermia for moderate or severe HIE on outcome. CI = confidence interval. (Data from Edwards D *et al.*, Neurological outcomes at 18 months of age after moderate hypothermia for perinatal hypoxic ischaemic encephalopathy: synthesis and meta-analysis of trial data. *BMJ* 2010; **340**: c363.)

Sick newborn infants have the same rights to life and access to care as any other person. Their care is totally dependent on a successful partnership between parents and the clinical team (Fig. 67.1).

Table 67.1 Definitions of the principles of medical ethics.

Beneficence	Do good
Non-maleficence	Do no harm
Justice	Legal justice, respect for rights, fair distribution of resources
Respect for autonomy	Respect for the individuals' right to make informed and thought-out decisions for themselves
Trust	Parents need to develop trust in their physician, who has a responsibility to ensure that this trust is not misplaced

Question

What is the role of clinical ethics committees?

These are increasingly being developed as a resource for doctors and other health-care professionals and parents facing difficult ethical problems. In the US hospitals are required to have mechanisms in place to address ethical issues in patient care. Ethics committees are often diverse, including physicians, nurses, lay members, pastoral care, and others. In the US and some centers in the UK, the committee can be rapidly constituted to discuss an individual problem proactively. Ethics committee decisions are generally advisory. In those circumstances where there is continued conflict after ethics committee involvement, referral to court may be required. In addition to assisting with individual cases, institutional ethics committees are becoming more involved in organizational ethical issues such as conflict of interest and the impact of performance incentives on patient care.

The withholding or withdrawal of life-saving medical treatment

There are a number of situations in neonatal practice where withholding or withdrawal of life-saving medical treatment is considered appropriate. Their management is influenced by the parents' religious beliefs and cultural background, the laws of the country and national guidelines (e.g. American Academy of Pediatrics, Royal College of Paediatrics and Child Health) (Tables 67.2 and 67.3) These decisions are stressful not only for the parents but also for the health-care team, amongst whom consensus and an agreed management plan should be reached. Consent must be obtained from the parents, but the extent to which they may wish to be

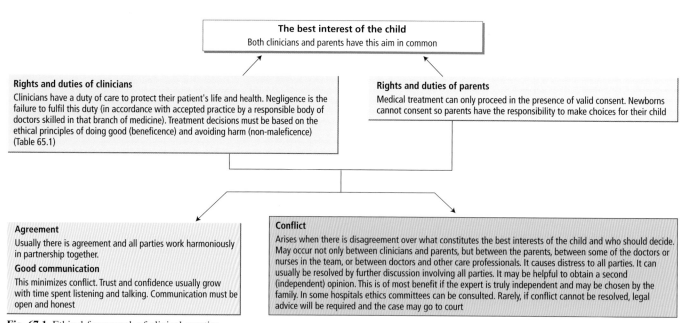

The best interest of the child
Both clinicians and parents have this aim in common

Rights and duties of clinicians
Clinicians have a duty of care to protect their patient's life and health. Negligence is the failure to fulfil this duty (in accordance with accepted practice by a responsible body of doctors skilled in that branch of medicine). Treatment decisions must be based on the ethical principles of doing good (beneficence) and avoiding harm (non-maleficence) (Table 65.1)

Rights and duties of parents
Medical treatment can only proceed in the presence of valid consent. Newborns cannot consent so parents have the responsibility to make choices for their child

Agreement
Usually there is agreement and all parties work harmoniously in partnership together.
Good communication
This minimizes conflict. Trust and confidence usually grow with time spent listening and talking. Communication must be open and honest

Conflict
Arises when there is disagreement over what constitutes the best interests of the child and who should decide. May occur not only between clinicians and parents, but between the parents, between some of the doctors or nurses in the team, or between doctors and other care professionals. It causes distress to all parties. It can usually be resolved by further discussion involving all parties. It may be helpful to obtain a second (independent) opinion. This is of most benefit if the expert is truly independent and may be chosen by the family. In some hospitals ethics committees can be consulted. Rarely, if conflict cannot be resolved, legal advice will be required and the case may go to court

Fig. 67.1 Ethical framework of clinical practice.

Neonatology at a Glance, 2nd edition. Edited by Tom Lissauer & Avroy A. Fanaroff. © 2011 Blackwell Publishing Ltd.

Table 67.2 Examples of situations in neonatal practice where withholding or withdrawal of intensive care may be appropriate in the UK.

The no hope situation

The child has such severe disease that life-sustaining treatment simply delays death without significant alleviation of suffering, e.g. a child with trisomy 13 or 18 needing mechanical ventilation for congenital abnormalities

The no purpose situation

The patient may be able to survive with treatment, but it is expected that the degree of physical or mental impairment will be devastating. The child in this situation will never be capable of taking part in decisions regarding treatment or its withdrawal. An example is a newborn with profound neurologic damage following severe hypoxic–ischemic brain damage, in whom microcephaly, profound developmental delay, blindness and quadriplegia are believed to be inevitable

The unbearable situation

There is progressive and irreversible illness where further treatment is more than can be borne by the infant and family caregivers. An infant with progressive and severe deteriorating respiratory failure from bronchopulmonary dysplasia (chronic lung disease) might be considered in this category

---

involved in the decision-making depends on the individual family. Repeated discussion without coercion may be necessary.

If life-saving support is going to be withheld or withdrawn, all aspects of palliative care including symptom management and psychosocial support should be in place. Many parents will accept the appropriateness of withdrawal of mechanical ventilation and appreciate the opportunity to spend time with their baby away from the technology of intensive care, but with staff to support them. The baby's comfort should be a priority and appropriate analgesia and anxiolytics given. Analgesia using opioids should be maintained. Parents need to know that the infant may continue to breathe for some time after disconnection from the ventilator.

If clinical situations do not fit the categories described in Table 67.2 or where there is dissent or uncertainty about the degree of future impairment, the child's life should be safeguarded and full care provided by *all* in the health-care team.

Questions

What is the difference between withholding and withdrawing intensive care?

There is no ethical or legal distinction between them, though emotionally it may be easier not to start treatment than to withdraw it. If there is uncertainty, provide intensive care and subsequently withdraw it after full assessment.

Is euthanasia allowed?

Giving a medicine with the primary intent to hasten death is unlawful in both North America and Europe (though in the Netherlands it is accepted on a carefully regulated basis). Giving a medicine to relieve pain, which as a side effect may hasten death (the principle of double effect), is ethically appropriate if its primary purpose is to alleviate distress or suffering.

Table 67.3 Situations where treatment of disabled infants can be withheld in the US.

The legislation regarding the treatment of infants with birth defects was introduced following the case of Baby Doe who was born in 1982 with Down syndrome (trisomy 21) and esophageal atresia. Partly on the advice of their obstetrician, the parents refused to consent to life-saving surgery to repair the esophageal defect. They felt that a 'minimally acceptable quality of life was never present for a child suffering from such a condition'. Without the surgery, the infant was unable to eat.

Legal dispute

The hospital disagreed with the parent's refusal to consent and filed in court an emergency petition seeking authorization to perform the surgery.

The trial court felt that the parents had a right to choose a medically recommended course of treatment. The obstetrician had recommended against surgery. The court did not give permission for surgery. The hospital appealed the decision, but the baby died when 6 days old.

Political consequences

The case drew widespread media attention, and ignited a national debate over the treatment of infants with birth defects.

President Reagan disagreed with the decision –'The judge let Baby Doe starve and die.'

The Surgeon General, C. Everett Koop, a pediatric surgeon, became involved in getting Congress to pass the Baby Doe Amendments.

The Child Abuse Prevention and Treatment Act (CAPTA) 1973, reauthorized 2003

This prevents the withholding of 'medically indicated treatment' from disabled newborns with life-threatening conditions.

Five circumstances under which treatment can be withheld are:

1. Chronically and irreversibly comatose
2. Treatment would merely prolong dying
3. Treatment would not be effective in ameliorating or correcting all of the infant's life-threatening conditions
4. Treatment would be futile in terms of survival
5. Treatment would be virtually futile and the treatment itself under such circumstances would be inhumane

Research

Health professionals wish to provide the best possible care for newborn infants. This should be evidenced-based, but this is only possible when evidence is available from properly conducted research. It is therefore unethical for properly conducted research on newborn infants **not** to be performed. Failure to do research leads to stagnant and second-rate medical care.

Research may be interventional, e.g. evaluation of a new therapy, or non-interventional, e.g. descriptive or observational (Table 68.1).

There are a number of obstacles to overcome in order to perform research in newborn infants. These are practical and ethical.

Practical difficulties in conducting research in infants

These include:
- The number of newborn infants who are preterm or have a specific problem or condition is small and usually requires trials to be multicentered, which adds enormously to the complexity and cost of each study. However, a number of networks have been established to facilitate this, such as the Vermont–Oxford and NICHD (National Institute of Child Health and Human Development) Neonatal Networks, and many multicentered trials have been performed throughout the world (see Cochrane neonatal reviews).
- Funding is difficult to obtain as the number of newborn infants with a specific problem is small, making pharmaceutical companies less likely to develop new products or conduct trials.
- In order to proceed with a trial, the information required about a potential new drug or therapy is becoming ever more stringent. This also applies to pilot studies, making it increasingly difficult to obtain the data required to conduct a larger study.

Ethical difficulties in conducting research in infants

All research must be peer-reviewed and sanctioned by an independent ethics advisory committee – Institutional Review Board in North America, appropriate research ethics committee (REC) in the UK.

Parents must be able to make informed choices when asked for consent for their infant to take part in research. This can be problematic when decisions need to made rapidly, e.g. when a baby suddenly becomes ill, especially immediately after delivery, when parents are emotionally stressed. The differences between assent and informed consent are outlined in Table 68.2.

Criteria for informed consent for research include:
- **Competence** of the person giving consent.
- **Information** – sufficient for informed choice, including a written information sheet for parents and the use of an interpreter if there are concerns about the parents' understanding of English.
- **Understanding** – parents must have understood the research sufficiently to be able to evaluate choices. In the US and UK, consent can be provided by one parent; in some countries in Europe both parents must agree.

Table 68.1 Differences between interventional and non-interventional research.

Interventional (therapeutic) research
Research which directly affects the treatment an individual receives. They may receive a new treatment or, in a randomized trial, a new or conventional treatment or placebo. At the start of the project the answer to the question of which is better will not be known (equipoise). Use of a placebo instead of treatment is unethical if there is an accepted treatment. The new and potentially better therapy should be compared with accepted treatment.

Non-interventional (non-therapeutic) research
Research that will *not benefit directly* the person involved. This is observational research – e.g. the normal levels of vitamin A in a particular group of infants. The infants themselves will in no way benefit – so the invasiveness of obtaining the information must be minimal (a small extra volume of blood when venepuncture is required for other reasons, or a single venepuncture, well performed with analgesia).

Table 68.2 Informed consent and assent in research.

Informed consent	Agreement in principle (assent)
This comes from the ability to evaluate options in the exercise of choice. It is based on judgment of risk and benefit, which must be made clear by the researcher. It is acknowledged that time (in most normal situations 24 hours) should be allowed between the provision of the information and the decision-making by the parents. *Fully informed consent* is probably never truly possible, but consent should be *sufficiently informed*. Parents should be informed about minor side effects if common and serious ones even if rare. The amount of information exchanged should be appropriate for the situation. An excessive amount of information may confuse.	Patients for certain clinical trials must be recruited within minutes or hours of presentation, e.g. research into the best way to ventilate a newborn infant or hypothermia after hypoxic–ischemic encephalopathy. It will be impossible in these situations for parents to assess the trial in a fully informed way. At this emergency stage they should be asked to assent to the trial and their acceptance or otherwise should be recorded in the notes. Formal consent should be obtained over the next hours or days. Assent should only be used where a 24-hour assimilation period cannot be used, and should be sanctioned specifically by the review board/ethics committee when considering the trial protocol.

Neonatology at a Glance, 2nd edition. Edited by Tom Lissauer & Avroy A. Fanaroff. © 2011 Blackwell Publishing Ltd.

- **Written consent** should be obtained, with one copy for the parents and another filed in the case record.
- **Voluntary** – parents must be aware that they can decline or withdraw from the research without jeopardizing their baby's care.

Consent in clinical practice

Health professionals are under pressure to allow parents greater involvement in decision-making and enable them to give consent to treatment.

Parental consent should be obtained for complex procedures or treatment and for all surgical procedures. Documentation about the communication with the parents explaining the basis, benefits and risks of the procedure or treatment is more important than obtaining a signature on a consent form. Consent for a surgical procedure must be obtained by someone fully conversant with it. However, with infants receiving intensive or special care in a neonatal unit, it would be impractical to obtain detailed consent from parents for the multitude of low-risk procedures performed on their baby. However, parents should be given an overview about what the care of their infant involves and what range of procedures will be performed, both verbally and in an information booklet.

In clinical practice, consent is most problematic about the initial resuscitation and immediate management of extremely premature infants at the limit of viability and when withdrawal of treatment is being considered. The former is considered in Chapter 12 on neonatal resuscitation, the latter in Chapter 67 on ethics.

Question

Is consent required for treatment of acute life-threatening situations?

No, but the clinician must believe that the treatment is in the patient's best interests.

In the newborn nursery, most deaths are of extremely preterm infants receiving intensive care, but some are term infants with hypoxic–ischemic encephalopathy, major congenital malformations or metabolic disorders. In the past many of these deaths occurred shortly after birth, but now they often occur after many difficult days or weeks, making the death even more stressful for both parents and staff. When it is expected that the baby is going to die, a management plan is required to ensure optimal symptom control for the infant and psychologic and spiritual support for the parents, siblings and family, and also that practical needs before and after death are addressed. Pediatric palliative care services may assist with this as they become increasingly involved in perinatal palliative care.

Whenever death is expected, the baby should be in a private area with the family. Occasionally, if desired by the family and community support is available, babies may be taken to die in the family's home or children's hospice.

Symptom control

The aim is to allow the baby to die free of pain and discomfort and with dignity. Analgesia should not be reduced or discontinued for fear that it might contribute to the infant's death. If mechanical ventilation is withdrawn, extremely preterm infants usually die shortly afterwards, but mature infants may continue to breathe for some time. The parents and family need to be forewarned.

Psychologic and spiritual support for the parents, siblings and family

Frequent and honest discussions should be held about the impending death of the baby between the family and health-care team. This may include grandparents, siblings and other family members. It is now uncommon for people to have seen a dead person and many have fears about what will happen.

Grief is the normal response to an infant's death. Parents and staff need to know that it is normal to show their emotions at such a sad time and be given the opportunity to explore their feelings.

Arrange for religious leaders to visit if wanted. Parents may want the baby blessed or baptized.

Practical care after death

Allow parents and family members to hold the baby before death and afterwards, if desired (but do not force them). Many parents value photos of them and their baby at this time, especially if this is the first occasion they can hold their baby free of tracheal tubes and lines and monitors.

Give unhurried, sympathetic care of the body after death, and provide unrestricted access for parents and visitors.

After the infant has died, provide the family with pictures and personal items – name tags, locks of hair, footprints, etc., of the baby.

Provide information about registering the baby's death and funeral arrangements.

Inform family practitioner, health visitor, obstetrician and other health professionals involved.

Some units have remembrance books and hold memorial services.

Grief

Grief may manifest with shock and disbelief, often followed by anger and guilt. There may be associated physical symptoms of anxiety, depression, tearfulness, loss of appetite, fatigue, insomnia and inability to concentrate. It may last many years but is usually most intense in the first few months. Parents may need advice about supporting siblings, grandparents and other family members in their grief. The two parents may also have different patterns of grief and this may place additional stress on their relationship. Provide information about professional resources and self-help groups for bereavement support and counseling.

Families often find it helpful to have ongoing communication with the health-care team. A meeting is usually arranged shortly after the child has died to provide an opportunity to discuss again the circumstances around the infant's death and to answer any questions about their baby's care, as well as covering any unresolved issues. It may be helpful if the obstetrician is also present. Health-care providers must be good listeners, not lecturers, at these meetings in order to learn how the family is feeling.

If there are concerns about abnormal grieving, referral for professional assessment and assistance can be recommended.

Caring for the staff

The death of a baby can also be distressing for staff. Many babies who die on neonatal units have needed protracted periods of intensive care, during which time the staff and parents become closely involved in the infant's day-to-day care. They are also likely to have encountered critical periods in the infant's condition which they have overcome together. The infant's death may be perceived as a failure, staff often feeling that the baby might have survived if something had been done differently.

Open discussion between all members of staff both before and after the baby's death is crucial, so that all are fully informed and aware of the situation and are able to express their feelings and concerns. Close dialogue is especially important when withdrawal of care is being considered. Many units also provide personal psychologic support for staff if desired.

Neonatology at a Glance, 2nd edition. Edited by Tom Lissauer & Avroy A. Fanaroff. © 2011 Blackwell Publishing Ltd.

Autopsy

Why is it performed?

In some situations, autopsy is a legal requirement, e.g. after a sudden unexpected death, surgery, or if any unnatural causes are implicated. Usually, it is performed to provide feedback for:
• parents, to help them understand why their baby died, and for genetic counseling and planning future pregnancies
• clinicians – to audit their management with a view to future improvement; it may confirm the clinician's diagnosis or identify diagnoses that were missed.

Autopsy also contributes to medical education and research.

It should be performed by a pediatric pathologist.

Comparing clinical and autopsy findings reveals major differences are present in 10–12% and lesser differences in 17–32%.

What is involved in an autopsy?

Autopsy examination involves:
• Photographs and imaging
  – Photographs form permanent documentation for the patient record. Particularly helpful for dysmorphology.
  – X-rays (and MRI if indicated) for bone and other pathology not evident on clinical examination.
• External and internal examination
  – Involves full-length incision from neck to pubis and over back of head; when sutured afterwards not visible when clothed. All organs are removed and inspected and weighed.
• Histology
  – Widespread samples taken for tissue blocks and slides. Traditionally archived for future reference and studies.
• Organ retention
  – Retained for fixing – mainly brain and heart. Can be reviewed with relevant clinicians. Some retained for teaching and research.

Consent

Detailed consent must be obtained unless the autopsy is legally required. All procedures involved must be described, and agreement reached about whether tissues, slides and organs are retained, disposed of in a lawful and respectful way, or when and how the tissues can be returned for burial. Even if autopsy is legally required, parents should be informed about the procedure.

Why has the autopsy rate fallen?

In the UK and US the autopsy rate has fallen dramatically over the past 20 years. Reasons for this include increasing reluctance by parents to consent to autopsy as they feel that their baby has had enough medical intervention, doctors are more reluctant to ask for consent, obtaining consent has become more complex, increased numbers of babies are Muslims and from other religions where autopsy is not accepted for religious reasons, lack of finance for the service and difficulty in obtaining autopsies performed by perinatal pathologists.

Are there alternatives to autopsy?

MRI-assisted biopsy of target organs has been advocated, but some causes are likely to be missed, e.g. infection and metabolic disorders. Limited autopsy or biopsy confined to specific tissues may be performed, but conventional autopsy remains the gold standard.

Taking home a preterm baby who required intensive care and many weeks in a neonatal unit is often daunting for parents (Fig. 70.1). Their fears are shared by parents of term infants who became seriously ill or have complex problems.

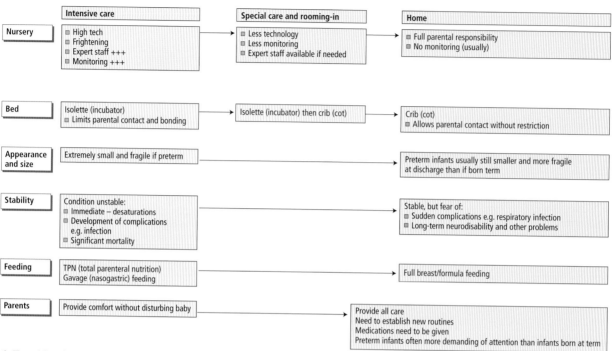

Fig. 70.1 Transition from intensive care to home.

Questions

When can babies go home?

Most go home when their condition is stable and they have established feeding. Parents must be able to care for the baby and provide health-care needs.

Some babies requiring long-term oxygen therapy, e.g. for BPD (bronchopulmonary dysplasia, chronic lung disease), or gavage (tube) feeding can be managed at home (Fig. 70.2).

This depends on the infant's medical condition (likely time course, if otherwise stable, etc.), the parents, home circumstances and community support available.

Should babies with bronchopulmonary dysplasia (chronic lung disease) have a 24-hour saturation recording done before going home?

This is performed in some units a few days after oxygen therapy is stopped to confirm the absence of significant desaturations. Its value has not been established.

All infants who were preterm should be checked to ensure that they are able to maintain their airway and saturations when placed in a car seat.

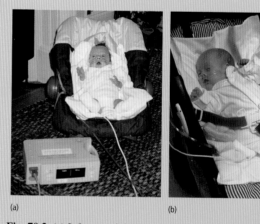

(a) (b)

Fig. 70.2 (a) Infant receiving oxygen therapy at home, and an oxygen saturation monitor. (b) Same infant receiving oxygen therapy in a stroller.

Neonatology at a Glance, 2nd edition. Edited by Tom Lissauer & Avroy A. Fanaroff. © 2011 Blackwell Publishing Ltd.

Discharge planning

Good discharge planning aims to minimize parental anxiety and ensure seamless transfer of care between professionals in the hospital and community. This can be achieved by:

• having a named nurse with this responsibility

• considering discharge arrangements (Fig. 70.3) during regular updates with parents and, if necessary, arranging predischarge meetings with the parents and other professionals involved, e.g. the family's pediatrician or family practitioner, community nurses, health visitors, therapists, child development team.

Facilities where parents can room in with their baby for several days or longer ('step-down units') before going home are helpful, especially when establishing full breast-feeding.

Some units have specialist nurses who provide care in the family's home and liaise with community-based services. Some of these nurses may also work on the unit and know the baby and family before discharge.

Health promotion
i) SIDS (sudden infant death syndrome)
   prevention:
   ▪ Lie on back not prone
   ▪ Avoid overheating
   ▪ Avoid smoking near baby
ii) Resuscitation training:
   ▪ Demonstration, may be complemented by video

Medications
What to give, how often, how to give them and for how long

Immunizations
Which have been given, when are the next ones due? Is RSV (respiratory syncytial virus) prophylaxis (palivizumab, a monoclonal antibody) indicated? If so, who will give it and when?

Follow-up arrangements
Who, when and where

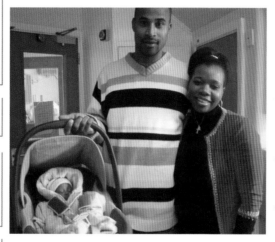

Past and potential medical problems
Check that parents have good understanding Parents should have a copy of the discharge summary in case professional help is needed

Ongoing or new medical problems
Who to contact and how to manage them Awareness of most likely problems requiring hospitalization, e.g. respiratory infections, inguinal hernias

Feeding
Is breast milk fortifier or a preterm formula feed required? If so, how can they be obtained and for how long?

Vision and hearing
Have they been checked? Are further checks required?

Parent support group
Would it be helpful, e.g. multiple births, etc? If so, do parents have contact address or is there a helpful internet site?

Fig. 70.3 Parents and their baby leaving the neonatal unit. The items that need to be considered prior to discharge are listed.

Goals

The goals of high-risk follow-up are:
- early identification of disability or developmental or behavior problems
- management of ongoing medical issues
- facilitation of early intervention, with referral if necessary
- family support
- monitoring of neonatal outcomes.

Criteria

High-risk infants include:
- very preterm (usually <1500 g or <32 weeks of gestation)
- neurologic abnormality, including:
  - neonatal seizures
  - hypoxic–ischemic encephalopathy
  - neonatal meningitis
- mechanical ventilation/nitric oxide therapy/ECMO
- severe IUGR (intrauterine growth restriction)
- congenital malformations (significant)
- maternal drug abuse
- significant parental psychosocial problems.

Organization and timing

Timing of visits will vary with different programs and with the extent of pediatric neurodevelopmental expertise available to the family locally. It will also depend on whether neurodevelopmental outcome is being monitored at standard times. A typical program for clinic visits and reason for their timing is shown in Fig. 71.1.

Who should conduct neonatal follow-up?

Many neonatologists provide neonatal follow-up with or without support from other physicians. This has the advantage of continu-

ity of care for the parents. It also gives direct feedback on the sequelae of neonatal care.

Good follow-up programs are multidisciplinary and include:
- developmental specialists – particularly for older children, when developmental assessment and management become more specialized and complex; in some programs all follow-up is performed by developmental specialists
- community nursing team – if involved with the family following discharge
- dietitian
- therapists
- psychologist
- social services.

The family practitioner/pediatrician provides general pediatric care and other pediatric specialists may be required for specific problems such as pulmonary, ophthalmology, etc.

Components

- Growth.
- Neurologic assessment.
- Developmental assessment including behavior.
- Vision and hearing.
- Social/family integration.

Outcome measures

Evaluation is tailored to the child's age. Most follow-up programs conduct formal data collection at 18-24 months of age corrected for prematurity including a disability assessment, neurologic evaluation and a developmental assessment using a standardized assessment.

Widely used developmental assessments at this age are the Bayley Scales (3E) or the Griffiths Scales (Table 71.1). They are standardized to a population mean of 100 and with a standard deviation of 15 points. Children with scores <55 (−3 standard

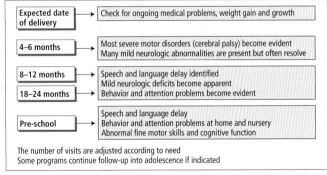

Fig. 71.1 An example of a high-risk follow-up program.

Table 71.1 Widely used developmental assessments.

Bayley scales of infant development (3rd edition)	Griffiths Mental Development Scales – Revised
Age range 0–42 months	Age range: 0–24 months (Baby scales) 24–96 months (Extended)
Subscales:	Subscales:
• Fine motor	• Locomotor
• Gross motor	• Personal social
• Receptive language	• Hearing and language
• Expressive language	• Eye hand coordination
• Cognitive scale	• Performance
	• Practical reasoning (from 2 years)

Neonatology at a Glance, 2nd edition. Edited by Tom Lissauer & Avroy A. Fanaroff. © 2011 Blackwell Publishing Ltd.

deviations) have severe developmental impairment likely to persist, children with scores 55–70 have moderate impairment and are highly likely to have low scores at later ages, while children with scores 70–85 have milder impairment and may catch up.

A formal classification of disability at 2 years is shown in Table 37.1. Such a series of definitions is useful for comparing outcomes between centers and for use in evaluating the results of randomized trials.

Follow up of older children requires formal IQ and behavioral screening. School evaluation by the class teacher is valuable for identifying need for support.

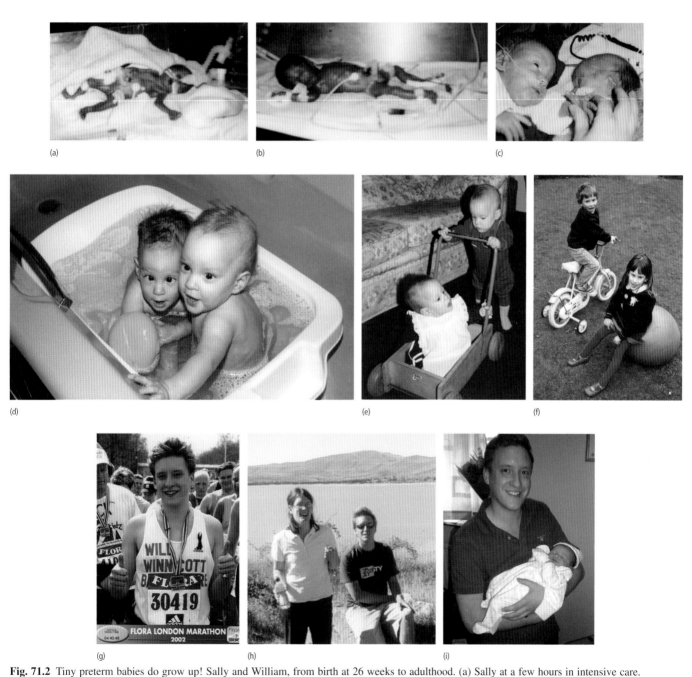

Fig. 71.2 Tiny preterm babies do grow up! Sally and William, from birth at 26 weeks to adulthood. (a) Sally at a few hours in intensive care. (b) William shortly after extubation. (c) Together at last at 4 weeks! (d) At a year. (e) Just walking. (f) At 5 years. (g) At 18 years, William completing the London marathon. (h) At 19 years, Sally and William on vacation in New Zealand. (i) The next generation has arrived, rather larger at birth than her father! (With thanks to Sally and William for permitting the use of these photographs.)

Globally, every year there are about:
- 135 million births
- 3.6 million neonatal deaths.

Enormous efforts are being made in developing countries to achieve Millennium Goal 4, a two-thirds reduction in child mortality from 1990 to 2015.

The mortality rate for children <5 years old has declined markedly since 1990 (particularly from immunization, early treatment and prevention of malaria and HIV) (Fig. 72.1) but:
- neonatal mortality (first 28 days) has declined much more slowly
- no measurable reduction in early neonatal deaths (first week of life), when 75% of neonatal deaths occur, with up to 40% in the first 24 hours.

Geography of newborn deaths

Only 1.3% of neonatal deaths occur in high income countries. About three-quarters of all newborn deaths occur in sub-Saharan Africa and South Asia (Fig. 72.2). The same regions have the highest risk and numbers of maternal deaths.

Ten countries account for two-thirds of the world's neonatal deaths (Table 72.1). They are – India, Nigeria, Pakistan, China, DR Congo, Ethiopia, Bangladesh, Indonesia, Afghanistan and Tanzania. India alone has one million neonatal deaths a year. Almost all now have a national plan for Maternal, Newborn and Child Health, although in many cases the plan for the newborn is the weakest part.

Causes of newborn deaths

The main causes of neonatal death are shown in Fig. 72.3.

Table 72.1 Neonatal mortality by region.

Region	Neonatal mortality rate per 1000 live births (2008)	Annual number of neonatal deaths
Sub-Saharan Africa	41	1 230 000
Middle East and North Africa	21	209 000
South Asia	37	1 571 000
East Asia and Pacific	13	346 000
Latin America and Caribbean	11	117 000
Central and Eastern Europe and the countries of the former Soviet Union	12	66 000
High-income	4	44 000
Middle-income	26	2 382 000
Low-income	37	1 149 000
World	26	3 575 000

Data source: UN databases and WHO NMR estimates for 2008.

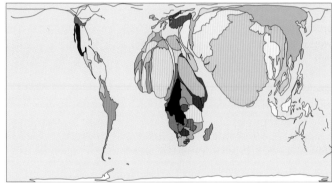

Fig. 72.2 Global burden of neonatal deaths. Territory size shows the proportion of early neonatal deaths worldwide that occurred there in 2000. (Source: worldmapper.org.)

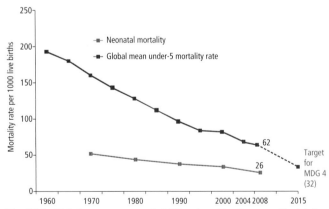

Fig. 72.1 Global progress towards Millennium Development Goal 4 for child survival. (Source: Lawn, J. Newborn survival in low resource settings – are we delivering? *BJOG* 2009; **116**(Suppl 1): 49–59; updated 2010 for data to 2008.)

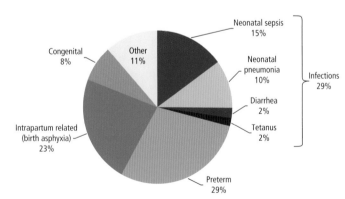

Fig. 72.3 Direct causes of neonatal death in 192 countries in 2008. (Black, RE *et al.* for the Child Health Epidemiology Reference Group of WHO and UNICEF. Global, regional, and national causes of child mortality in 2008: a systematic analysis. *Lancet* 2010; **375**: 1969–1987.)

In low income, high mortality countries the main causes are:
- infection
- preterm births complications – also contributes to infection deaths
- intrapartum-related neonatal deaths (previously more loosely called 'birth asphyxia').

For preterm infants, antenatal steroids could halve deaths from respiratory distress syndrome globally but remain underused.

Neonatal sepsis and pneumonia kill about one million babies each year (more than child deaths from malaria but they receive much less attention). An important success story is the dramatic reduction in deaths from neonatal tetanus over the last decade due to maternal tetanus toxoid immunization.

Timing of newborn deaths – birth and the first few days are critical

The birth of a baby should be a time of celebration yet, all too often it is a time of tragedy. Globally, the risk of dying during the first day of life is high. Almost 10 per 1000 (1%) babies die, there are around 1 million intrapartum stillbirths and almost half of the world's 343 000 maternal deaths (2008) occur around the time of delivery.

The first few days after birth also have ongoing high risk for death and long-term disability. Yet currently less than 20% of mothers and babies receive postnatal care in the first 2 days.

Maternal health and obstetric care

Maternal health and obstetric care have a substantial impact on neonatal morbidity and mortality. Priorities in developing countries are:
- before conception:
  - birth spacing – considerable health advantages for infant and mother if 3-year birth intervals and mother over 18 years of age
  - nutrition – including calories, protein, iodine, folic acid, iron
  - infection control – malaria, tetanus, sexually transmitted diseases, HIV
- during pregnancy – antenatal care, testing and treatment of maternal infections, and management of complications of pregnancy
- labor and delivery – skilled attendance, management of complications.

Notable features are:
- Only 10 of the 68 highest burden countries have increased the provision of skilled care at birth by more than 10% between 1990 and 2010. In some countries such as Ethiopia, only 5% of births are in health facilities. Globally 60 million births are at home each year. Urgent attention is required to improve access to health facilities able to deal with obstetric emergencies.
- Education of groups of mothers about how to care for their newborn babies has been shown to increase the use of skilled birth attendants and improve newborn survival (Fig. 72.4).

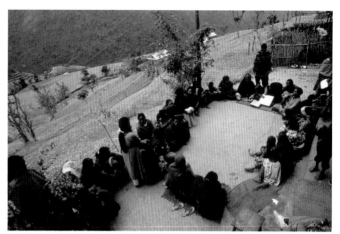

Fig. 72.4 Health education classes for mothers in rural Nepal. Shown to reduce neonatal mortality. (Courtesy of Prof. Anthony Costello.)

HIV infection

Maternal HIV-positive prevalence (see Chapter 43) is as high as 30–40% in some sub-Saharan African countries, resulting in around 280 000 child deaths each year following vertical transmission. They are mainly between 1 month and 1 year of age. In addition, the non-infected siblings suffer from their parents becoming ill and dying, and having to be cared for by relatives or friends or in institutions. In many high HIV prevalence countries there has been rapid progress in providing antiretroviral therapy to HIV-positive pregnant women which reduces vertical transmission.

In developing countries, it is recommended that HIV-positive mothers should breast-feed unless formula feeds can be given safely. Mixed formula and breast-feeding should be avoided, as the risk of transmission appears greater than breast-feeding alone. Even if formula feeding can be provided safely, if the mother is taking combination antiretroviral therapy, the transmission rate when breast feeding is only around 1%. Alternatively, where the mother does not require therapy for her own health, the infant may be given antiretroviral therapy for protection from breast milk transmission. These new options have been adopted by WHO to promote breast-feeding in resource poor-settings.

Breast-feeding

Plays a crucial role in prevention of infection and should be strongly encouraged in all countries (Fig. 72.6).

Breast milk should also be used for low birthweight infants.

Key point

The promotion and marketing of formula is restricted by the International Code of Marketing of Breast Milk Substitutes (WHO, UNICEF).

Question

Why are over 400 thousand infants throughout the world still acquiring HIV infection?

Reducing transmission to infants requires:

(i) identifying that the mother has HIV by testing

(ii) giving a short course of antiretroviral therapy to the mother before delivery, intrapartum and to the infant after birth (even a single maternal dose halves the transmission rate)

(iii) delivery by cesarean section

(iv) ability to safely feed infants of infected mothers, either by breast-feeding together with antiretroviral therapy to the mother or infant or by formula feeding.

Unfortunately, this is still not available universally in many developing countries.

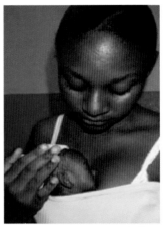

Fig. 72.5 Kangaroo mother care for a preterm infant. (Photo courtesy of Save the Children, South Africa.)

Saving newborn lives – what works?

It is estimated that two-thirds of neonatal deaths globally could be prevented with low cost care that does not include intensive care units and high-tech machines. Over 1 million could be saved each year even with simple care possible outside hospitals. An example of how the need for essential newborn care remains unmet in many resource-poor countries such as Nepal is shown in Table 72.2.

Newborn survival for babies born at home or in a health clinic would be improved by:

• Trained birth attendant present and able to provide care for not only the mother but also the newborn.

• Baby assessed at birth and basic resuscitation with bag and mask provided if necessary.

• Baby's temperature maintained – by drying baby at birth, keeping warm with skin-to-skin contact, having a warm environment, covering the baby, including head

• Infection control – clean cutting and tying of cord to prevent neonatal tetanus.

• Exclusive breast-feeding – starting within 1 hour of birth and avoiding any formula milk.

• Early detection of problems and appropriate care-seeking. This is impeded in some cultures where there is strong pressure on mothers and newborn babies not to go outside their home for the

Table 72.2 Summary of survey of newborn care in rural Nepal, where the neonatal mortality is 50/1000 live births.

90%	Gave birth at home
6%	Skilled attendant at delivery
11%	Alone at delivery
33%	Cord cut with household sickle
64%	Wrapped baby only at 30 minutes of age
92%	Bathed in first hour (high risk of hypothermia)
99%	Breast-fed

Adapted from Osrin D *et al.*, Cross sectional, community based study of care of newborn infants in Nepal. *BMJ* 2002; **325**: 1063.

first 4–6 weeks, or by cost or distance. In addition, the hospital or health facility must be able to provide quality care for sick babies. When this is not available, home-based treatment may be an alternative. Several studies in South Asia have shown that community health workers can provide home injection treatment for infections with reductions of 30% or more in neonatal deaths.

Kangaroo mother care (Fig. 72.5) is highly effective, yet in many countries is available only in the teaching hospital; it could be scaled up at district hospital or even health center level.

Priorities for doctors working on newborn care in low income settings

Find as much data as you can about your setting – What are newborns dying of? What is working already and could be strengthened? Are there key policies that need advocacy support, e.g. regarding formula milk marketing and use, or for postnatal home visits? What staff training is available for newborn care? Are basic equipment and drugs available and if not who could influence this?

If you are based in a hospital:

• Is basic neonatal resuscitation available? Life support courses are increasingly available.

• Does it have baby-friendly status from UNICEF?

If you work in a neonatal unit:

• Are there measures to prevent infection, e.g. hand hygiene and gloves?

• Thermal regulation – warm nursery, clothing and hat for infants?

• Guidelines for the most common conditions?

• Provision of feeding support for preterm babies – help for mothers to express milk, cup feeding, gavage (nasogastric) tube feeding if needed?

• Is there effective kangaroo mother care? For stable babies <2 kg it reduces crowding and hospital stay as well as mortality.

• Availability of basic equipment and investigations? Tactfully approach key people if not.

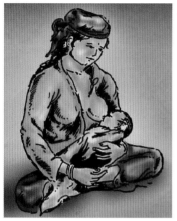
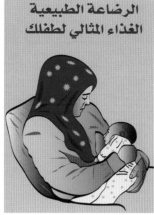

الرضاعة الطبيعية
الغذاء المثالي لطفلك

(a)   (b)

Fig. 72.6 Examples of the promotion of breast-feeding. a) Nepal b) Oman. (Courtesy of Dr Saleh Al-Khusaiby.)

• Adequate disposable items, e.g. feeding tubes, cannulae?

• Oxygen therapy? Is there adequate monitoring with pulse oximeter?

• Nasal CPAP for respiratory support? Is it available? If not, would it be appropriate and feasible? If available, optimally used?

However, initial emphasis is often on ventilators. Artificial ventilation may be appropriate depending on the level of care available but should be considered carefully as requires:

– a lot of time from skilled doctors and nurses
– consistently functioning equipment and power supplies
– adequate monitoring, both laboratory and in the nursery
– careful infection control.

Basic life saving care for *all* babies should be the first step.

Questions

Why has neonatal mortality in resource poor countries failed to decline?

Many reasons, including:

• Neonatal care is wrongly considered too 'high-tech'.

• Neonatal care depends on both maternal and child health teaching and training programs and often falls between them.

• Lack of experience or interest of some pediatricians in newborn care.

How can neonatologists in developed countries help developing countries?

They can help by:

• advocacy – promoting newborn care in resource-poor countries

• participating in collaborative programs or partnerships. These need to be appropriate for local conditions but still retain scientific rigor and evidence base. Program must also be aligned to local and national strategy.

Additional reading and resources

• The Lancet Neonatal series 2005: http://www.who.int/child_adolescent_health/documents/lancet_neonatal_survival/en/index.html

• Opportunities for Africa's newborns: http://www.who.int/pmnch/media/publications/africanewborns/en/index.html

• Health Newborn Network: http://www.healthynewborn network.org/

Transport

The infrastructure
- Training – physicians, nurses, respiratory therapists (in US).
- Maintain dedicated equipment.
- A 'transport hotline' – for communication with referring hospitals. Mobile phones for the team on the move.
- Contracts and protocols for transport – ambulance, helicopter (Fig. 73.1), fixed-wing plane (Fig. 73.2).
- Insurance liabilities to cover adverse events.
- Outreach training to less specialized units.

Why transfer?
Higher level of care:
- Prematurity, low birthweight.
- Respiratory distress/failure.
- Total parenteral nutrition.
- Sepsis/shock.
- Severe congenital anomalies.
- Hypoxic–ischemic encephalopathy.
- Seizures.
- Hemolytic disease/jaundice.
- Resistant hypoglycemia.
- Metabolic disease.
- Undefined sick infant.
   For subspecialty care:
- Cardiac, surgery, neurosurgery, orthopedic.

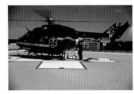

Fig. 73.1 Helicopter transfer in northern Canada.

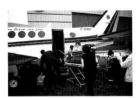

Fig. 73.2 Transport incubator being loaded into fixed-wing plane.

Equipment
- Transport incubator.
- Airways – mask, oral, nasal, tracheal.
- Respiratory support – ventilator, air, oxygen, nitric oxide.
- Full ICU monitoring.
- IV access – infusions, pumps.
- Chest and pericardial tubes.
- Medications.
- Hand-held blood testing – glucose, electrolytes, hemoglobin, blood gases.
- Power source – ambulance, aircraft, hospital wall supply. Battery if nothing else.
   All this is heavy: needs handling skills and equipment to assist.

Initial communication
- Record all clinical details necessary to plan the retrieval.
- Give appropriate advice for ongoing care:
   – Ensure current vital signs, laboratory tests and blood gases are appropriate.
   – Request respiratory support, vascular access, infection treatment, specialist care for cardiac or surgery to be initiated if necessary.
- Request that referring hospital prepares:
   – full documentation of pregnancy, birth and postnatal course; radiographs; laboratory results; vitamin K status.
   – names of baby, parents and contact details
   – consent for planned procedures
   – maternal blood for cross-match.
- Record exact location of patient, city, hospital, ward.
- Estimate arrival time and inform referring hospital.
- Provide ongoing contact number for clinical advice from specialist if needed.

Documentation
- Use standardized clinical assessment and treatment records.
- Necessary for debriefing, audit, legal records.

Key points

Parents need information, support, transport, accommodation, finance, child care and counseling.
   They will remember this experience for the rest of their lives.

Managing the infant

Diagnosis and assessment

- Identify problems and diagnoses needing pretransport therapy.
- Determine the appropriate destination for the identified specialist care needs.

Stabilize before *not during* transport

Baby should have:
- normal temperature
- secure airway and breathing
- optimized blood pressure, circulation, urine output
- optimized blood results – glucose, electrolytes, complete blood count (CBC), blood gases, etc.

Neonatology at a Glance, 2nd edition. Edited by Tom Lissauer & Avroy A. Fanaroff. © 2011 Blackwell Publishing Ltd.

- immediate treatment given, e.g. antibiotics, transfusion, prostaglandin (Prostin), anticonvulsants
- status rechecked after transfer to transport incubator.

Access

Tailor to the infant's needs:
- secure airway
- IV access – two lines preferable
- arterial access
- naso/orogastric tubes
- monitoring attached.

Transport

Plan the transfer of the infant over to the transport equipment. Check infant is stable.
- Continuous monitoring, record vital signs regularly as in ICU (Fig. 73.3).
- Keep emergency medications, chest tubes, airways and IV lines accessible.
- Avoid all unnecessary interventions.

Arrival at receiving hospital

Full report to receiving staff.
- Ensure stable transfer to ICU monitoring and therapy.
- Complete documentation.

Specific diagnoses

Some conditions have special requirements before and during transport. Examples are:
- extremely low birthweight – thermal regulation
- pneumothoraces (chest tubes)
- choanal atresia (oral airway)
- esophageal atresia and tracheoesophageal fistula
- diaphragmatic hernia
- bowel obstruction, omphalocele, gastroschisis
- infant of diabetic mother
- congenital cardiac disease (prostaglandin)
- patients needing ECMO (extracorporeal membrane oxygenation)
- patients on high-frequency ventilation
- treatment with nitric oxide.

Aeromedical considerations

- May be faster if ground transport takes more than 2 hours.
- Helicopter maximum distance is about 300 miles, then use fixed-wing plane. Local conditions will determine the choice.
  Problems:
- Expensive.
- Multiple transfers between vehicles.
- Cramped space/difficult access to baby (Fig. 73.4).
- Noise and vibration.
- Decreased barometric pressure:
  - Fixed-wing planes are pressurized at 8000 ft (2500 m), so, for example, 50% FiO$_2$ at ground level will require 67% at 8000 ft (2500 m). Prone position may help.
  - There will be expansion of closed air-filled cavities, so:
    - stomach and bowel need a gastric tube
    - pneumothoraces may become more severe
    - blood pressure cuffs may cause occlusion of blood vessels.

Pitfalls

- Extreme weather.
- Vehicle failure.
- Equipment failure.
- Battery or medical gas failure.
- Accidents.
- Travel sickness.
- *Be prepared!*

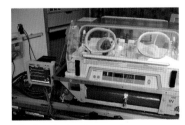

Fig. 73.3 Full monitoring during transport.

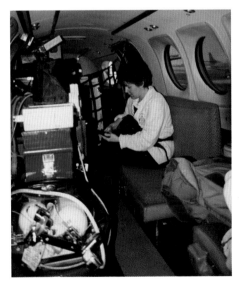

Fig. 73.4 Cramped space in fixed-wing plane.

Endotracheal intubation

Indications

- Neonatal resuscitation (see Chapter 12):
  - Failure to respond to Airway (clearing of airway), Breathing (with mask ventilation) and Circulation (circulatory support)
  - Aspiration of meconium.
- Mechanical ventilation for respiratory failure:
  - Apnea – prolonged/recurrent not responding to mask ventilation.
  - Increasing respiratory distress on CPAP.
  - Inadequate oxygenation (hypoxemia) and/or in carbon dioxide elimination (hypercarbia) on CPAP.
- Replace blocked or dislodged tracheal tube.
- Administration of surfactant.
- Upper airway obstruction – to provide a secure airway.
- Congenital diaphragmatic hernia – to avoid bowel distension.

Procedure

- Ensure you have trained assistance.
- Place head in neutral position (head in midline and neck slightly extended with the chin in a 'sniffing' position). Avoid over-extension of neck as view of cords obscured.
- Pre-oxygenate with mask ventilation. Monitor oxygen saturation and heart rate continuously.
- Insert laryngoscope with left hand to just beyond base of tongue.
- Lift entire blade and identify glottis and epiglottis (Fig. 74.1). Suction to clear secretions if needed.
- Insert tracheal tube (Table 74.1) with right hand into right side of infant's mouth and pass through the vocal cords (Fig. 74.2) to the level of the cord guide (a black line near the tube tip). A stylet may help in directing the tube through the cords.
- Note depth of insertion from gum or lip.
- Verify placement by positive pressure ventilation:

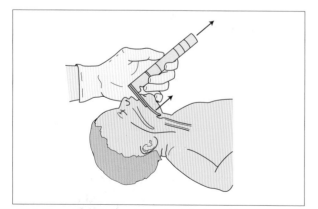

Fig. 74.1 Place tip of blade at base of epiglottis or lift epiglottis. Lift the entire blade to visualize the vocal cords. Cricoid pressure may help.

Table 74.1 Endotracheal tube size.

Size (mm)	Weight (kg)	Gestation (weeks)	Depth of insertion (cm from upper lip)
2.5	<1	<28	6–7
3.0	1–2	28–34	7–8
3.5	2–3	35–38	8–9
3.5–4	>3	>38	9–10

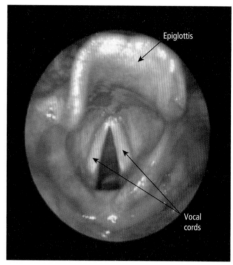

Fig. 74.2 View of vocal cords at intubation.

- a CO_2 detector attached to the endotracheal tube shows presence of end-tidal CO_2 (change in color) if the endotracheal tube is placed in the trachea.
- auscultating over upper lungs and stomach. Watch for chest rise with no gastric distension and improvement in oxygen saturation, heart rate and clinical condition. If air entry greater on right side than left, tube is in right main bronchus; withdraw tube until breath sounds equal.
- Secure tube, noting any change in tube depth of insertion. Confirm position with chest X-ray.
- **Limit attempts to 20–30 seconds.**
- Mask-ventilate and oxygenate infant between attempts.

Nasotracheal intubation

- Advantage – tube stability.
- Disadvantage – risk of nasal damage.

Procedure

- As for endotracheal intubation.
- Insert lubricated nasotracheal tube into nostril to back of throat.

Neonatology at a Glance, 2nd edition. Edited by Tom Lissauer & Avroy A. Fanaroff. © 2011 Blackwell Publishing Ltd.

- Insert laryngoscope to visualize vocal cords.
- To advance tracheal tube through vocal cords, move head to adjust neck flexion/extension so that tracheal tube is aligned to pass through the cords directly or lift the tracheal tube with McGill forceps.

Elective tracheal intubation

Infants should be given propofol, a short-acting anesthetic or rapid sequence induction before elective intubation:
- anesthesia – fentanyl
- vagal tone blockade – with atropine
- muscle relaxant – suxamethonium.
  Fentanyl may rarely cause stiff chest syndrome.

Chest tubes (chest drain)

Indications

- Pneumothorax.
- Pleural effusion.

Technique

- Site: lateral – 3rd to 5th intercostal space, anterior axillary line.
- Avoid nipple and breast bud.
- Sterile technique.
- Approach – upper edge of rib.
- Local anesthesia – 1% lidocaine to whole area; intravenous analgesia/fentanyl as indicated.
- Small incision along skin line. Blunt dissection of intercostal muscle with forceps.
- Use either an 8FG or 10FG chest tube or a pigtail catheter.
- Insert with trocar; grip trocar firmly at desired insertion depth to avoid inserting too far. Direct trocar towards clavicle on opposite side of chest.
- Connect tube to three-way tap and underwater seal, observing air bubbles and swinging with respiration, or to valve if prior to transport.
- Fix the tube to chest wall with sterile strips and adhesive dressing. Avoid suturing round the tube as may leave scars (see Fig. 65.7).
- X-ray to check tube position and lung re-expansion (Fig. 74.3).

Complications

- Hemothorax.
- Surgical emphysema.
- Scarring of skin or breast tissue.

Pleural tap

Indications

- Pleural fluid.

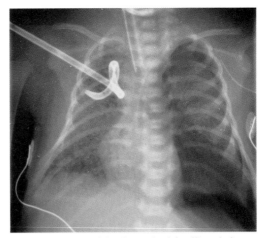

Fig. 74.3 X-ray showing a right chest tube (pigtail) to drain a pneumothorax. Pulmonary interstitial emphysema (PIE) is present in the right lung. There is a left pneumothorax with lung collapse and mediastinal shift to the right.

Technique

- Sterile.
- Ultrasound-guided to identify fluid.
- Local anesthesia – 1% lidocaine and intravenous analgesia/fentanyl if indicated.
- Small incision along skin line. Blunt dissection of intercostal muscle with forceps.
- Insert a 22G cannula just above the rib.
- Attach to three-way tap.
- Aspirate fluid with a syringe.

Complications

- Pneumothorax.
- Hemothorax.

Chest needling

Indication

- Tension pneumothorax – if immediate treatment is required.

Technique

- Site – 2nd or 3rd intercostal space, mid-clavicular line.
- Insert butterfly needle. Create underwater seal or aspirate air from chest with syringe via three-way tap.
- Usually followed by chest tube insertion.

Neonatal care involves a large number of practical procedures. Each has specific advantages and risks. Training and preparation are the key to success and avoiding complications. Consider how to minimize discomfort or pain with sucrose, gentle wrapping, positioning and consider what is the optimal time from the baby's perspective in relation to feeds and other procedures. Also make certain to obtain the necessary consents and perform a 'time-out' prior to the procedure. Some common procedures are shown in Table 75.1.

Table 75.1 Some common procedures.

Procedure	Preparation and equipment	Comments	Technique	Advantages	Potential complications
Capillary blood sampling (heelstick)	Clean procedure Gloves, sterile alcohol swab, automatic mini-lancet, tubes, gauze	Autostylets less painful than stylets inserted by hand. Avoid undue squeezing of heel, as painful and gives misleading results	**Fig. 75.1** Shaded areas show site for capillary sampling.	Simple technique for blood glucose, hematocrit, complete blood count, electrolytes and blood gases	If results are abnormal, confirm with venepuncture Bruising Infection Rarely osteomyelitis
Venous sampling of blood	Clean procedure Gloves, sterile alcohol swab, needle, tubes for blood sample, gauze	Use venepuncture needle. Avoid potential sites for central venous access	**Fig. 75.2** Venous blood sampling from back of the hand.	Good flow of blood – avoids hemolysis of sample	Bruising Infection Difficult access in some infants
Peripheral venous cannulation	Clean procedure Gloves, sterile alcohol swab, cannulae, flushed T-piece, stopper, syringe, tape, clear dressing, splint if necessary	Fiber-optic light may facilitate visualization of veins Leave site of cannula tip visible for inspection	**Fig. 75.3** Peripheral venous cannulation. When blood flows back, advance cannula over stylet.	Usually achieved relatively quickly	Bruising Inflammation Infection Extravasation injury

Neonatology at a Glance, 2ⁿᵈ edition. Edited by Tom Lissauer & Avroy A. Fanaroff. © 2011 Blackwell Publishing Ltd.

Table 75.1 (*continued*)

Procedure	Preparation and equipment	Comments	Technique	Advantages	Potential complications
Peripheral arterial cannulation	Clean procedure Gloves, sterile alcohol swab, cannulae, flushed T-piece, stopper, tape, dressing	Hand: radial artery Foot: posterior tibial, dorsalis pedis Do not use temporal artery Infuse heparinized saline	Fig. 75.4 Peripheral arterial cannulation. (a) Check collaterals (Allen test) – hand blanches when both arteries occluded; color returns when occlusion of one artery is released. (b) Cannula insertion is facilitated by a fiber-optic light.	Access for repeated blood sampling Accurate BP measurement unless poor peripheral circulation	Short functioning time (hours to few days) Variable success at insertion Blood loss if line disconnected If poor perfusion of fingers/toes –**REMOVE** Rarely ischemia or gangrene
Urinary catheter	Sterile procedure Gloves, sterile towel, cleaning fluid, urinary catheters 4 or 5 FG	To obtain sterile urine Also for monitoring urinary output in renal failure		Simpler and more reliable in obtaining a specimen than suprapubic aspirate and no needlestick	Urethral damage Hemorrhage Contaminated urine sample
Suprapubic aspirate (bladder tap)	Sterile procedure Gloves, sterile alcohol swab, needle, syringe, sterile pot, gauze	To obtain sterile urine Higher success rate if ultrasound abdomen to check if bladder is full	Fig. 75.5 Suprapubic aspiration under ultrasound guidance. In an infant the bladder extends into the abdomen. (Adapted from Lissauer, T and Clayden, G, *Illustrated Textbook of Paediatrics*, Elsevier Ltd, 2007.)	Sterile sampling for reliable diagnosis of urinary tract infection	Rare – hemorrhage or needlestick injury to bowel
Lumbar puncture	Sterile procedure Gloves, sterile towels, cleaning fluid, gauze, LP needles, containers for CSF samples	Position infant lying on side or sitting with spine flexed Minimize discomfort (Chapter 62) Slowly advance needle with stylet in direction of umbilicus. May feel a give when entering subarachnoid space	Fig. 75.6 Lumbar puncture. Back curved.	Identifies meningitis Treatment of post-hemorrhagic hydrocephalus Rarely, screening for metabolic disorder	Blood-stained CSF – trauma or hemorrhage (intraventricular or subarachnoid) Contraindicated: • bleeding diathesis, e.g. thrombocytopenia • cardiorespiratory instability • Local skin infection

Umbilical catheters

Umbilical artery catheter (UAC)

Indications
- Continuous measurement of arterial blood pressure.
- Frequent blood gases and other blood samples.
- Exchange transfusion – to remove blood.

Contraindications
- Vascular compromise in the lower extremities or gluteal area.
- Necrotizing enterocolitis, peritonitis.
- Omphalitis.
- Omphalocele.

Insertion
Easiest on first day, possible on first 3–4 days.
- Length catheter is inserted (cm) for a high placement – use formula 3 × weight (kg) + 9 + stump length (cm).
- Monitor baby during procedure.
- Prime catheter with saline.
- Sterile technique, identify artery (Fig. 76.1). Dilate the artery with fine forceps or a dilator.
- Insert gently a 3 or 4.5 French gauge catheter to predetermined position and check that blood can be withdrawn (Fig. 76.2).

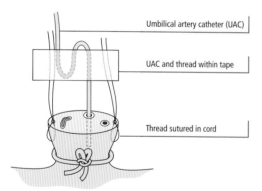

Fig. 76.1 Two arteries and one vein in umbilicus. The arteries are small, circular and have a muscular wall; the vein is larger, thin-walled and irregular.

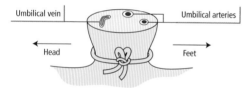

Fig. 76.2 Insertion and fixation of umbilical artery catheter. Transverse cutting of cord as shown here or cut-down onto artery. Dilate with fine forceps or dilator. Magnification may be helpful. The umbilical cord is tied to a strip of tape to avoid tape on the skin. Alternatively, tape placed in H shape on abdominal wall to incorporate catheter and tie suture to tape.

Position of catheter (Fig. 76.3)
- High: T6–10.
- Low: L3–4.
- The high position is above the diaphragm, so is above the celiac axis (T12), the superior mesenteric artery (T12–L1) and the renal arteries.
- The low position is below these structures and below the level of the inferior mesenteric artery but above the aortic bifurcation.
- The high position is generally preferred as it is associated with fewer vascular complications and a longer catheter life.
- Check position with X-ray (Fig. 76.4) or ultrasound.

Management
- Secure catheter (Fig. 76.3).
- Heparinize line and flush.
- Label line arterial or use red 3-way tap.
- Remove as soon as no longer required.

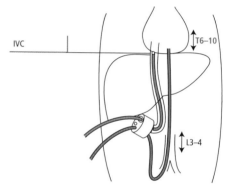

Fig. 76.3 Correct position of umbilical and venous catheters. IVC, inferior vena cava.

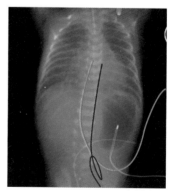

Fig. 76.4 X-ray to confirm position of the umbilical artery (red) and umbilical vein (blue) catheters, which need to be withdrawn. The artery first goes towards the groin before going towards the head between the vertebrae. Also check position of tracheal tube (satisfactory) and nasogastric tube (missing).

Neonatology at a Glance, 2nd edition. Edited by Tom Lissauer & Avroy A. Fanaroff. © 2011 Blackwell Publishing Ltd.

Complications

- False track by catheter or resistance at stump of cord – may be overcome by pulling cord towards infant's head to straighten artery.
- Poor perfusion of lower limbs – withdraw catheter, consider volume support; if does not resolve directly, immediately **REMOVE**.
- May withdraw significant blood volume from sampling – keep an accurate record of volume of blood samples.
- Blood loss if line disconnects.
- Aortic thrombosis and emboli.
- Infection.

Umbilical vein catheter (UVC)

Indications

- Resuscitation – for intravenous access.
- Inotropes.
- Total parenteral nutrition.
- Exchange transfusion.

Contraindication

- Omphalitis
- Omphalocele
- Peritonitis

Insertion

- Insert umbilical arterial catheter first if also required.
- Length to be inserted (cm) for UVC in inferior vena cava = 2 × weight (kg) + 5 cm + stump length (cm).
- Sterile technique.
- Single or double lumen.
- Prime catheter with saline (or seal end if emergency use).

Position of line

- High (preferred) – in inferior vena cava, just above diaphragm and below right atrium (T9–10).
- Avoid tip in portal vein or opposite renal veins or right atrium.
- Check position with X-ray (Fig. 76.4) or ultrasound.

Management

- Label clearly that it is a venous line.
- Remove as soon as no longer essential.

Complications

- Thrombosis or emboli.
- Hepatic damage.

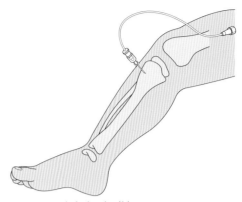

Fig. 76.5 Intraosseous infusion in tibia.

- Infection.
- Pleural or pericardial effusion (if in right atrium).

Intraosseous cannulation

Indication

- Emergency infusion of fluids and medications and no venous access possible (not sodium bicarbonate).

Preparation

- Sterile procedure.
- Position infant with knee flexed and supported.

Insertion

- Proximal tibia 1–3 cm below tibial tuberosity – medial flat surface (Fig. 76.5).
- Use neonatal intraosseous needle.
- Insert needle at 10–15 degrees from vertical towards foot (avoids growth plate).
- Use twisting motion.
- Dressing.

Infusion

- By syringe.

Complications

- Fracture.
- Cellulitis/osteomyelitis.

Central venous catheters

In neonatal units, central catheters are usually peripherally inserted (PICC lines), but sometimes a surgically placed subclavian catheter is required for long-term management.

Peripherally inserted central catheters (PICC lines)

Indications
- Total parenteral nutrition – often in preterm infants or after surgery.
- Inotropes.
- Hyperosmolar infusions, e.g. glucose >12.5%.
- Prolonged administration of antibiotics.

Vein
- Common sites – brachial, saphenous, sometimes scalp.

Insertion (Figs 77.1–77.4)
- Prepare infant – place in optimal position, consider how to minimize discomfort (see Chapter 62), temperature control, monitoring, measure length of line from cannulation site to inferior or superior vena cava.
- Prepare equipment – gauze, polyurethane catheter, cannula for insertion, T-piece and connection, dressing, saline flush.
- Sterile procedure – wear two sets of gloves and remove outer gloves once placement area cleaned and sterile.

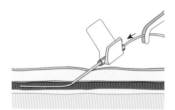

Fig. 77.1 An example of placing a peripherally inserted central catheter (PICC line). A tourniquet is made out of sterile gauze and applied to the upper arm. Needle is inserted into vein. The central line is threaded through the cannula. Non-toothed forceps may be used. The limb may need to be maneuvered to enable the line to be threaded centrally.

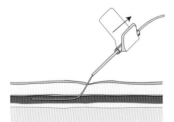

Fig. 77.2 Withdraw needle from vein over the central line. Pressure is applied over insertion site to stop bleeding.

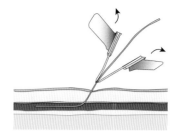

Fig. 77.3 The cannula is split and removed, leaving the long line in place.

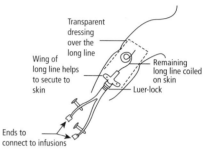

Fig. 77.4 Securing the line but allowing visibility of insertion site. Sterile strips are applied over puncture sites and line secured with clear adhesive dressing, incorporating loops of the central line. Ensure that infusion site is visible, that the infant is comfortable, that the dressing is not constricting the line or arm and is easy to redress if required (Figs 77.1–4 courtesy of Dr Sunit Godambe).

Position of line
- Ideal position of the tip is in the inferior or superior vena cava just distal to but **not in** the right atrium.
- Position of the long line should be checked initially by X-ray (Fig. 77.5) and subsequently by ultrasound scans or X-ray to check not migrated to right atrium.
- If line inserted in upper arm, perform X-ray for position with arm abducted.

Management
- Lines usually last 10 days to 2 or more weeks.

Complications
- Infection.
- Thrombus and emboli.
- Extravasation – pleural effusion, pericardial effusion causing tamponade, tissue edema.
- Superior vena caval obstruction.
- Blockage.
- Leakage at connection sites.
- Line breaking off on removal.

Neonatology at a Glance, 2nd edition. Edited by Tom Lissauer & Avroy A. Fanaroff. © 2011 Blackwell Publishing Ltd.

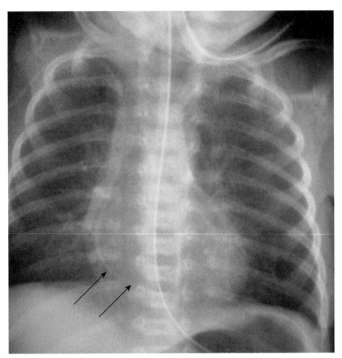

Fig. 77.5 X-ray demonstrating importance of confirming catheter position. Central line may be radio-opaque or need contrast flushed into it. The central venous catheter is in the right atrium (arrows) and must be withdrawn.

Subclavian

Indications
- Long-term central access.
- Peripheral insertion not possible.

Insertion
- Usually by a pediatric surgeon or interventional radiologist under general anesthetic in operating theater.
- Tunneled under skin.

Position
- Superior vena cava.

Complications
- Pneumothorax.
- Surgical scar.
- Superior vena caval obstruction.
- Blockage.
- Infection.

Exchange transfusion

Indications
- Severe hyperbilirubinemia – exchange with fresh blood (CMV-negative), 2 × blood volume.
- Polycythemia – exchange with normal saline, to reduce hematocrit to 0.55 (approx. 20 mL/kg).

Technique

Blood withdrawn via umbilical or peripheral arterial line; infused via umbilical or peripheral vein
- Infuse blood at a constant rate through the vein via a blood warmer.
- Withdraw blood from arterial line in aliquots (5 mL extremely preterm, 20 mL term).

Via umbilical venous catheter (if only access available)
- Alternate between withdrawing and infusing aliquots (5–20 mL) of blood.

Monitoring
- Vital signs throughout.
- Volume infused and withdrawn.
- Glucose, electrolytes, calcium, acid–base before, during and after procedure
- Allow time for equilibration – perform over 1 hour for double volume exchange.
- No feeds during procedure.

Complications
- Technical problems.
- Air embolization or thrombosis.
- Volume overload or depletion.
- Electrolyte imbalance – hyperkalemia, hypocalcemia, acidosis or alkalosis.
- Hypoglycemia.
- Infection.
- Hypothermia.
- Mortality – possibly up to 1%.

The anterior fontanel provides an ideal window for obtaining cranial ultrasound images. Ultrasound is especially helpful in identifying brain injury in preterm infants. The examination is non-invasive and can be performed at the bedside with minimal disturbance to the infant. Serial imaging allows monitoring of progression or resolution of lesions, which is much more informative than an individual scan.

Ultrasound images of the brain vary with gestational and post-natal age. At early gestation, the cortex is relatively smooth with few cerebral fissures, sulci and gyri. By term, the surface of the cortex appears convoluted and sulci and gyral patterns are well developed.

Indications

- Infants <1500 g birthweight or <32 weeks' gestation.
- Infants requiring intensive care.
- Neurologic abnormality – clinical, seizures, encephalopathy.
- Antenatally detected abnormality.

Lesions that can be identified

Preterm infants

- Hemorrhage.
- Ventricular dilatation.
- Periventricular leukomalacia.

All infants

- Range of CNS congenital abnormalities.
- Ventricular dilatation.
- Cerebral edema.
- Calcification from congenital infection.
- Basal ganglia lesions in hypoxic–ischemic encephalopathy.
- Strokes.
- Hematomas.

Standard views for scans

Coronal views (Fig. 78.1**)**

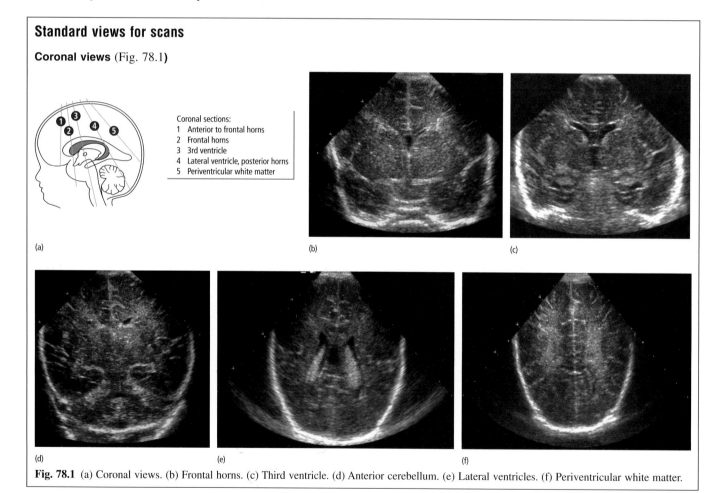

Coronal sections:
1 Anterior to frontal horns
2 Frontal horns
3 3rd ventricle
4 Lateral ventricle, posterior horns
5 Periventricular white matter

(a) (b) (c)

(d) (e) (f)

Fig. 78.1 (a) Coronal views. (b) Frontal horns. (c) Third ventricle. (d) Anterior cerebellum. (e) Lateral ventricles. (f) Periventricular white matter.

Neonatology at a Glance, 2nd edition. Edited by Tom Lissauer & Avroy A. Fanaroff. © 2011 Blackwell Publishing Ltd.

Sagittal views (Fig. 78.2)

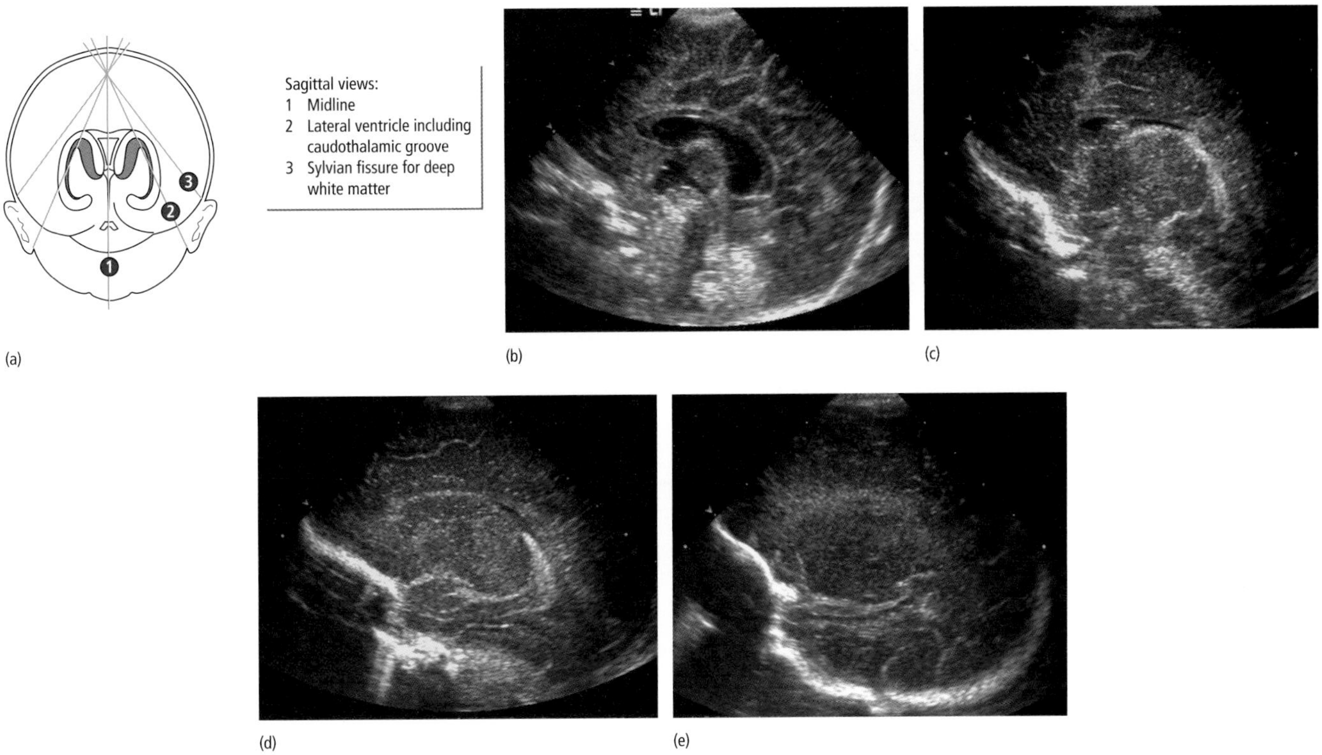

Sagittal views:
1 Midline
2 Lateral ventricle including caudothalamic groove
3 Sylvian fissure for deep white matter

(a)

(b)

(c)

(d)

(e)

Fig. 78.2 (a) Sagittal views. (b) Midline. (c) Caudothalamic groove. (d) Body of lateral ventricle. (e) Sylvian fissure.

Hemorrhage, ventricular dilatation

Germinal matrix hemorrhage (Grade 1) (Fig. 78.3)

Intraventricular hemorrhage (Grade 2 – no ventricular dilatation) (Fig. 78.4)

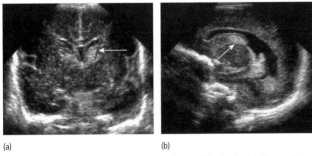

(a)

(b)

Fig. 78.3 Left germinal matrix hemorrhage (Grade 1). (a) Coronal view. (b) Sagittal view.

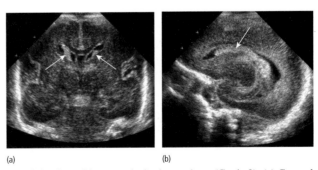

(a)

(b)

Fig. 78.4 Bilateral intraventricular hemorrhage (Grade 2). (a) Coronal view. (b) Sagittal view.

(continued)

Intraventricular hemorrhage (Grade 3 – ventricular dilatation) (Fig. 78.5)

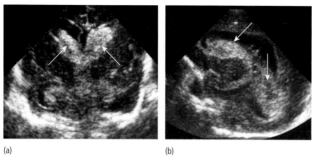

(a) (b)

Fig. 78.5 Bilateral intraventricular hemorrhage (Grade 3). (a) Coronal view. (b) Sagittal view.

Hemorrhagic parenchymal infarct (Grade 4) (Fig. 78.6)

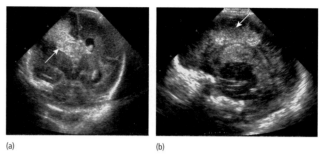

(a) (b)

Fig. 78.6 Right hemorrhagic parenchymal infarct (Grade 4). (a) Coronal view. (b) Sagittal view.

Ventricular dilatation (Figs 78.7–78.9)

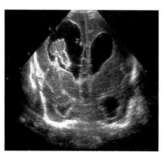

Fig. 78.7 Marked bilateral ventricular dilatation and hemorrhage in right ventricle on coronal scan.

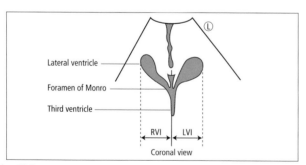

Fig. 78.8 Ventricular index, measured from the midline to the lateral border of the ventricle on a coronal scan in the plane of the third ventricle. Other indices can be used. (LVI, left ventricular index; RVI, right ventricular index.)

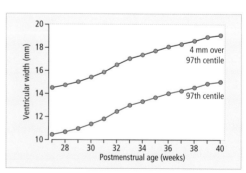

Fig. 78.9 Centiles for ventricular index showing 97th centile. The upper line is when treatment is likely to be required. (Levene MI, *Arch Dis Child* 1981; **56**: 900–904.)

Periventricular leukomalacia (PVL) (Figs 78.10 and 78.11)

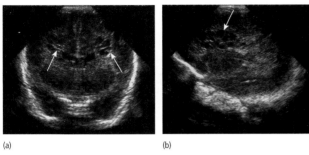

(a) (b)

Fig. 78.10 Widespread periventricular cysts on day 55 in (a) coronal and (b) sagittal views. Initial scans were normal and then showed some increased periventricular echogenicity.

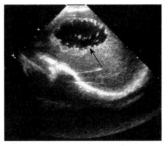

Fig. 78.11 Porencephalic cyst at site of a unilateral hemorrhagic parenchymal infarct.

Limitations of ultrasound

- Cannot reliably distinguish between hemorrhage and infarction.
- Poor sensitivity in identifying:
  - cerebral white matter injury in preterm or after hypoxic-ischemic encephalopathy
  - cerebral edema
  - subdural, subgaleal (subaponeurotic) hemorrhage.

  MRI imaging is more sensitive in identifying these lesions.

Practical issues

- Always clean the probe before and after use with each infant.
- Record images.
- Never report an abnormality unless visible on both coronal and sagittal views.
- Enter written report by experienced neonatologist or radiologist into patient record.

Question

When can the lesions in very low birthweight infants be identified?

Shortly after birth – identifies antenatal and early injury – small cysts, flares, hemorrhage.

During first week – hemorrhage, early ventricular dilatation, flares.

Next few weeks – ventricular dilatation, cysts from PVL and if lesions progress or resolve.

At discharge or term – prognosis is good if ventricles are normal, there is no excess intracerebral space between the brain and the skull and head circumference is increasing at normal rate; if not, prognosis is variable.

Targeted neonatal echocardiography (functional echocardiography) is a limited assessment of the ductus arteriosus, myocardial performance and pulmonary and systemic hemodynamics. It enables one to:
- identify and evaluate shunting across a patent ductus arteriosus
- assess cardiac function to determine the need and efficacy of inotropes and volume support
- identify the position of umbilical and central venous lines
- exclude major cardiac defects
- identify pulmonary hypertension
- exclude pericardial effusion.

It may be performed by a pediatric cardiologist or trained neonatologist working in close collaboration with a pediatric cardiac center, increasingly using telemedicine to review ultrasound images. However, echocardiography of complex congenital heart disease is the realm of the pediatric cardiologist or trained ultrasonographer.

Views

The standard views (Figs 79.1 and 79.2) in a neonate are:
- four-chamber and five-chamber
- parasternal short-axis
- parasternal long-axis
- subcostal.

High-quality images must be obtained.

Four-chamber view

- Confirms (Figs 79.3 and 79.4):
  - there are four chambers – appropriate size
  - there are normal mitral and tricuspid valves, and tricuspid is offset, i.e. lower position
  - ventricular septum is intact.
- Quantifies the degree of tricuspid regurgitation – useful for estimating pulmonary artery pressure.
- If the probe is angled more anterior to the four-chamber view the five-chamber view is obtained, which allows direct visualization of the left ventricular outflow tract. This allows indirect measurement of left ventricular output.

Short-axis view

This view (Figs 79.5 and 79.6) allows identification of:
- patent ductus arteriosus
- perimembranous ventricular septal defect (VSD)
- usual arrangement of pulmonary artery and aorta
- structural defects, e.g. transposition of the great arteries, pulmonary stenosis.

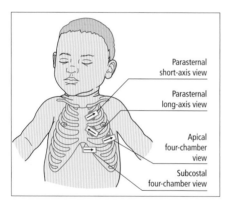

Fig. 79.1 Positions of probe and views obtained.

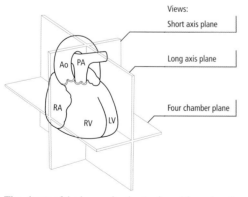

Fig. 79.2 The planes of the long axis, short axis and four-chamber apical or subcostal views. The five-chamber view is obtained by aiming the probe anterior to the subcostal view to visualize the left ventricular outflow tract.

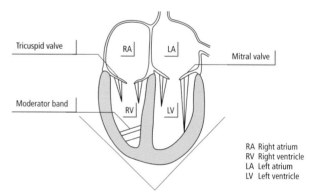

Fig. 79.3 Four-chamber view. The right ventricle can be identified from a band of tissue, the moderator band.

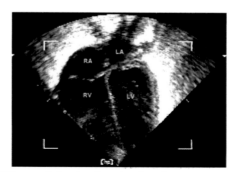

Fig. 79.4 Ultrasound showing four-chamber view.

Neonatology at a Glance, 2nd edition. Edited by Tom Lissauer & Avroy A. Fanaroff. © 2011 Blackwell Publishing Ltd.

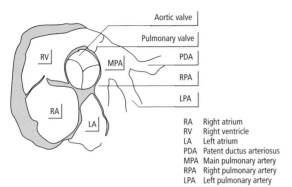

Fig. 79.5 Short-axis view.

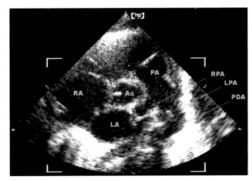

Fig. 79.6 Ultrasound of short-axis view.

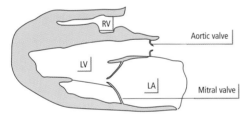

Fig. 79.7 Long-axis view.

Long-axis view

This view (Figs 79.7 and 79.8) is used to:
• identify correct position of pulmonary artery and aorta
• detect structural defects, e.g. tetralogy of Fallot
• assess volume overload in a patent ductus arteriosus (left atrial:aortic root ratio).

Subcostal view

This view is used to:
• check liver on right and aorta on left side, i.e. situs solitus
• obtain high-quality images if other views affected by lung hyperinflation or high-frequency oscillation (HFOV)
• check position of central lines in inferior vena cava or aorta.

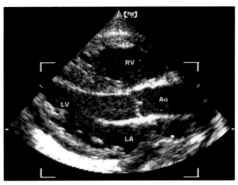

Fig. 79.8 Ultrasound showing long-axis view.

Patent ductus arteriosus

See Chapter 32.

Assessment of left ventricular function in critically ill neonates

Is there poor cardiac contractility or volume depletion? Functional echocardiography can provide this information in critically ill infants, which clinical examination alone cannot provide reliably. Echocardiography can provide this information from:
• subjective assessment of cardiac contractility from the variation in left ventricle size
• estimation of systolic function (from the left ventricular shortening fraction)
• intravascular volume estimation from inferior vena caval filling – it is collapsed with hypovolemia; however, assessment of cardiac volume loading is particularly difficult in the first few days of life, when the transitional circulation is present
• calculating left ventricular output – to determine whether impaired systolic performance or hypovolemia is leading to compromised systemic blood flow.

Three-dimensional echocardiography and reconstructive magnetic resonance imaging are being developed to quantify cardiac chamber size and provide more accurate functional assessments.

Assessment of persistent pulmonary hypertension (PPHN) in critically ill neonates

Functional echocardiography may be used to diagnose increased pulmonary artery pressure and its impact on right and left ventricular performance. The magnitude of the pulmonary hypertension may also be estimated from the direction of blood flow across the ductus arteriosus:
• pure right-to-left (from pulmonary artery to aorta) transductal flow implies suprasystemic pulmonary artery pressure
• bidirectional transductal flow (right-to-left during systole and left-to-right during diastole) implies that pulmonary artery pressure approximates systemic arterial pressures
• left-to-right transductal flow implies that pulmonary artery pressure is less than systemic arterial pressure.

Gestational age assessment: Ballard exam

Gestational age can be assessed clinically (±2 weeks) from the changes in neuromuscular and physical maturity with gestation. The most widely used scoring systems are the Dubowitz and the somewhat shorter Ballard score shown in Fig. 80.1 and Table 80.1.

Maturity rating

Add up the individual neuromuscular and physical maturity scores for the 12 categories, then obtain the estimated gestational age from Table 80.2. The neuromuscular maturity score may be unreliable if the infant is sedated or ill.

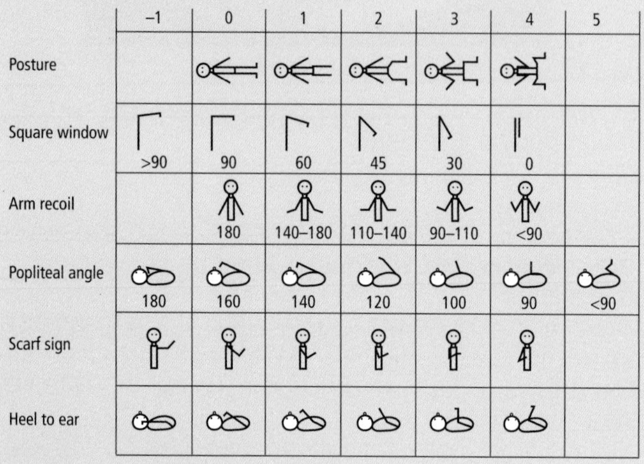

Fig. 80.1 Neuromuscular maturity.

Table 80.2 Gestational age estimated from summed neuromuscular and physical maturity scores.

Total score	Gestational age (weeks)
–10	20
–5	22
0	24
5	26
10	28
15	30
20	32
25	34
30	36
35	38
40	40
45	42
50	44

Table 80.1 Physical maturity scores.

Sign	–1	0	1	2	3	4	5
Skin	Sticky, friable, transparent	Gelatinous red, translucent	Smooth pink, visible veins	Superficial peeling and/or rash, few veins	Cracking, pale areas, rare veins	Parchment, deep cracking, no vessels	Leathery, cracked, wrinkled
Lanugo	None	Sparse	Abundant	Thinning	Bald areas	Mostly bald	
Plantar creases	Heel–toe 40–50 mm = –1 <40 mm = –2	Heel–toe >50 mm, no creases	Faint red marks	Anterior transverse crease only	Creases over anterior 2/3	Creases over entire sole	
Breast	Imperceptible	Barely perceptible	Flat areola, no bud	Stippled areola, bud 1–2 mm	Raised areola, bud 3–4 mm	Full areola, bud 5–10 mm	
Eye and ear	Lids fused loosely = –1, tightly = –2	Lids open, pinna flat, stays folded	Slightly curved pinna, soft with slow recoil	Well-curved pinna, soft but ready recoil	Formed and firm, with instant recoil	Thick cartilage, ear stiff	
Genitalia, male	Scrotum flat, smooth	Scrotum empty, faint rugae	Testes in upper canal, rare rugae	Testes descending, few rugae	Testes down, good rugae	Testes pendulous, deep rugae	
Genitalia, female	Clitoris prominent, labia flat	Prominent clitoris, small labia minora	Prominent clitoris, enlarging minora	Majora and minora equally prominent	Majora large, minora small	Majora cover clitoris and minora	

Neonatology at a Glance, 2nd edition. Edited by Tom Lissauer & Avroy A. Fanaroff. © 2011 Blackwell Publishing Ltd.

Blood pressure charts (Figs 80.2 and 80.3)

There is consensus neither on the definition of hypotension nor when low blood pressure should be corrected. Blood pressure spontaneously increases in extremely low birthweight infants during the first 24 hours. Infants hypotensive on gestational age criteria but with clinical evidence of good perfusion have as good an outcome as normotensive patients. A stepwise approach to correction of hypotension with evidence of poor perfusion includes fluid boluses, administration of dopamine, dobutamine or catecholamines and thereafter administration of corticosteroids (see Fig. 24.4). Echocardiography can provide information about left ventricular function and volume depletion (see Chapter 79). Its use is being evaluated.

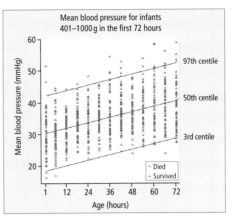

Fig. 80.3 Mean blood pressure in infants weighing 401–1000 g in first 72 hours of life. (Courtesy of Dr Jon Fanaroff, 2003.)

Severity of illness scores

Scores have been devised in order to be able to compare and predict morbidity and mortality whilst allowing for severity of illness. They incorporate measures of physiologic instability in the first 12 postnatal hours.

The most widely used in neonatology are:
- SNAP-PE II score
- CRIB II score.

The SNAP-PE II (Score Neonatal Acute Physiology Perinatal Extension) is based on the physiologic derangement in a number of organ systems (urine output, mean blood pressure, worst PaO_2/FiO_2 ratio, lowest serum pH, occurrence of seizures) in the first 12 hours after admission to the NICU (neonatal intensive care unit), birthweight, Apgar score at 5 minutes, and whether there is IUGR (intrauterine growth restriction).

The CRIB (Clinical Risk Index for Babies) score is for very low birthweight (VLBW) infants and is based on birthweight, gestation, maximal base excess in the first 12 hours of life and temperature on admission.

The use of the SNAP-PE is limited by the complexity of the data required and the CRIB score by the overwhelming effects of birthweight and gestational age on outcome.

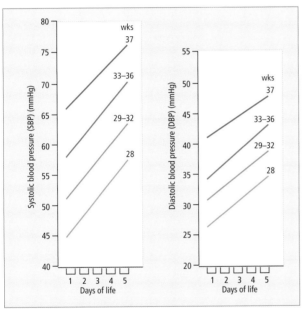

Fig. 80.2 Systolic and diastolic blood pressure by age and gestational age. (From Zubrow AB *et al.* Determinants of blood pressure in infants admitted to neonatal intensive care units: A prospective multicenter study. Philadelphia Neonatal Blood Pressure Study Group. *J Perinatol* 1995; **15**: 470.)

Index

Page numbers in *italics* represent figures, those in **bold** represent tables.

Neonatology at a Glance, 2ⁿᵈ edition. Edited by Tom Lissauer & Avroy A. Fanaroff. © 2011 Blackwell Publishing Ltd.

neonatal care
  levels of 15, *15*
  low income settings 174–5
neonatal infection 102–3, *102*, 104–5
neonatal infection *continued*
  bacterial sepsis 102
  clinical presentation 102–3
  conjunctivitis 105, *105*
  Gram-negative 105
  group B streptococcus 104, *104*
  investigations 103
  laboratory investigations 103
  Listeria monocytogenes 104–5
  risk factors 102
  sites of *105*
  skin 105, *105*
  viral 106–7
neonatal intensive care 11
neonatal mortality 12, *12*, 172–3, *172*, **173**
  and birthweight **13**
  causes 173, *173*
  global burden *172*
  prevention 174, *174*, **174**
  timing 173
neonatal resuscitation 34–7, *34*
  airway 35, *35*
  breathing 35–6, *35*, *36*
  circulation 36, *36*
  drugs 36, **37**
  ethical decisions 37, *37*
  initial assessment *34*
  intubation 36
  preparation 34
  special cases 37
  warmth/stimulation 34
neonatal unit 58–9
  assisting attachment 59, *59*
  communication 58–9
  developmental care 60–1, *60*, **60**, *61*
  family-friendly environment 59
  open access 58, *58*
  welcoming parents and families 58
neonatal withdrawal syndrome 26–7, **26**
neural tube defects 142
neurologic examination 48–9
neutropenia 134
neutrophilia 134, *134*
nevus flammeus 139, *139*
newborn
  behavior of 60, **60**, *61*
  common problems 56–7, **56**, *57*
  definition of 12
  medical problems 57, *57*
    see also individual conditions
  minor abnormalities 54–5, *54*, *55*
  neurologic examination 48–9
  routine care 44–5
    discharge 45
    health promotion 45, *45*
    screening 44–5

routine examination 46–7, *46*, *47*, **47**
sick, transport of 176–7, *176*, *177*
skin lesions 55, *55*
see also neonatal
nitric oxide, inhaled 67, *67*
non-nutritive feeding 77
NSAIDs, congenital anomalies **27**
nuchal translucency *16*
nutrition 10, 76–7
  breast-feeding 44, 52–3, *52*, *53*, **76**
  formula milks 52, **76**
  supplements 76

obstetric care 173, *173*
omphalocele *15*, 114–15, *114*
opiates, congenital anomalies **27**
opisthotonus 98
Ortolani maneuver 46
osteogenesis imperfecta 147, *147*
osteomyelitis 147
osteopenia of prematurity 83, *83*
oxygen dissociation curve *132*
oxygen saturation 63, *63*
oxygen supplementation *64*

pain 150–1
  minimization of 151, *151*
pain assessment 150–1, **151**
pain pathways 150, *150*
pain response 150, *150*
pallor 57
parents
  communication with 51, **51**
  support for 50–1, *50*
parvovirus B19, congenital 31
Patau syndrome (trisomy 13) 25, *25*
patent ductus arteriosus 80–1, *80*
  clinical features 80–1, *80*, *81*
  ductal closure 80
  investigations 81, *81*
  management 81
  morbidity 81
  risk factors 80
patient-triggered ventilation 65
pericentricular leukomalacia *189*
perinatal medicine 14–15, *14*
  neonatal involvement 14–15, *15*
perinatal mortality 12
peripheral artery cannulation *181*, **181**
  ischemic damage 157–8, *158*
peripheral venous cannulation *180*, **180**
periventricular leukomalacia 78–9
  clinical features 79
  diagnosis 78–9, **79**
  incidence **78**
  laboratory findings 79
  management 79, *79*
  pathogenesis 78
  prevention 79
  prognosis 79

persistent pulmonary hypertension of
  newborn 94, *94*
  echocardiography 191
pharmacology 152–3, *152*
phocomelia 27
phosphate balance 125
phototherapy 100–1, **101**
physical maturity scores 192, *192*
Pierre Robin sequence 97, *97*
plethora 57
pleural tap 179
pneumatosis intestinalis 87
pneumonia 93
  aspiration 159
pneumothorax 73, 94
polycystic kidney disease 123, *123*
polycythemia 18, 133, *133*
polyhydramnios 116
porencephalic cyst *189*
port wine stain 139, *139*
portal vein thrombosis 158, *158*
positive pressure ventilation 65–6
  indications 65
  intermittent 65, *65*
  patient-triggered 65–6
  synchronous intermittent mandatory 65
post-neonatal mortality 12
posterior urethral valves 123, *123*
posture 48, *48*
potassium balance 125
Potter syndrome *123*
Prader–Willi syndrome 145, *145*
prenatal screening 16
prepregnancy care 16
preterm delivery 22–3, *22*
preterm infants 68–9
  anemia 82–3
  characteristics of *68*
  complications *69*
  discharge from hospital 168–9, *168*, *169*
  evaporative heat loss 74, *75*
  growth 76
  hydrocephalus 143
  infection 82, *82*
  jaundice 82
  morbidity 69
  mortality 69, *69*
  necrotizing enterocolitis 86–7
  nutrition 76–7, **76**
  osteopenia 83, *83*
  retinopathy of prematurity 84–5, *85*, **85**
  very low birthweight *see* very low
    birthweight infants
procalcitonin 103
protein C deficiency *135*
pulmonary haemorrhage 73
pulmonary interstitial emphysema 73
pulse oximetry 45
pustular melanosis, transient 55
pyloric stenosis 116–17

vision 149, *149*, **149**
visual fixing and following 48
vitamin K 44, 76
    deficiency **137**
volume expanders **37**

volume-limited ventilation 67
vomiting *57*, 112–13, *112*, *113*, **113**
    bile-stained 112
    blood-stained 113
von Willebrand disease **137**

weight loss *57*
Werdnig–Hoffman syndrome 145
withholding treatment 162–3, **163**